MIDWIFERY AND OBSTETRICAL NURSING

MIDWIFERY AND OBSTETRICAL NURSING

Piyush Sharma

genNEXT Publication

Midwifery and Obstetrical Nursing

Rs. 890

ISBN: 978-81-908675-4-2

Published in 2010 in India by
Gennext Publication
23 Main Ansari Road, Darya Ganj,
New Delhi-110002
E-Mail:GenNextpublication@hotmail.com
Phone: 23282060

Printed at: Singhal Print Media, Delhi

Contents

Preface

Midwifery is now a major public health issue. Nurses are working in new and innovative ways in this field. Many nurses are working in advanced and specialized clinical roles as independent practitioners. With this important concept in mind, this book provides a valuable resource for nurses working towards, and at advanced level in Midwifery and Obstetrical Nursing, also the book is relevant to nurses working in normal hospital settings.

This book also provides a skill base for student nurses who aspire to excel in Midwifery and Obstetrical Nursing. Using this book, nursing students could develop their practice to an advanced level.

This book has been written primarily in response to the increasing concern expressed about the lack of ability in both student nurses and newly qualified nurses to perform clinical skills in this field. The intention of this book is to outline the elements of essential nursing procedures, providing the principle for the recommended actions

This book is unique in that it encourages the students to achieve clinical skill competence. It also differs from existing books in that it is presented in accessible and user-friendly format. Further, this text is also of benefit to lay persons interested in this field.

The selection of topics for inclusion is based on extensive consultation with experienced clinicians, students, practitioners as well as teachers of nursing. Each topic has been carefully researched to provide a contemporary foundation for practice.

1

Introduction

The simplest definition of midwifery is "with woman", but truly, midwifery means different things to different people. For many, the Midwifery Model is an attitude about women and how pregnancy and birth occur, and view that pregnancy and birth are normal events until proven otherwise. It is an attitude of giving and sharing information, of empowerment, and of respecting the right of a woman and her family to determine their own care.

The attitude of midwifery, or the Midwifery Model can be contrasted with the Medical Model. In general, the Medical Model is an attitude that there is potential pathology in any given situation, and that medicine can assist to improve the situation. Medicine is also about teaching, informing, and prevention, but the power seems to be more with the provider rather than with the woman.

Historically, midwives have always been around to help women give birth. Before physicians, midwives were the primary healers in their communities. They were the medicine women of their own cultures, and assisted families and women throughout their lives. In the Old Testament they were described as examples of the strength and faith in God. Midwives were once the nutritionists, herbalists, doctors, ministers, counselors all rolled into one 'profession'. Many feel they were the first holistic practitioners. Midwives were always available to help the poor, the women without medical care or the women who were the outcasts of their culture. Today, midwives take care of anyone who wishes to see them, but practice within the constraints of their medical and legal systems.

There are two main divisions of modern midwifery: nurse-midwives and direct-entry midwives:

Nurse-midwives are advanced practice nurses who have specialized in the practice of obstetrical and gynecological care of relatively healthy women. Many registered nurse-midwives have a master's degree in nursing. Nurse-midwives practice in hospitals and medical clinics, and may also deliver in birth centres and at home. They are able to prescribe medications. Nurse-midwives provide care to women from puberty through menopause and may work closely with obstetricians who provide consultation and assistance in births which develop complications. Women with high risk pregnancies can receive the benefits of midwifery care from a nurse-midwife in collaboration with a physician.

Direct-entry midwives learn midwifery through self-study, apprenticeship, a midwifery school, or a college or university-based program that does not require nurse certification. A direct-entry midwife is trained to provide the "Midwives Model of Care" to healthy women and newborns throughout the childbearing cycle primarily in out-of-hospital settings.

Obstetrics (from the Latin obstare, "to stand by") is the medical surgical specialty dealing with the care of a woman and her offspring during pregnancy, childbirth and the puerperium (the period shortly after birth). Most obstetricians are also gynaecologists. Obstetrics and Gynaecology (often abbreviated to OB/GYN or O&G) form a single medical specialty. All gynaecologists are trained obstetricians, and vice versa, having completed postgraduate medical training and residency programs. OB/GYN specialists work to ensure that pregnancy culminates in the delivery of a healthy baby, without impairing the health of the mother.

Midwives are trained to recognize and deal with deviations from the norm during the term of pregnancy and during the birth and refer to obstetricians when a woman requires care beyond the areas of the midwife's expertise. In many cases, these professions work together to provide all necessary care to childbearing women and their families. The midwife and the OB/GYN have a crucial role in health counseling and education, not only for the woman, but also within the family and community. They offer education involving antenatal education and preparation for parenthood and may extend to women's health, sexual or reproductive health and childcare.

A healthy pregnancy leading to a healthy birth is the first gateway to a life of opportunity and a crucial time for the newborn to embody a sense of acceptance and fulfillment- physically, mentally, emotionally and spiritually. The cultural values, personal preferences of the women and families in their care, honouring the delicate choice of home birth, birthing centre or hospital birth and to what extent medical intervention is appropriate are all of paramount importance in holistically honouring every birth experience as the precious foundation of one's entire life experience.

Today midwives are as diverse as the populations they serve. Midwives are willing to take care of anyone who wishes to see them. Over 70% of births in the world are attended by midwives. Each country worldwide has a slightly different view of midwifery, and of how midwives work within their communities.

INTRODUCTION TO CONCEPTS OF MIDWIFERY AND OBSTETRICAL NURSING

Midwives teach, educate and empower women to take control of their own health care. In most communities, they provide prenatal care, or supervision of the pregnancy, and then assist the mother to give birth. They manage the birth, and guard the woman and her newborn in the postpartum period. Most midwives encourage and monitor women throughout their labour with techniques to improve the labour and birth. Reassurance, positive imaging and suggestions to change positions and walk helps labours progress.

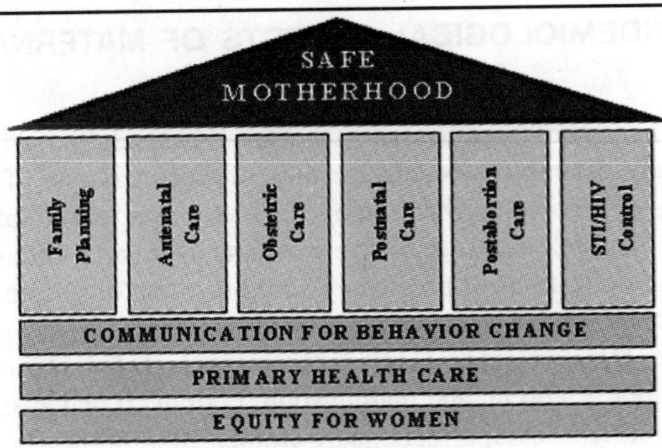

Pillars of Sale Motherhood

Fig. Concepts of Midwifery and Obstetrical Nursing

Many midwives provide family planning services and routine women's health examinations such as pap smears and physical examinations. They teach women about sexually transmitted infections, and focus on prevention of the spread of infections. What specifically midwives do will depend upon: her training, her licensure, and what is allowed in the state, province, or country in which she practices. For example, in the United States some midwives can prescribe medications, provide women's health care throughout the menopause years. Midwives worldwide attend births in the home, hospital or birthing centre, depending upon their education and licensure, and the rules governing their practice. Midwives believe it is especially important to provide time for questions, teaching, and time to listen to the concerns and needs of the women they care for.

The WHO definition of the midwife gives us the following information:

She must be able to give the necessary supervision, care and advice to women during pregnancy, labour and the postpartum period, to conduct deliveries on her own responsibility and to care for the newborn and the infant. This care includes preventative measures, the detection of abnormal conditions in mother and child, the procurement of medical assistance and the execution of emergency measures in the absence of medical help. She has an important task in health counseling and education, not only for the woman, but also within the family and the community. The work should involve antenatal education and preparation for parenthood and extends to certain areas of gynecology, family planning and child care. She may practice in hospitals, clinics, health units, domiciliary conditions of in any other service.

EPIDEMIOLOGICAL ASPECTS OF MATERNAL AND CHILD HEALTH

The delivery of a healthy baby who survives to adulthood is not only a potentially desirable outcome for any mother, it is one of the most valuable assets a community can enjoy. Each year over ten million children in the world die below the age of five years and over half a million women die from complications of pregnancy, child-bearing, or unsafe abortion. Most of these deaths occur in developing countries, where poverty is widespread, effective public-health programmes and clinical care services are often poor or absent, and malnutrition, both overt and at subclinical and micronutrient level, affects many women of child-bearing age and their infants. The health of both is jeopardized by resulting impaired immunity to infectious disease and the suboptimal physical and mental development that ensues.

MAGNITUDE OF MATERNAL AND CHILD PROBLEMS

The mental health of mothers and children are closely linked. Efforts to improve Maternal and child nutrition have always been a major focus of India's health and nutrition research scientists. In the first forty years after independence maternal and child undernutrition were the major public health problems. Epidemiologists defined the magnitude of the problems and nutrition scientists identified major factors responsible and how to combat them. Based on these studies, Government of India initiated intervention programmes to combat undernutrition in women and children.

The nineties witnessed a change in this scenario. While undernutrition remained the unfinished agenda, overnutrition emerged as a public health problem. Indian research studies highlighted the possibility that during the ongoing nutrition transition, undernutrition may be a predisposing factor for overnutrition in later life. Epidemiological studies showed that micronutrient deficiencies continue to be widespread in all income groups and they could have adverse effect on growth and development. Several investigators are currently exploring the intergenerational effect of micro and macro nutrient deficiencies in different periods of life.

TRENDS IN MIDWIFERY AND OBSTETRICAL NURSING

In recent years there has been a change in obstetrical nursing and midwifery. Obstetrical nurses and midwives have started to employ a range of data collection methods that are relatively new to the profession. Predominantly quantitative research, which concentrates on reduction, objectivity, manipulation, categorisation, passivity, control, prediction, causality and generalisability, is starting to be replaced by other approaches perhaps more congruent with nursing, midwifery and caring.

There is probably a multitude of reasons for the move away from using the previously dominant quantitative paradigm approaches to the study of nursing and midwifery. In identifying four patterns of knowing in nursing, Carper (1978) highlighted that in addition to the empirical; nurses could also pay attention to aesthetic, moral and personal knowledge. In order to allow this, less emphasis needed to be placed on the "hard science" experimental design approach and more emphasis on different ways of knowing and on different forms of knowledge. Nurses were beginning to identify the "complexity of nursing knowledge" and that the concern of nursing was and is "complex human phenomena", that often require differing methods of conducting nursing research. Nursing was being challenged to develop and utilise research methods as expansive as the subjects they study.

The reducing dependence on reductionistic approaches that often failed to acknowledge the existence or importance of personal and contextual factors could improve the much cited failure to implement research findings in practice. For example, if research is conducted in context and is emancipatory and relevant, then it is much more likely to succeed in bringing about change. With so many research results not being used and resulting in an 'application gap', nursing and midwifery research must look to methods that involve the personal and contextual experience of practitioners in the identification of research questions.

In recent years there has been a move away from the reductionistic medical models of nursing and midwifery towards a more holistic nursing and midwifery paradigm. In the era of holism, the appropriateness or adequacy of the traditional scientific mode of enquiry in nursing and midwifery has been increasingly questioned. The same questions need to be asked when studying the effects of complementary therapies. In nursing and midwifery, as in complementary therapies, new and exciting methods of research are needed that are "congruent with the belief systems".

LEGAL AND ETHICAL ASPECTS

Medicine as a profession is very hierarchical, and so too is health care delivery with doctors generally located at the top of the pecking order. In turn, this means that obstetricians sometimes feel that they have the professional autonomy to override the professional judgement of a midwife; indeed, they may feel that they have a duty to override what they perceive as an incorrect judgement. They may also believe that it is best way to have systems in place that ensures that they have the final say where the boundaries of professional responsibility are blurred. This is understandable and even justifiable where their legal responsibilities are greater. However because of the existence of the overall hierarchy, it is possible for this process to be much more casual than it needs to be, and than one would otherwise expect it to be when the judgement of two professionals is at issue. For instance, two consultants from different specialities would automatically expect that where there was a difference of professional judgement about a patient in their dual care this would be open for courteous professional discussion that led to shared agreement, not one consultant overriding or disregarding the views of another. This would be expected not just as a matter of professional etiquette but also as a matter of ethical responsibility when the best interests of the patient are at stake, and uncertain to the extent that there is room for professional disagreement.

Similarly, where a midwife's professional judgement is overridden in a way that is casual and disrespectful there is cause for legitimate complaint where there are systems in place that limit legitimate professional judgement. There is less cause for complaint when legal responsibility is not equally shared, unless the midwife has the greater responsibility. Similarly midwives must be cautious to distinguish between professional autonomy and the autonomy that they have as persons.

PRECONCEPTION CARE AND PREPARING FOR PARENTHOOD

Preconception care is recognized as a critical component of health care for women of reproductive age. The main goal of preconception care is to provide health promotion, screening, and interventions for women of reproductive age to reduce risk factors that might affect future pregnancies. Preconception care is part of a larger health-care model that results in healthier women, infants, and families.

A substantial number of definitions for preconception care have been used. Preconception care is defined as a set of interventions that aim to identify and modify biomedical, behavioral, and social risks to a woman's health or pregnancy outcome through prevention and management. Certain steps should be taken before conception or early in pregnancy to have a maximal effect on health outcomes. Preconception care is more than a single visit to a health-care provider and less than all well-woman care, as defined by including the full scope of preventive and primary care services for women before a first pregnancy or between pregnancies (i.e., commonly known as interconception care).

Improving preconception health and pregnancy outcomes will require more than effective clinical care for women. Changes in the knowledge and attitudes and behaviours related to reproductive health among both men and women need to be made to improve preconception health. Despite several health promotion campaigns aimed at reducing smoking, misuse of alcohol, intimate partner violence, obesity, human immunodeficiency virus (HIV)/acquired immunodeficiency syndrome (AIDS), reduction of vaccine-preventable diseases, and exposure to occupational hazards. Preconception health promotion, therefore, should focus on a general awareness among men and women regarding reproductive health and risks to childbearing.

THEORIES, MODELS AND APPROACHES APPLIED TO MIDWIFERY PRACTICE

Development of midwifery theory which started in the late 1970s has occurred on several fronts. The adaptation of nursing models to midwifery, the development of local models and care plans, the continued use of midwifery process applied to the individual and the introduction of standard setting and quality assurance have all played a part in creating a theoretical framework for midwives.

Birth Territory Theory: The theory of Birth Territory describes, explains and predicts the relationships between the environment of the individual birth room, issues of power and control, and the way the woman experiences labour physiologically and emotionally.

The theory was synthesised inductively from empirical data generated by the authors in their roles as midwives and researchers. It takes a critical post-structural feminist perspective and expands on some of the ideas of Michel Foucault. Theory synthesis was also informed by current research about the embodied self and the authors' scholarship in the fields of midwifery, human biology, sociology and psychology.

In order to demonstrate the significance of the theory, it is applied to two clinical stories that both occur in hospital but are otherwise different. This analysis supports the central proposition that when midwives use 'midwifery guardianship' to create and maintain the ideal Birth Territory then the woman is most likely to give birth naturally, be satisfied with the experience and adapt with ease in the post-birth period. These benefits together with the reduction in medical interventions also benefit the baby. In addition, a positive Birth Territory is posited to have a broader impact on the woman's partner, family and society in general.

ROLE OF NURSE IN MIDWIFERY AND OBSTETRICAL CARE

A nurse-midwife is an advanced practice nurse with additional training around delivering babies and providing prenatal and postpartum care to women.

Nurse-midwives are very involved in labour and delivery, sometimes never leaving the mother during the entire labour process. They are trained to recognize signs and symptoms that deviate from normal conditions and will consult with a physician who may become involved in the delivery if needed.

Although qualified to administer drugs and to perform medical procedures, those interventions are not routine for nurse-midwives, and they are used only when the mother requests them.

Most nurse-midwives deliver babies in hospitals and in homes. They also provide both prenatal and postpartum care for both mothers and newborns. In addition, nurse-midwives provide family planning and birth control counseling, and normal gynecological services such as: physical and breast exams, pap smears, and preventive health screening. In most states, nurse-midwives may prescribe medications.

The nurse-midwife assumes two professional roles: one of the registered nurse and one of the nurse-midwife. These roles may require different activities and may provoke different expectations. It may be assumed that role conflict exists both within the nurse-midwife (intrarole conflict) and between the nurse-midwife and the obstetric nurse (interrole conflict).

Midwives have the lead professional role and are present at over 75% of the births. They have an important role in making decisions about appropriate care in pregnancy, labour and after the birth and are thus in a very privileged position. They make a positive contribution to the health and well being of the mother and the unborn child and is therefore a very highly skilled profession.

Unlike other healthcare professions, midwives are responsible for a client-group, who are on the whole healthy and free from disease or injury. A further difference is the fact that midwives deliver continuous care over several months and are therefore able to develop more effective relationships with their client-group. Midwives are caring and understanding individuals, who need to have a sensitive nature and are willing to look after women from a range of social and ethnic backgrounds.

INDEPENDENT NURSE MIDWIFERY PRACTICE

The concept of autonomous practice does not figure largely within the framework of hospital policy. Many midwives feel much more comfortable working in a place where medical back-up is a constant presence. Some midwives are not even aware of independent midwifery, and seem to think that hospital based practice is the only option. In reality, a midwife can actually start practicing independently as soon as she qualifies, although very few do that.

Those currently practicing independently have many reasons, but the prime reason for all seems to be that they are unable to practice fully as a midwife within the confines of current hospital systems. Often it appears that women's needs come second to the needs of the institution. Staffing requirements dictate that women may have to wait for hours in antenatal clinics; may have to share their midwife on labour ward with one, two or even three other women; and that their time on the postnatal ward is characterized by heat, noise, conflicting advice and meals at all the wrong times! Even community midwives are bound by policies on who they may or may not accept for a homebirth - not realizing, or choosing to mislead women about, the fact that it is the woman's right to choose where and how compel, or coerce, or blackmail women into doing as we think best. There is evidence, however, that these tactics are being used all too often.

There are uncertainties in independent practice, as in any self-employed occupation. The positive side of independent practice is based upon the knowledge that the service provided at least gives women the opportunity make their own decisions, in possession of the information necessary to make those decisions. Independents are often perceived as mavericks; natural rebels against authority, iconoclasts, boat rockers. Well, yes, to an extent that may be so. However, without challenge, there is no change; without grit, there is no pearl; without independents, there would be nothing for the hospital-based system to measure itself against. If the system feels itself threatened, then there must be something in the system that is capable of being threatened. That something is contained in the way in which institutions treat pregnant women, regarding them, in general, as unfit vessels for the task of childbearing.

Independent midwives do not, however, do it alone. Although some midwives do practice single-handed, the majority work in partnerships, or practices of three or more. This enables midwives to have time off, and to remind themselves of what their own family looks like, and where they live. These little points tend to get forgotten when practices get really busy.

NATIONAL POLICY AND LEGISLATION IN RELATION TO MATERNAL HEALTH AND WELFARE

Maternal health is almost always seen as a technical and health issue which means that the medical establishment is regarded as best qualified to speak on it. Policy making on maternal health has therefore never consulted those who are directly affected, that is the women who undergo pregnancy. Policies and Five Year Plans set ambitious targets to reduce maternal mortality, but programmes continue to look away from women. Women have never been consulted on where they prefer to give birth, what support they need for their choices, what happens when they seek help, and what their experience have been in seeking abortions. Neither have women been asked whether all their pregnancies are of choice, whether they need more support in making reproductive decisions and whether they can actually exercise sexual choices and sexual health protection.

Article 3

1. In all actions concerning children, whether undertaken by public or private social welfare institutions, courts of law, administrative authorities or legislative bodies, the best interests of the child shall be a primary consideration.
2. States Parties undertake to ensure the child such protection and care as is necessary for his or her well-being, taking into account the rights and duties of his or her parents, legal guardians, or other individuals legally responsible for him or her, and, to this end, shall take all appropriate legislative and administrative measures.
3. States Parties shall ensure that the institutions, services and facilities responsible for the care or protection of children shall conform with the standards established by competent authorities, particularly in the areas of safety, health, in the number and suitability of their staff, as well as competent supervision.

Article 2

1. States Parties shall respect and ensure the rights set forth in the present Convention to each child within their jurisdiction without discrimination of any kind, irrespective of the child's, parent's or legal guardian's race, colour, sex, language, religion, political or other opinion, nationality, ethnic or social origin, property, disability, birth or other status.
2. States Parties shall take all appropriate measures to ensure that the child is protected against all forms of discrimination or punishment on the basis of the status, activities, expressed opinions, or beliefs of the child's parents, legal guardians or family members.

Article 6

1. States Parties recognise that every child has the inherent right to life.
2. States Parties shall ensure to the maximum extent possible the survival and development of the child.

Article 12

1. States Parties shall assure to the child who is capable of forming his or her own views the right to express those views freely in

all matters affecting the child, the views of the child being given due weight in accordance with the age and maturity of the child.

2. For this purpose, the child shall in particular be provided the opportunity to be heard in any judicial and administrative proceedings affecting the child, either directly, or through a representative or an appropriate body, in a manner consistent with the procedural rules of national law.

MATERNAL MORBIDITY, MORTALITY AND FERTILITY RATES

Infant Mortality Rate (IMR) is regarded as an important and sensitive indicator of the health status of a community. It also reflects the general standard of living of the people and effectiveness of interventions for improving maternal and child health in a country.

Compared to other indicators like crude birth rate, maternal mortality rate and under-five mortality rate etc, this indicator has always been accorded greater importance by the public health specialists because infant mortality is the single, largest category of mortality. Moreover, deaths during infancy are due to a particular mix of diseases and conditions to which the adult population is less exposed and less vulnerable. Changes in specific health interventions affect IMR more rapidly and directly and hence it may change more dramatically than the crude death rate in a population. This is clearly demonstrated in a developing country like India. In the 1960s, IMR in India used to hover around the 100 mark in the country. However, due to rapid strides that the country has taken in socio-economic development, health and education, average IMR is currently estimated to be around 60/1000 live births/year (SRS 2003). IMR has declined in both urban areas (40/1000 live births/yr) and rural areas (69/1000 live births/yr). Compared to an IMR of as low as 5/1000 lb/yr in countries such as Japan and Sweden the IMR in India is still quite high. However, it is close to the world average of IMR of 56/1000 (yr 2002).

In fact, not only in India but in the developing world in general, the fall in IMR has been greater than in the developed world. Despite these successes, IMR is still in the unacceptable range and a lot needs to be done. To make matters worse, in a country like India, there are wide inter-state variations. We have extremely low IMR states states like Kerala (14/1000) while in 3-4 states IMR < 50 (T. Nadu, A.P., Maharashtra and Pb) but we also have high IMR states like Uttar Pradesh (83/1000) and

Orissa (96/1000), Bihar, M.P. within each state also, there are wide rural-urban variations.

PERINATAL MORBIDITY AND MORTALITY RATES

Globally, child mortality rates have been halved over the last few decades, a developmental success story. Nevertheless, progress has been uneven and in recent years mortality rates have increased in some countries. The major causes of childhood mortality are also reviewed and strategic options for the different states of India are proposed that take into account current mortality rates and the level of progress in individual states. The slowing decline in childhood mortality rates in India calls for new approaches that go beyond disease-, programme- and sector-specific approaches.

In 1998, about 2.5 million under-5-year-olds died in India, the highest total of any country (1). India's health goals for the year 2000 included reducing the national mortality rate for children under 5 years of age to less than 100 per 1000 live births; the infant mortality rate to less than 60 per 1000 live births; and the perinatal mortality rate to less than 85 per 1000 live births. Between the mid-1980s and early 1990s, significant progress was made toward these goals and national targets appeared to be within reach, despite large disparities in mortality levels, rates of decline and child health determinants among the various Indian states. However, recent data indicate that the decline in child mortality rates is slowing. In this study we examine, inter alia, the trend in infant mortality rates since 1981. The data support the hypothesis that the decline in child mortality rates is slowing.

REFERENCES

Ament LA and Hanson L. A Model for the Future: Certified nurse-midwives replace residents and house staff in hospitals. Nursing and Health Care Prospectives 1998;19:1 26-33.

Baldwin LM, et. al. Do providers adhere to ACOG standards? The case of prenatal care. Obstetrics and Gynecology 1994;84:549-55

Bell K and Mill JI. Certified nurse-midwife effectiveness in the health maintenance orginization obstetric team. Obstetrics and Gynecology 1989; 74:112-16.

Brown SA and Grimes DE. A meta-analysis of nurse practitioners and nurse-midwives in primary care. Nursing Research 1995;44: 332-39.

Butler J, et, al. Supportive nurse-midwife care is associated with a reduced incidence of cesarean section. American Jouran of Obstetrics and Gynecology 1993; 168:1407-13.

Capan P, et al. Nurse-managed clinics provide access and improved health care. Nurse practitioner 1993; 18:50-5.

Haire D and Elsberry C. Maternity care and outcomes in a high-risk service: the North Central Bronx Hospital experience. Birth 1991; 18:33-7.

MacDorman, M and Singh, GK. Midwifery care, Social and Medical Risk factors, and birth outcomes in the USA. Journal of Epidemiology and Community Health. 1998; 52(5): 310-317.

Murphy, PA and Fullerton, J. Outcomes of Intended Home Births in Nurse-Midwifery Practice: A Prospective Descriptive Study. Obstetrics & Gynecology 1998 92:3; 461-470.

Paine L. The role of nurse-midwife in primary ob/gyn. The Female Patient 1992; 17:129-145.

Paine L. Primary care for women An overview of the role of the nurse-midwife. The Journal of Nurse-Midwifery 1995; 40:65-73.

Turnbull D, et. al. Randomized, controlled trial of efficacy of midwife-managed care. Lancet 1996; 348:213-18.

Nielsen I. A midwife-physician team in private practice. American Journal of Nursing 1975; 75:1693-95.

2

Anatomy & Physiology of Reproductive System

The major function of the reproductive system is to ensure survival of the species. Other systems in the body, such as the endocrine and urinary systems, work continuously to maintain homeostasis for survival of the individual. An individual may live a long, healthy, and happy life without producing offspring, but if the species is to continue, at least some individuals must produce offspring.

Within the context of producing offspring, the reproductive system has four functions:

- To produce egg and sperm cells.
- To transport and sustain these cells.
- To nurture the developing offspring.
- To produce hormones.

These functions are divided between the primary and secondary, or accessory, reproductive organs. The primary reproductive organs, or gonads, consist of the ovaries and testes. These organs are responsible for producing the egg and sperm cells, (gametes), and for producing hormones.

These hormones function in the maturation of the reproductive system, the development of sexual characteristics, and have important roles in regulating the normal physiology of the reproductive system.

All other organs, ducts, and glands in the reproductive system are considered secondary, or accessory, reproductive organs. These structures transport and sustain the gametes and nurture the developing offspring.

FEMALE PELVIS

BONY PELVIS

The bony pelvis is formed by the hip bones in front and at the sides and by the sacrum and coccyx behind. When a subject is in the anatomical position, the anterior superior iliac spines and the pubic tubercles are in the same coronal plane. The pelvic surface of the body of the pubis, on which the bladder rests, faces more upward than backward. The pelvic surface of the sacrum faces more downward than forward.

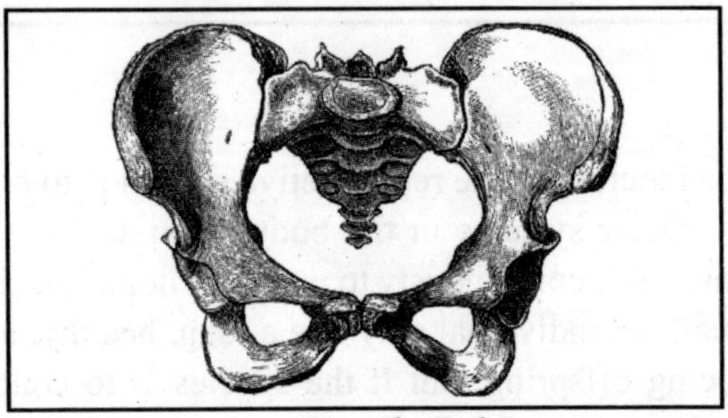

Fig. Female Pelvis

The (lesser) pelvis has an inlet, a cavity, and an outlet, each of which has three main diametres: anteroposterior (or conjugate), oblique, and transverse.

The Pelvic Inlet

The pelvic inlet, or brim (upper pelvic aperture), is indicated by the lineae terminales, the iliac parts of which are the arcuate lines. The inlet is at about half a right angle to the horizontal. The anteroposterior (or true) conjugate diametre extends from the upper margin of the pubic symphysis to the middle of the sacral promontory. The obstetrical conjugate diametre, which is measured from the back ofthe pubic symphysis, is the shortest diametre through which the foetal head must pass in its course through the inlet. The diagonal conjugate diametre, between the lower margin of the pubic symphysis and the sacral promontory, is measured per vaginam. Inability to palpate the sacral promontory suggests that the conjugate diametre of the inlet is adequate for parturition, whereas palpation indicates a contracted pelvis.

The Pelvic Cavity

The pelvic cavity extends backward and downward from the inlet to the outlet. It curves with the sacrum and coccyx, and hence is longer behind than in front.

The Pelvic Outlet

The pelvic outlet (lower pelvic aperture) extends from the pubic symphysis to the tip of the coccyx (its anteroposterior, or conjugate, diametre) and, from side to side, between the ischial tuberosities; hence it is diamond shaped. The outlet is at a slight angle (10 to 15 degrees) to the horizontal.

The pubic arch formed by the conjoined rami of the pubes and ischia has its apex at the symphysis, where it forms the subpubic angle.

The path taken through the pelvic cavity by the foetal head is known as the axis of the birth canal. The axis intersects the inlet at a right angle, turns forward at the uterovaginal angle (level of ischial spines), and follows the axis of the vagina. During parturition, the foetal head (usually the suboccipitobregmatic diametre) occupies successively the inlet (transverse diametre), cavity (oblique diametre, and outlet (anteroposterior diametre).

Classification of Pelvises

Although pelvises can be arranged by the measurements of their diametres, it is usual in obstetrics and radiology to classify pelves according to the shape of the pelvic inlet. Four main types are recognized: (1) gynecoid, a rounded inlet; (2) android, a heart-shaped inlet; (3) anthropoid, a long, narrow, oval inlet; and (4) platypelloid, an ovoid inlet with its long axis transverse, like a flat bowl. A female pelvis may belong to any of the four types (only about half are gynecoid), but intermediate types are more frequent. The female pelvis tends to have thinner and lighter bones with less prominent muscular markings, and the subpubic angle is less acute (approximating a right angle). Pelvic diametres and shape can be determined in vivo by radiographic pelvimetry.

JOINTS OF PELVIS

The joints of the pelvis include the lumbosacral, sacrococcygeal, and sacro-iliac, and the pubic symphysis. Associated ligaments include the sacrotuberous, sacrospinous, and iliolumbar.

The lumbosacral joint is that between L.V.5 and the sacrum. It includes an intervertebral disc and joints between the articular processes. The sacrococcygeal joint, which may undergo bony fusion, consists of an intervertebral disc between the sacrum and coccyx and accessory ligaments.

The sacro-iliac joints are synovial articulations between the auricular surfaces of the sacrum and ilium on each side. The surfaces may be smooth and flat or reciprocally curved and irregular. The joint is strengthened posteriorly by interosseous and dorsal sacro-iliac ligaments. The weight of the body is transmitted through the sacrum and ilia to the femora during standing and to the ischial tuberosities in sitting.

The pubic symphysis is a cartilaginous joint between the bodies of the pubic bones in the median plane. The symphysial surfaces, each covered by hyaline cartilage, are united by an interpubic disc of fibrocartilage, which may present a cleft. The ligaments around the joint become relaxed during pregnancy.

The sacrotuberous ligament extends from the dorsal surface of the sacrum (as well as from the ilium and coccyx) to the ischial tuberosity. The sacrospinous ligament extends from the lateral margin of the sacrum (and coccyx) to the ischial spine. The sacrotuberous ligament converts the sciatic notches into foramina, which are separated from each other by the sacrospinous ligament. The greater sciatic foramen transmits the piriformis muscle, superior and inferior gluteal vessels and nerves, (internal) pudendal vessels and nerve, sciatic and posterior femoral cutaneous nerves, and the nerves to the obturator intemus and quadratus femoris muscles. The lesser sciatic foramen transmits the obturator intemus tendon, the nerve to the obturator intemus, and the (internal) pudendal vessels and nerve.

WALLS OF PELVIS

The wall of the pelvic cavity includes (1) superficial muscles, such as the glutei; (2) the hip bones, the sacrum and coccyx, and their associated ligaments; and (3) deep muscles, blood vessels, nerves, and peritoneum. For descriptive purposes, the pelvic wall can be subdivided into two lateral walls, a posterior wall, and a floor.

Each lateral wall, limited by the hip bone below the linea terminalis, is lined by the obturator internus muscle, medial to which are the obturator nerve and vessels and other branches of the internal iliac artery. Rarely, the intestine may protrude through the obturator canal (obturator hernia) and lie under cover of the pectineus. The lateral wall of the pelvis is crossed behind by the ureter and in front by the round ligament or the ductus deferens. The ovary lies in a slight depression on the lateral wall. The lateral and posterior walls are separated by the sacrotuberous and sacrospinous ligaments and by the greater and lesser sciatic foramina.

The posterior wall, formed by the sacrum and coccyx, is lined laterally by the piriformis and coccygeus muscles. The lumbosacral trunk and sacral plexus are situated in front of the piriformis. In the median plane is the median sacral artery (from the aorta), which ends in a vascular mass, the coccygeal body or glomus.

The pelvic floor (a term variously defined) may conveniently be considered as the main structures that support the abdominal and pelvic viscera, i.e., the peritoneum and the pelvic and urogenital diaphragms. The peritoneum descends to be reflected from the front of the rectum to the bladder (rectovesical pouch in the male) or to the uterus and vagina (rectouterine and rectovaginal pouches in the female). The pouches are bounded laterally by peritoneal elevations that are frequently termed sacrogenital folds. In front, the peritoneum is reflected from the uterus to the bladder (uterovesical pouch). The blood vessels and neural plexuses to the viscera (as well as the ureter and ductus deferens) are situated in the connective tissue between the peritoneum and the pelvic diaphragm. Localized thickenings of this extraperitoneal tissue form ligaments. The pelvic floor has two median openings, one for the rectum and the other for the urethra (and vagina).

LIGAMENTS

The female pelvis has a wider diametre and a more circular shape than that of the male. The wider inlet facilitates head engagement and parturition. The wider outlet predisposes to subsequent pelvic floor weakness. Numerous projections and contours provide attachment sites for ligaments, muscles, and fascial layers. Of note is the thin and triangular sacrospinous ligament, which extends from the ischial spines to the lateral margins of the sacrum and coccyx anteriorly to the sacrotuberous ligament. Its anterior surface is muscular and constitutes the coccygeus; the ligament is often regarded as the degenerate part of the muscle. The greater and lesser sciatic foramina are above and below the ligament.

MUSCULAR SUPPORTS OF THE PELVIC FLOOR

Pelvic Diaphragm

The levator ani and coccygeus muscles that are attached to the inner surface of the minor pelvis form the muscular floor of the pelvis. With their corresponding muscles from the opposite side, they form the pelvic diaphragm. The levator ani is composed of 2 major muscles from medial to lateral: the pubococcygeus and iliococcygeus muscles.

The bulkier medial portion of the levator ani is the pubococcygeus muscle that arises from the back of the body of the pubis and anterior portion of the arcus tendineus. The arcus tendineus of the levator ani is a dense connective tissue structure that runs from the pubic ramus to the ischial spine and courses along the surface of the obturator internus muscle. The muscle passes back almost horizontally to behind the rectum. The inner border forms the margin of the levator (urogenital) hiatus, through which passes the urethra, vagina, and anorectum.

Various muscle subdivisions have been assigned to the medial portions of the pubococcygeus to reflect the attachments of the muscle to the urethra, vagina, anus, and rectum. These portions are referred to by some investigators as the pubourethralis, pubovaginalis, puboanalis, and puborectalis-or collectively as the puboviscerals, because of their association and attachment to the midline viscera. The urethral portion forms part of the periurethral musculature, and the vaginal and anorectal portions insert into the vaginal walls, perineal body, and external anal sphincter muscle. The puborectalis portion passes behind the rectum and fuses with its counterpart from the opposite side to form a sling behind the anorectum. Other more posterior parts of the pubococcygeus attach to the coccyx.

The thin lateral part of the levator ani is the iliococcygeus muscle, which arises from the arcus tendineus of the levator ani to the ischial spine. Posteriorly it attaches to the last 2 segments of the coccyx. The fibers from both sides also fuse to form a raphe and contribute to the anococcygeal ligament. This median raphe between the anus and the coccyx is called the levator plate and is the shelf on which the pelvic organs rest. It is formed by the fusion of the iliococcygeus and the posterior fibers of the pubococcygeus muscles. When the body is in a standing position, the levator plate is horizontal and supports the rectum and upper two thirds of vagina above it. Weakness of the levator ani may loosen the sling behind the anorectum and cause the levator plate to sag. This opens the urogenital hiatus and predisposes to pelvic organ prolapse. Women with prolapse have been shown to have an enlarged urogenital hiatus on clinical examination.

The coccygeus muscle that extends from the ischial spine to the coccyx and lower sacrum forms the posterior part of the pelvic diaphragm. It sits on the anterior surface of the sacrospinous ligament. Three-dimensional magnetic resonance imaging (MRI) of the pelvic diaphragm shows its peripheral attachments and demonstrates the urogenital hiatus.

Direct innervation of the levator ani muscle on its cranial surface is primarily from the third and fourth sacral nerve roots via the pudendal nerve. The puborectalis may derive some if its innervation from a pudendal branch on the caudal side. Regarding the type of the striated muscle, it has been reported that the majority of the muscle fibers in the levator ani are slow-twitch fibers that maintain constant tone (type I), with an increased density of fast-twitch (type II) fibers distributed in the periurethral and perianal areas. This suggests that the normal levator ani maintains tone in the upright position to support the pelvic viscera. Furthermore, voluntary squeezing of the puborectalis may increase the tone to counter increased intra-abdominal pressure.

Urogenital Diaphragm (Perineal Membrane)

Another musculofascial structure, the urogenital diaphragm, is present over the anterior pelvic outlet below the pelvic diaphragm. However, there is controversy over whether this structure contains a transverse sheet of muscle extending across the pubic arch (deep transverse perinei muscle) sandwiched between superior and inferior fascia or 3 contiguous striated muscles (compressor urethrae, sphincter urethrae, and urethra-vaginalis) and an inferior fascial layer called the perineal membrane. Despite the controversy, MRI scans clearly depict the structure.

The more superficial ischiocavernosus and bulbocavernosus muscles, as well as the thin slips of the superficial transverse perinei, complete the inferior aspect of the urogenital diaphragm. The structure bridges the gap between the inferior pubic rami bilaterally and the perineal body. It closes the urogenital (levator) hiatus; supports and has a sphincter-like effect at the distal vagina; and, because it is attached to periurethral striated muscles, contributes to continence. It also provides structural support for the distal urethra. The posterior triangle around the anus does not have a corresponding diaphragm or membrane. The ischiorectal fossae are the spaces lateral to the anus below the pelvic diaphragm.

Perineal Body

The perineal body is a pyramidal fibromuscular structure in the midline between the anus and vagina with the rectovaginal septum at its cephalad apex. Below this, muscles and their fascia converge and interlace through the structure. Attached to the perineal body are the rectum, vaginal slips from the pubococcygeus, perineal muscles, and the anal sphincter; it also contains smooth muscle, elastic fibers, and nerve endings. During childbirth, the perineal body distends and then recoils. It is an important part of the pelvic floor; just above it are the vagina and the uterus. Acquired weakness of the perineal body gives rise to elongation and predisposes to defects such as rectocele and enterocele.

The bladder and urethra and the vagina and uterus are attached to the pelvic walls by a system of connective tissue that has been called the endopelvic fascia. This structure lies immediately beneath the peritoneum and is one continuous unit with various thickenings or condensations in specific areas.

The endopelvic fascia is continuous with the visceral fascia, which provides a capsule containing the organs and allows displacements and changes in volume. The distinct regions of this structure are given individual names, specifically ligaments and fascia, with variable internal structure. Endopelvic fascia and ligaments are a mesh-like group of collagen fibers interlaced with elastin, smooth muscle cells, fibroblasts, and vascular structures. The structures that attach the uterus to the pelvic wall, the cardinal ligaments, derive strength from the supportive collagen forming the walls of arteries and veins. Other structures, such as the pelvic sidewall attachment of the endopelvic fascia (arcus tendineus of the pelvic fascia), are predominantly fibrous collagen.

Anterior Supports

There is agreement among investigators that the connective tissue supports of the urethra, bladder, and vagina extend to the arcus tendineus of the pelvic fascia on the pelvic diaphragm. There is also agreement that a "hammock" of anterior vaginal wall tissue, bridging the gap medially in the urogenital hiatus, supports the vesical neck and urethra. There is controversy, however, focusing on the connective tissue structures that are associated with this hammock.

The pubourethral ligaments are connective tissue structures that extend from the urethra to the pubic bone. Various authors have described them as structures responsible for supporting the urethra and keeping the vesical neck closed. However, other authors have described connective tissue between the proximal urethra (and vesical neck) and the pubis as containing smooth muscle and cholinergic nerves that make the structures more suited to vesical neck opening during micturition than to urethral support. Because there is an attachment of the lower third of the urethra to the pubis, it is postulated that there are 2 separate structures-one for support at the mid-or distal urethra and one near the bladder neck that may open it during voiding. The distal support has been described as connective tissue that joins the vaginal wall and periurethral tissue to the arcus tendineus of the pelvic fascia and the levator muscles. Since the arcus tendineus inserts into the pubic bone, these are the ligaments that are palpable during a retropubic dissection. These ligaments are important for urethral support.

There is controversy regarding the amount of supportive tissue or fascia in the anterior vaginal wall. Although the wall is composed of mucosa, muscularis, and adventitia and abuts a similar arrangement in both the urethra and bladder, various authors have attributed to it a vaginal fascial layer. Weber and Walters cited many articles on both sides of the controversy and reported no specific fascial layer, whereas DeLancey demonstrated a fascial layer suburethrally on the anterior vaginal wall. With or without the suburethral fascial layer, the anterior vaginal wall supports the urethra by its lateral attachment to the levators (pubococcygeus) and to the endopelvic fascia from the arcus tendineus of the pelvic fascia. In essence, it is a double hammock. Paradoxically, the more advanced the prolapse, the more thickened and hypertrophied is the vaginal submucosal layer.

Urethropelvic ligaments from the suburethral fascia at the bladder neck and proximal urethra to the levators and arcus tendineus have been described and demonstrated on MRI scans. The existence of these ligaments as separate entities apart from the hammock of tissue supporting the proximal urethra has been disputed.

At the level of the bladder base, there is little actual endopelvic fascia between the bladder and vaginal muscularis. Here, the support comes from the lateral attachment of the vagina to the arcus tendineus of the pelvic fascia. The pubocervical fascia has been described as extending from the symphysis along the anterior vaginal wall to blend with the fascia that surrounds the cervix. It is continuous laterally with the pubococcygeus and also suspended to the arcus tendineus of the pelvic fascia. Its existence as a separate and discernable entity is also in dispute.

Middle Supports

The paracolpium and parametrium are the connective tissues surrounding the vagina and the uterus, respectively. In the midvagina, the paracolpium fuses with the pelvic wall and fascia laterally. The cardinal ligaments (also called the transverse cervical ligaments of Mackenrodt) extend from the lateral margins of the cervix and upper vagina to the lateral pelvic walls. They originate over a large area from the region of the greater sciatic foramen over the piriformis muscles, from the pelvic bones in the region of the sacroiliac joint, and from the lateral sacrum. They are condensations of the lowermost parts of the broad ligaments. Laterally, the cardinal ligaments are continuous with the connective tissue surrounding the hypogastric vessels. Medially, they are continuous with the paracolpium and parametrium as well as the connective tissue in the anterior vaginal wall, the so-called pubocervical fascia.

The uterosacral ligaments are attached to the cervix and upper vaginal fornices posterolaterally. Posteriorly, they attach to the pre-sacral fascia in front of the sacroiliac joint. The connective tissue of the uterosacral ligaments is continuous with that of the cardinals around the cervix.

Posterior Supports

The posterior vaginal wall, below the cardinals, is supported from the sides by the paracolpium, which is attached to the endopelvic fascia (referred to as rectovaginal fascia in this area) and pelvic diaphragm. The anterior and posterior fascial layers unite along the sides of the vagina. According to DeLancey, the rectovaginal fascia is found mostly at the sides and is extremely thin in the midline of the vaginal wall. However, a posterior rectovaginal septum, consisting of fibromuscular elastic tissue, extending from the peritoneal reflection to the perineal body has been described. During foetal life, the peritoneal cavity extends to the cranial part of the perineal body, but it becomes obliterated in early life. Its fused layers (Denonvillier's fascia) probably become part of the rectovaginal septum adherent to the undersurface of the posterior vaginal wall. This fascia forms the anterior margin of another potential space, the rectovaginal space. The rectovaginal septum, if intact and normal, permits independent mobility of the rectal and vaginal walls.

In the distal vagina, 2 cm to 3 cm above the hymeneal ring, the vaginal wall is directly attached to surrounding structures without any intervening paracolpium. Anteriorly, the vagina fuses with the urethra and the connective tissue of the perineal membrane and muscles (urogenital diaphragm). Laterally, it blends with the levator ani muscles and, posteriorly, it fuses with the perineal body. The rectovaginal fascia is thickest in this region, and the vagina in this area has no mobility separate from its adjacent structures.

The fascial supports for the rectum, the lateral rectal ligaments, extend from the posterolateral pelvic side wall (level with the third sacral vertebra) to the rectum and surround the middle rectal arteries. Additional prerectal and pararectal fascial elements are frequently described.

The urethra is a complex tubular structure extending below the bladder to the external meatus. It has distinct muscular elements associated both within and without to permit its functioning for storage (continence) and voiding.

The smooth muscle of the urethra is contiguous with that of the trigone and detrusor. It has a prominent inner longitudinal and a thin outer circular layer. The layers lie inside the outer striated urogenital sphincter muscle and are present throughout the upper four fifths of the urethra. The configuration of the circular muscle implies a role in constricting the lumen, and the longitudinal muscle may aid in shortening the urethra during voiding.

The outer layer of the urethra is formed by the muscle of the striated urogenital sphincter that is found in the middle three fifths of the length. In its upper two thirds, the sphincter-like fibers are circular. In the distal part, the fibers exit the urethra and surround the vaginal wall as the urethrovaginal sphincter or extend along the inferior pubic rami above the perineal membrane as the compressor urethra. The muscle is composed mainly of slow-twitch fibers, well suited for maintaining constant tone. Voluntary muscle activation can also increase the constriction of the urethra when needed.

The urethral mucosa extends from the bladder transitional epithelium to the external meatus and is primarily nonkeratinizing squamous epithelium. It is derived from the urogenital sinus along with the lower vagina and vestibule. It is hormonally sensitive and undergoes changes with stimulation. The hormonally sensitive submucosal tissue contains a rich and prominent vascular plexus. Several specialized types of arteriovenous anastomoses have been demonstrated, and it is thought that they provide a watertight closure of the mucosal surface with an increase in blood flow that may occur with an increase in pressure on abdominal vessels.

In addition to the muscular and vascular tissue of the urethra, there is a considerable quantity of connective tissue interspersed within the muscle and submucosa. This tissue contains collagen and elastin fibers and is thought to add to urethral closure passively. Lastly, a series of glands are found in the submucosa, mainly along the vaginal surface of the urethra. They are most predominant in the middle and lower third of the urethra.

It is the admixture of the smooth and striated muscle, connective tissue, mucosa, and submucosa that accounts for a functional sphincter. A functional urethral sphincter has intact neural control and provides watertight apposition of the urethral lumen, compression of the wall around the lumen, and a means of compensating for abdominal pressure changes.

The "hammock hypothesis" is a readily understood way to explain the continence mechanism. The requirements for continence include a quiescent bladder, functioning musculofascial supports, and a functional urethral sphincter mechanism. The fascial attachments connect the periurethral tissue and anterior vaginal wall to the arcus tendineus at the pelvic sidewall, whereas the muscular attachments connect the periurethral tissue to the medial border of the levator ani. Urethral support is provided by a coordinated action of fascia and muscles acting as an integrated unit under neural control.

This musculofascial support provides a hammock onto which the urethra is compressed during increases in intra-abdominal pressure. One can surmise that the urethral sphincter mechanism is operative and adds to the process. Furthermore, failure of one of the support components will not invariably produce stress incontinence, because of the compensatory effect of the other component. This may explain why some women with hypermobility have no incontinence. It may also explain why injectable agents can be used in women with hypermobility: the bulking agent may improve urethral sphincter function.

VARIATIONS IN PELVIS SHAPE

The shape of the female pelvis may vary considerably from woman to woman. Some pelves are eminently suitable for child-bearing, whilst others are not. They may be classified into four groups according to the shape of the brim.

Gynaecoid: The gynaecoid pelvis has a round brim and is the most suitable shape for child bearing. This type of pelvis is found in the woman of average build with hips broader than her shoulders, with a height of over 1.5, and taking size 4 (british sizing) or larger in shoes.

Android: The android pelvis has a heart-shaped brim morphologically resembling the male pelvis; posterior vertex positions of the foetus (where the foetus turns with its back towards its mother's spine) producing back labour are more common in women with this type of pelvis. Forceps and episiotomy are often necessary for delivery.

Anthropoid: The anthropoid pelvis has an oval brim with narrow transverse (across the widest part) diametre. Posterior vertex positions of the foetus with back-ache in labour are not uncommon and delivery may take longer than that of a woman with a gynaecoid pelvis.

Platypelloid: The platypelloid or flat pelvis has a kidney-shaped brim which is narrow in the antero-posterior (from back to front) diametre. Labour is likely to be lengthy because of the shallow brim and a Caesarian section is often necessary. However, if the baby's head passes successfully through the brim of the pelvis, the remainder of the labour is usually very rapid.

FEMALE ORGANS OF REPRODUCTION

Each sex has its own unique reproductive system. They are different in shape and structure, but both are specifically designed to produce, nourish, and transport either the egg or sperm.

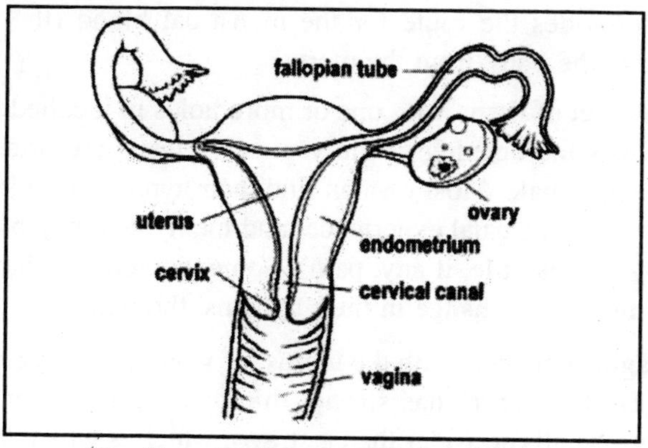

Fig. Female Organs of Reproduction

Unlike the male, the human female has a reproductive system located entirely in the pelvis. The external part of the female reproductive organs is called the vulva, which means covering. Located between the legs, the vulva covers the opening to the vagina and other reproductive organs located inside the body.

The fleshy area located just above the top of the vaginal opening is called the mons pubis. Two pairs of skin flaps called the labia (which means lips) surround the vaginal opening. The clitoris, a small sensory organ, is located toward the front of the vulva where the folds of the labia join. Between the labia are openings to the urethra (the canal that carries urine from the bladder to the outside of the body) and vagina. Once girls become sexually mature, the outer labia and the mons pubis are covered by pubic hair.

A female's internal reproductive organs are the vagina, uterus, fallopian tubes, and ovaries.

The vagina is a muscular, hollow tube that extends from the vaginal opening to the uterus. The vagina is about 3 to 5 inches (8 to 12 centimetres) long in a grown woman. Because it has muscular walls, it can expand and contract. This ability to become wider or narrower allows the vagina to accommodate something as slim as a tampon and as wide as a baby. The vagina's muscular walls are lined with mucous membranes, which keep it protected and moist.

The vagina serves three purposes:

1. It's where the penis is inserted during sexual intercourse.
2. It's the pathway that a baby takes out of a woman's body during childbirth, called the birth canal.
3. It provides the route for the menstrual blood (the period) to leave the body from the uterus.

A thin sheet of tissue with one or more holes in it called the hymen partially covers the opening of the vagina. Hymens are often different from female to female. Most women find their hymens have stretched or torn after their first sexual experience, and the hymen may bleed a little (this usually causes little, if any, pain). Some women who have had sex don't have much of a change in their hymens, though.

The vagina connects with the uterus, or womb, at the cervix (which means neck). The cervix has strong, thick walls. The opening of the cervix is very small (no wider than a straw), which is why a tampon can never get lost inside a girl's body. During childbirth, the cervix can expand to allow a baby to pass.

The uterus is shaped like an upside-down pear, with a thick lining and muscular walls - in fact, the uterus contains some of the strongest muscles in the female body. These muscles are able to expand and contract to accommodate a growing foetus and then help push the baby out during labour. When a woman isn't pregnant, the uterus is only about 3 inches (7.5 centimetres) long and 2 inches (5 centimetres) wide.

At the upper corners of the uterus, the fallopian tubes connect the uterus to the ovaries. The ovaries are two oval-shaped organs that lie to the upper right and left of the uterus. They produce, store, and release eggs into the fallopian tubes in the process called ovulation. Each ovary measures about 1½ to 2 inches (4 to 5 centimetres) in a grown woman.

There are two fallopian tubes, each attached to a side of the uterus. The fallopian tubes are about 4 inches (10 centimetres) long and about as wide as a piece of spaghetti. Within each tube is a tiny passageway no wider than a sewing needle. At the other end of each fallopian tube is a fringed area that looks like a funnel. This fringed area wraps around the ovary but doesn't completely attach to it. When an egg pops out of an ovary, it enters the fallopian tube. Once the egg is in the fallopian tube, tiny hairs in the tube's lining help push it down the narrow passageway toward the uterus.

The ovaries are also part of the endocrine system because they produce female sex hormones such as estrogen and progesterone.

EXTERNAL GENITALIA

The function of the external female reproductive structures (the genital) is twofold: To enable sperm to enter the body and to protect the internal genital organs from infectious organisms. The main external structures of the female reproductive system include:

- Labia majora: The labia majora enclose and protect the other external reproductive organs. Literally translated as "large lips, " the labia majora are relatively large and fleshy, and are comparable to the scrotum in males. The labia majora contain sweat and oil-secreting glands. After puberty, the labia majora are covered with hair.
- Labia minora: Literally translated as "small lips, " the labia minora can be very small or up to 2 inches wide. They lie just inside the labia majora, and surround the openings to the vagina (the canal that joins the lower part of the uterus to the outside of the body) and urethra (the tube that carries urine from the bladder to the outside of the body).
- Bartholin's glands: These glands are located next to the vaginal opening and produce a fluid (mucus) secretion.
- Clitoris: The two labia minora meet at the clitoris, a small, sensitive protrusion that is comparable to the penis in males. The clitoris is covered by a fold of skin, called the prepuce, which is similar to the foreskin at the end of the penis. Like the penis, the clitoris is very sensitive to stimulation and can become erect.

INTERNAL GENITAL ORGANS AND THEIR ANATOMICAL RELATIONS

The internal reproductive organs include:

- Vagina: The vagina is a canal that joins the cervix (the lower part of uterus) to the outside of the body. It also is known as the birth canal.
- Uterus (womb): The uterus is a hollow, pear-shaped organ that is the home to a developing foetus. The uterus is divided into two parts: the cervix, which is the lower part that opens into the vagina, and the main body of the uterus, called the

corpus. The corpus can easily expand to hold a developing baby. A channel through the cervix allows sperm to enter and menstrual blood to exit.

- Ovaries: The ovaries are small, oval-shaped glands that are located on either side of the uterus. The ovaries produce eggs and hormones.
- Fallopian tubes: These are narrow tubes that are attached to the upper part of the uterus and serve as tunnels for the ova (egg cells) to travel from the ovaries to the uterus. Conception, the fertilization of an egg by a sperm, normally occurs in the fallopian tubes. The fertilized egg then moves to the uterus, where it implants to the uterine wall.

HORMONAL CYCLES

The female Hormonal or reproductive cycle is an example of a real biological oscillating system where the periodic nature of the system may be described by a set of difference equations. The model is developed using blood-level of three different ovarian and gonadotropic hormones, estrogen, progesterone, and luteinizing hormone. We construct this model using actual sample data describing the levels of these hormones present in the body throughout the month, then discuss the applications of such research.

The female reproductive cycle is an intricate series of chemical secretions and reactions, and delicate changes in physical anatomy, which produce the ultimate potential for fertility and birth. These chemicals, known as hormones, are human proteins with the capacity to affect and regulate human growth and function. The female reproductive cycle is a general term which encompasses the ovarian cycle, the uterine cycle, the hormonal changes that regulate them, and cyclical changes in the breasts and the cervix. The ovarian cycle is the term used to describe the series of events associated with a developing oocyte, or, egg cell, within the ovaries, while the uterine cycle is the preparation of the environment of the uterus for the reception of a fertilized ovum. The regulation of both the ovarian and uterine cycles is the function of several gonadotropic and ovarian hormones.

PHYSIOLOGY OF MENSTRUAL CYCLE

The female cycle is usually referred to as the menstrual cycle, menstruation being the most prominent event, however for our purposes, we will use the term fertility cycle, placing the emphasis on the cyclic changes of fertility. Cycles vary in length from 23 days or less in a short cycle, to over 35 days in a long cycle. Few women have an absolutely regular menstrual cycle, and a variation of up to 7 days is perfectly normal. For convenience, we will use an average length cycle of 28 days.

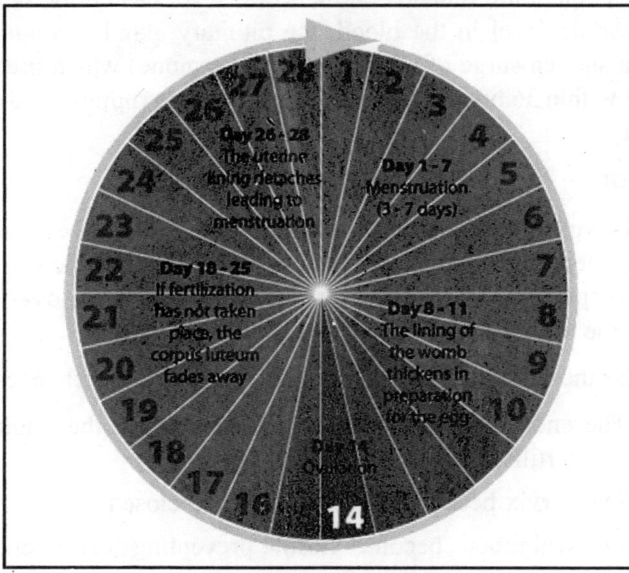

Fig. Menstrual Cycle

Hormonal changes in the fertility cycle: The fertility cycle is under the control of sex hormones. It may be conveniently divided into two phases - the phase before ovulation (pre-ovulatory) and the phase after ovulation (post-ovulatory)

Pre-ovulatory phase - controlled by FSH and oestrogen: The pituitary gland at the base of the brain secretes FSH (follicle-stimulating hormone) which, stimulates the ripening of follicles in the ovary. The ripening follicles produce increasing amounts of oestrogen. As the oestrogen levels rise approaching ovulation, certain changes take place:

- The endometrium (lining if the uterus) becomes thicker
- The cervix becomes higher and softer and open
- Cervical mucus produced by the glands or crypts in the cervix changes to a very 'sperm-friendly mucus':
- Increased salts, sugar and amino-acids - to nourish sperm
- Increased fluid (to keep cells isotonic). Up to 10x increase in mucus volume

- Highly-fertile mucus is 98% water - Transparent, glistening, slippery, stretchy - spinnbarkeit effect.
- The structure of fertile mucus using nuclear magnetic resonance shows a loose network aiding sperm penetration.

The temperature remains on the lower level. When the oestrogens reach a certain level in the blood, the pituitary gland is stimulated to produce a sudden surge of LH (luteinising hormone) which precipitates ovulation within 36 hours. The most mature follicle ruptures and releases the ovum.

Ovulation

Post-ovulatory phase - controlled by progesterone: Following ovulation, luteinising hormone or LH causes the ruptured follicle to develop into the corpus luteum, the flower-like structure in the ovary which produces the second ovarian hormone - progesterone.

Under the influence of progesterone, the following changes occur:

- The endometrium softens in preparation for the implantation of a fertilised ovum
- The cervix becomes lower, firmer and closed
- Cervical mucus becomes hostile preventing sperm penetration.
  — After ovulation there is a rapid reversion to the infertile state - A dense network of filaments forms a thick sticky mucus plug which impedes sperm penetration. Sperm are rapidly destroyed by the acidic vaginal secretions
- The temperature is raised by around 0.2°C or more.

The corpus luteum remains for around fourteen days, then it shrivels and dies; the level of progesterone falls; the temperature drops; and the endometrium disintegrates, so completing the cycle.

An average fertility cycle is of 28 days. The first day of menstruation is day 1 of the cycle. Subsequent days are numbered up to but not including the first day of the next menstrual period. A number of infertile days follow menstruation - this is the pre-ovulatory relatively infertile phase. The fertile phase occurs either side of ovulation. The first sign of cervical mucus designates the onset of the fertile phase, because sperm can survive in fertile mucus awaiting ovulation. After ovulation, time must be allowed for ovum survival and the possibility of a second ovulation occurring within 24 hours. The post-ovulatory infertile phase is confirmed by a combination of temperature and mucus signs about three days after ovulation. This phase lasts until the onset of the next menstrual period. The post-ovulatory infertile phase is the most effective in avoiding pregnancy.

Variations in Cycle Length

The post-ovulatory phase or interval between ovulation and the next menstrual period remains fairly constant - around 14 days. As cycles vary greatly in length, it follows that the interval between menstruation and ovulation (pre-ovulatory phase) must constitute the variable length of the cycle.

In a short cycle of 21 days, ovulation will occur around day 7 and there will be no pre-ovulatory infertile days. A normal length cycle (around 28 days) will have a few pre-ovulatory relatively infertile days and a long cycle (for example 35 days) where ovulation does not occur until around day 21, will have many pre-ovulatory relatively infertile days.

Monitoring Physiological Changes

A woman learns to monitor her fertility cycle subjectively by observing physiological changes in her body, using a combination of indicators of fertility. These indicators are scientifically proven to reflect changes in the ovarian hormone levels and to reflect fertility status accurately.

Indicators of Fertility

- The waking temperature
- Cervical mucus changes
- Changes in the cervix
- Calculation of cycle length
- Minor indicators of fertility for example abdominal pains and breast symptoms

The most effective method is a multiple indicator approach generally the sympto-thermal method combining temperature recordings with cervical mucus symptom.

First indicator - Temperature: Women are taught how to record, chart and interpret an accurate basal body or waking temperature, using specially-designed fertility charts and thermometres, preferably digital thermometres. The temperature rise or shift confirms ovulation. A sustained rise in temperature for 3 days indicates 48 hours past ovulation and determines the onset of the post-ovulatory infertile phase. Temperature readings give no indication of the onset of the fertile phase and the temperature is of no value in timing intercourse to achieve pregnancy.

Second indicator - Cervical mucus changes: Cervical mucus changes are observed at the vulva (vaginal entrance) and are recorded at the end of each day. Mucus changes can also be observed at the cervix where it may appear one day before its appearance at the vulva. Developing awareness of cervical mucus changes takes time and persistence. These changes may be masked by seminal fluid, spermicide or vaginal infections, so it is vital that a woman receives adequate teaching and support to monitor this sign.

- Dryness indicates the infertile phase.
- Sensation of moistness or dampness indicates potential fertility.
- Sensation of wetness, slipperiness and the presence of transparent, slippery, stretchy mucus indicates maximum fertility. This is the most valuable indicator for any woman experiencing difficulty conceiving.
- Peak day is the last day of highly fertile-type mucus recognised retrospectively. (coincides closely with ovulation).
- Following peak day there is a rapid return to dryness or moistness until the next menstruation.

Some NFP organizations teach cervical mucus changes as a single indicator method. This is known variously as the Ovulation method, Billings Ovulation Method or the Creighton Model (Hilgers Method)

Third indicator - Changes in the cervix: Detecting cervical changes can give additional information and is particularly useful for women with very long cycles, during breast-feeding or pre-menopausally. The first change in the cervix is frequently noted one or two days prior to changes in cervical mucus, and can give a very early warning of approaching fertility. It generally takes two or three cycles for women to be able to accurately detect these subtle changes in the level, position, consistency and the opening of the cervix.

- A low, long, tilted, firm, closed, dry cervix indicates infertility.
- A high, short, straight, soft, open, wet cervix indicates fertility.

Recording cycle length: The cycle length should be measured from the first day of a period (fresh red bleed) up to, but not including the first day of the next period. Any spotting prior to a period should be included in the previous cycle (pre-menstrual). This helps to determine the length of the pre and post-ovulatory phases more accurately.

A calculation can be made by taking the shortest cycle over the previous year and subtracting 20 to determine the last infertile day of the pre-ovulatory infertile phase.

Minor indicators of fertility: Ovulation or Mittelschmerz pain - A sharp pain or dull ache on one side of the lower abdomen for up to a few hours.

- Breast symptoms - A characteristic tenderness or tingling sensation may be experienced around ovulation.

HUMAN SEXUALITY

Human sexuality plays a major role in everyone's life. Regardless, whether we are young or old, man or woman, American or Japanese, it is an integral part of what we do and who we are. There has been much done by way of research and scholarly writing examining human sexuality. Of course, there are many emotions associated with human sexuality, but the primary aim of this particular paper will be a general overview of sexuality with special attention to the various perspectives, including the: (1) biological perspective, (2) cognitive perspective, and (3) learning perspective. All the while, the lens through which we summarize these perspectives will be with the understanding that human sexual behaviour is a motivation.

Next to sleeping and eating, it seems that it is one of the most important drives we have to deal with as humans. That is, it takes up so much of our time in thought and behaviour that it sometimes seems that every facet of our life revolves around this to a certain extent.

Human sexual behaviour is different from the sexual behaviour of other animals, in that, it seems to be governed by a variety and interplay of different factors. That is, while "lower" animals or species are driven by a "force" to reproduce and therefore partake in sexual behaviour. Humans are not sexually active just for the sake of reproduction, rather, there are a variety of complex factors that lead people to have sex.

Human sexuality is the way in which we experience and express ourselves as sexual beings. There are many factors that help develop our sexuality, arguably one of the most important, is our actual gender. Whether, I am a male or female will likely have a major influence on the development of my individual sexuality. Furthermore, sexuality is an integral part of our personalities whether we are aware of it or not.

This may seem like a rather simple-minded question, but one of the questions that should always be posed before any endeavor is, "why do it?" and "what do we hope to gain from it?" The former will be addressed here and the latter will hopefully become clear as we move along in our journey. An important reason to study human sexuality is that it is a primary source of motivation. Just consider the amount of time spent thinking and planning for sex, let alone the time spent in sexual behaviour itself. Sexual motivation does to some extent influence human behaviour. Another reason for studying human sexuality is that we may face various personal and social problems involving sexuality, such as, sexually transmitted diseases, unwanted pregnancies, and sexual harassment. This should sound especially timely during the times in which we live.

Biological Perspective

One cannot truly begin a dialogue about human sexuality without addressing the biological perspective, in particular, hormones. Hormones may be viewed as one of the major "driving forces" of sexual behaviour. Over the past several years, there has been much research examining the various roles that hormones play in the sexual behaviour of humans. Hormones are produced by the gonads (i.e., testes and ovaries), the adrenal cortex, the pituitary gland, and the hypothalamus. In addition, the hormones of androgens, estrogens, and progestins all exist in both males and females. They exist in different concentrations, however, within males and females. Males have a higher concentration of androgens and females have a higher concentration of estrogens and progestins. Incidentally, androgens are responsible for the sexual differentiation of the male reproductive system before birth and the sexual maturation of boys at puberty. Testosterone, a specific androgen, is associated with the male sexual drive and possibly with aggressive behaviour. Estrogens and progestins, found in higher concentrations within females, regulate the menstrual cycle and are essential for reproduction. The relationship of these hormones to the female sexual drive and behaviour are unclear. Hormone levels are usually correlated with sexual behaviour, but in humans this is not necessarily true because of intervening variables. Thus, an individual may be physiologically ready to participate in sexual behaviour, but does not because of factors that supercede any biological reason.

Cognitive Perspective

A comprehension of the processes of sexual arousal is an important element in understanding sexual responses. The notion that our most erogenous sex organ lies between our ears should not be dismissed. The cognitive activity of the brain can quickly either augment or inhibit a sexual response cycle. Perceptions and evaluations are the two major types of cognitive activity. That is, how a stimulus or situation is interpreted determines how the individual will respond to the stimulus. Perception includes at least three components: detection, labelling, and attribution. Detection is defined by an individual's ability to note the presence of a stimulus or to discriminate it from other stimuli. Next, labelling is the descriptors that an individual uses to categorize the stimulus event.

Learning Perspective

Even within the same society, family and personal experiences can shape unique sexual attitudes and behaviours. Learning theory focuses on environmental factors that shape behaviour. Within this context, learning theory examines the environmental factors that shape sexual behaviour. Behaviorism emphasizes the importance of rewards and punishments in the learning process. Events (such as rewards) that increase the frequency or likelihood of particular behaviour are termed reinforcements. When applied to sexual behaviour, children left to explore their bodies without parental condemnation will learn what feels good and tend to repeat it. However, when sexual behaviour (like masturbation) feels pleasurable, but parents connect it with feelings of guilt and shame, the child is placed in conflict. Conversely, punishment tends to suppress behaviour in circumstances in which it is expected to occur. Thus, if young people are severely punished for sexual exploration, we may come to associate sexual stimulation in general with feelings of guilt or anxiety. Social Learning Theory uses the concepts of rewards and punishment, but it also emphasizes the importance of cognitive activity (i.e., anticipations, thoughts, and plans) and learning by observation. Observational learning or modelling refers to acquiring knowledge and skills through observing others. Observational learning may also take place when exposed to certain films, books, or music. According to social learning theory children acquire the gender roles deemed appropriate in society through reinforcement of gender-appropriate behaviour. In addition, individuals duplicate behaviours of those they respect and hold as models.

Human sexuality is a very complex behaviour that is affected by many facets of our lives including our physiology, cognition, and learning. These are just a few of the components that this paper focused on for the sake of brevity. Otherwise, many other factors could have been discussed, such as, the culture, personal and general history, and the humanistic perspective. The point here is that human sexuality, like us, is multi-dimensional and one can only begin to get a sense of what it is by the inclusion of many perspectives and ideas. However, one particular point that this paper would like to get across to the reader is that it is a motivating factor. This is a bit over simplified but it seems that so much of what we do day in and day out as humans is in some way or another governed by our sexual self. While this makes us similar as humans, it is not necessarily the case that we condone the same behaviours or have overlapping norms from culture to culture. Thus, within this similarity there is still a great deal of diversity.

FOETAL DEVELOPMENT

Pregnancy begins with conception. Two cells, a sperm and an egg, come together inside the uterus to make one cell. In a few hours, this single cell will divide itself over and over. This makes a cluster of cells that will become a baby. The tiny cluster must attach to the lining of the uterus. This happens in the first 2 weeks.

The embryonic period in humans begins at fertilization (2nd week of gestation) and continues until the end of the 10th week of gestation (8th week of development).

The zygote spends the next few days travelling down the Fallopian tube. Meanwhile it divides several times to form a ball of cells called a morula. Further cellular division is accompanied by the formation of a small cavity between the cells. This stage is called a blastocyst. Up to this point there is no growth in the overall size of the embryo, so each division produces successively smaller cells.

The blastocyst reaches the uterus at roughly the fifth day after fertilization. It is here that lysis of the zona pellucida, a glycoprotein shell, occurs. This is required so that the trophectoderm cells, which give rise to extra-embryonic structures such as the placenta, of the blastocyst can come into contact with the luminal epithelial cells of the endometrium. (Contrast this with zona hatching, an event that occurs in vitro by a different mechanism, but with a similar result). It then adheres to the uterine lining and becomes embedded in the endometrial cell layer. This process is also called implantation. In most successful pregnancies, the conceptus implants 8 to 10 days after ovulation (Wilcox et al 1999). The inner cell mass forms the embryo, while the outer cell layers form the membranes and placenta. Together, the embryo and its membranes are referred to as a conceptus, or the "products of conception".

Rapid growth occurs and the embryo's main external features begin to take form. This process is called differentiation, which produces the varied cell types (such as blood cells, kidney cells, and nerve cells). A spontaneous abortion, or miscarriage, in the first trimester of pregnancy is usually due to major genetic mistakes or abnormalities in the developing embryo. During this critical period (most of the first trimester), the developing embryo is also susceptible to toxic exposures, such as:

- Alcohol, certain drugs, and other toxins that cause birth defects, such as Foetal alcohol syndrome
- Infection (such as rubella or cytomegalovirus)
- Radiation from x-rays or radiation therapy
- Nutritional deficiencies such as lack of folate which contributes to spina bifida

Generally, if a structure pre-dates another structure in evolutionary terms, then it often appears earlier than the other in an embryo; this general observation is sometimes summarized by the phrase "ontogeny recapitulates phylogeny." For example, the backbone is a common structure among all vertebrates such as fish, reptiles and mammals, and the backbone also appears as one of the earliest structures laid out in all vertebrate embryos. The cerebrum in humans, which is the most sophisticated part of the brain, develops last. The concept of recapitulation is not absolute, but it is recognized as being partly applicable to development of the human embryo.

CHANGES BY WEEKS OF GESTATIONAL AGE

Week 1 (Day 1-7 of Fertilization)

- Fertilization of the ovum to form a zygote. (day 1 of fertilization)
- The zygote undergoes mitotic cellular divisions, but does not increase in size. This mitosis is also known as cleavage. A hollow cavity forms marking the blastocyst stage. (day 1.5-3 of fertilization)
- The blastocyst contains only a thin rim of trophoblast cells and a clump of cells at one end known as the "embryonic pole" which include embryonic stem cells.
- The blastocyst hatches from its protein shell (zona pellucida) and performs implantation onto the endometrial lining of the mother's uterus. (day 5-6 of fertilization)
- If separation into identical twins occurs, 1/3 of the time it will happen before day 5.

Week 2 (8-14 Days from Fertilization)

- Trophoblast cells surrounding the embryonic cells proliferate and invade deeper into the uterine lining. They will eventually form the placenta and embryonic membranes. The blastocyst is fully implanted day 7-12 of fertilization.

- Formation of the yolk sac.
- The embryonic cells flatten into a disk, two cells thick.
- If separation into identical twins occurs, 2/3 of the time it will happen between days 5 and 9. If it happens after day 9, there is a significant risk of the twins being conjoined.
- Primitive streak develops. (day 13 of fertilization)
- Primary stem villi appear. (day 13 of fertilization)

Week 3 (15-21 Days from Fertilization)

- A notochord forms in the centre of the embryonic disk. (day 16 of fertilization)
- Gastrulation commences. (day 16 of fertilization)
- A neural groove (future spinal cord) forms over the notochord with a brain bulge at one end. Neuromeres appear. (day 18 of fertilization)
- Somites, the divisions of the future vertebra, form. (day 20 of fertilization)
- Primitive heart tube is forming. Vasculature begins to develop in embryonic disc. (day 20 of fertilization)

Week 4 (22-28 Days from Fertilization)

- The embryo measures 4 mm (1/8 inch) in length and begins to curve into a C shape.
- The heart bulges, further develops, and begins to beat in a regular rhythm. Septum primum appear.
- Branchial arches, grooves which will form structures of the face and neck, form.
- The neural tube closes.
- The ears begin to form as otic pits.
- Arm buds and a tail are visible.
- Pulmonary primordium, the first traits of the lung appear.
- Hepatic plate, the first traits of the liver appear.
- Buccopharyngeal membrane ruptures. This is the future mouth.
- Cystic diverticulum, which will become the gallbladder, and dorsal pancreatic bud, which will become the pancreas appear.

- Urorectal septum begins to form. Thus, the rectal and urinary passageways become separated.
- Anterior and posterior horns differentiate in the spinal cord.
- Spleen appears.
- Ureteric buds appear.

Week 5 (29-35 Days from Fertilization)

- The embryo measures 8 mm (1/4 inch) in length.
- Lens pits and optic cups form the start of the developing eye.
- Nasal pits form.
- The brain divides into 5 vesicles, including the early telencephalon.
- Leg buds form and hands form as flat paddles on the arms.
- Rudimentary blood moves through primitive vessels connecting to the yolk sac and chorionic membranes.

Week 6 (36-42 Days from Fertilization)

- The embryo measures 13 mm (1/2 inch) in length.
- Lungs begin to form.
- The brain continues to develop.
- Arms and legs have lengthened with foot and hand areas distinguishable.
- The hands and feet have digits, but may still be webbed.
- The gonadal ridge begins to be perceptible.
- The lymphatic system begins to develop.

Week 7 (43-49 Days from Fertilization)

- The embryo measures 18 mm (3/4 inch) in length.
- Nipples and hair follicles begin to form.
- Location of the elbows and toes are visible.
- Spontaneous limb movements may be detected by ultrasound.
- All essential organs have at least begun formation.

Foetal Period

The foetal period begins at the end of the 10th week of gestation (8th week of development). Since the precursors of all the major organs are created by this time, the foetal period is described both by organ and by a list of changes by weeks of gestational age.

Because the precursors of the organs are formed, foetus also is not as sensitive to damage from environmental exposures as the embryo. Instead, toxic exposures often cause physiological abnormalities or minor congenital malformation.

BY ORGAN

Changes by weeks of gestational age

From the 8th week until birth (around 38 weeks), the developing organism is called a foetus. The foetus is not as sensitive to damage from environmental exposures as the embryo, and toxic exposures often cause physiological abnormalities or minor congenital malformation. All major structures are already formed in the foetus, but they continue to grow and develop.

Week 8 (7th Week of Development)

- Embryo measures 30 mm (1.2 inches) in length.
- Intestines rotate.
- Facial features continue to develop.
- The eyelids are more developed.
- The external features of the ear begin to take their final shape.

Weeks 9 to 12 (8th to 11th Week of Development)

- The foetus reaches a length of 8 cm (3.2 inches).
- The head comprises nearly half of the foetus' size.
- The face is well formed
- The eyelids close and will not reopen until about the 28th week.
- Tooth buds, which will form the baby teeth, appear.
- The limbs are long and thin.
- The foetus can make a fist with its fingers.
- Genitals appear well differentiated.
- Red blood cells are produced in the liver.

Weeks 13 to 16 (12th to 15th Week of Development)

- The foetus reaches a length of about 15 cm (6 inches).
- A fine hair called lanugo develops on the head.
- Foetal skin is almost transparent.
- More muscle tissue and bones have developed, and the bones become harder.

- The foetus makes active movements.
- Sucking motions are made with the mouth.
- Meconium is made in the intestinal tract.
- The liver and pancreas produce fluid secretions.

Week 19 (18th Week of Development)

- The foetus reaches a length of 20 cm (8 inches).
- Lanugo covers the entire body.
- Eyebrows and eyelashes appear.
- Nails appear on fingers and toes.
- The foetus is more active with increased muscle development.
- "Quickening" usually occurs (the mother can feel the foetus moving).
- The foetal heartbeat can be heard with a stethoscope.

Week 23 (22nd Week of Development)

- The foetus reaches a length of 28 cm (11.2 inches).
- The foetus weighs about 725 g (1 lb 10 oz).
- Eyebrows and eyelashes are well formed.
- All of the eye components are developed.
- The foetus has a hand and startle reflex.
- Footprints and fingerprints continue forming.
- Alveoli (air sacs) are forming in lungs.

Week 27 (26th Week of Development)

- The foetus reaches a length of 38 cm (15 inches).
- The foetus weighs about 1.2 kg (2 lb 11 oz).
- The brain develops rapidly.
- The nervous system develops enough to control some body functions.
- The eyelids open and close.
- The cochleae are now developed, though the myelin sheaths in neural portion of the auditory system will continue to develop until 18 months after birth.
- The respiratory system, while immature, has developed to the point where gas exchange is possible.

Week 31 (30th Week of Development)

- The foetus reaches a length of about 38-43 cm (15-17 inches).
- The foetus weighs about 2 kg (4 lb 6 oz).
- The amount of body fat rapidly increases.
- Rhythmic breathing movements occur, but lungs are not fully mature.
- Thalamic brain connections, which mediate sensory input, form.
- Bones are fully developed, but are still soft and pliable.
- The foetus begins storing iron, calcium, and phosphorus.

Week 35 (34th Week of Development)

- The foetus reaches a length of about 40-48 cm (16-19 inches).
- The foetus weighs about 2.5 to 3 kg (5 lb 12 oz to 6 lb 12 oz).
- Lanugo begins to disappear.
- Body fat increases.
- Fingernails reach the end of the fingertips.
- A baby born at 36 weeks has a high chance of survival, but may require medical interventions.

Weeks 36 to 39 (35th to 38th Week of Development)

- The foetus is considered full-term at the end of the 37th week of gestational age.
- It may be 48 to 53 cm (19 to 21 inches) in length.
- The lanugo is gone except on the upper arms and shoulders.
- Fingernails extend beyond fingertips.
- Small breast buds are present on both sexes.
- Head hair is now coarse and thickest.

GENETICS

Reproductive genetics is a broad research area, and the topics discussed and listed below are not meant to be exclusive areas of interest, but rather a sampling of the types of problems that this program announcement intends to address.

Sex determination is the translation of the chromosomal sex (XX or XY) into the gender-appropriate internal and external reproductive structures. The initial events of sex determination are, therefore, genetically determined. Errors in the process can range in severity from complete sex reversal to gonadal dysgenesis or minor genital abnormalities. Sex determination, as an early embryological event, can help us address basic questions of the regulation of gene expression, cell-fate determination, and hormone signaling.

Approximately one in 1, 000 newborns has some abnormality of genital and/or gonadal development. In many cases, gonadal dysgenesis is part of a larger pathologic syndrome, such as Frasier syndrome, Deny-Drash syndrome, or campomelic dysplasia, to name a few. The known genes involved in sex determination often act as growth and/or differentiation factors and there is mounting evidence that they may be important in tumorigenesis in the gonads as well as other tissues.

Despite the identification of the Y-chromosome gene SRY as the "testis determining factor" almost 15 years ago, the mechanisms and pathways of normal sex differentiation are still not well understood. In particular, although some downstream effects of SRY are known, such as cellular proliferation, Sertoli cell differentiation, and testis-specific vascularization, the direct transcriptional targets of SRY remain unknown. The factors regulating SRY expression remain unknown as well. While genes such as SOX-9, WT-1, DAX-1, DMRT-1, GATA4, FOG2, and SF-1, among others, contribute to sex determination, the nature and timing of their interactions remain unclear, and there are clearly other unknown genes to be identified. A further level of complexity arises with gene dosage effects, such as XY sex reversal caused by duplication of Dax-1.

Sex determination can be divided into steps consisting of establishment of the bipotential gonad, formation of the primordial gonad, and differentiation of the gonad. Many of the sex determining genes act in multiple steps, but SRY mainly functions in shaping the primordial gonad into a testis. However, the classic view of SRY as a "switch" that confers maleness is an over- simplification as illustrated by the enormous potential for ambiguity in sex determination, and by evidence suggesting that steps in testis development that were once thought to be tightly coordinated, such as mesonephric cell migration and Leydig cell differentiation, or the formation of testis cords and the inhibition of male germ cell meiosis, can occur independently of each other. Additionally, ovarian development may not be the passive "default" process it was once thought to be. Estrogen may be necessary to maintain the ovarian phenotype, as mice unable to make estrogen (ArKO mice) or bind estrogen develop patches of Sertoli and Leydig cells within their ovaries postnatally.

Germ cells play a critical role in the formation of ovaries, although testes can form in their absence. The germ cells migrate into the gonad through the gut, through a process which has yet to be fully characterized. The presence of meiotic germ cells is critical for the formation and maintenance of ovarian follicles while, in contrast, in males the testis cords surround the germ cells and meiosis is inhibited. Germ cell migration and the progression into meiosis are not well understood.

There is clear evidence that the genes involved in sex determination have important roles beyond gonadal fate. Some, such as WT-1, are expressed in common embryonic precursors to different organ systems. Mutations in FOXL2, a gene deleted in polled intersex goats, cause the human syndrome BPES that often includes premature ovarian failure. The anti-mullerian hormone, known as Amh or MIS, causes regression of the female duct system in normal males, and in adult males, MIS has inhibitory effects on both Leydig cells and testosterone production. Such examples clearly demonstrate that the continued study of sex determination will not only benefit those born with gonadal

dysgenesis or ambiguous genitalia, but will also advance our knowledge of the physiology of the adult reproductive system, and the development and regulation of other organ systems.

GENETIC COUNSELLING

Genetic counselling is a communication process which deals with human problems associated with the occurrence, or the risk of occurrence of a genetic disorder in a family. This process involves an attempt by one or more appropriately trained persons (genetic counsellors) to help the individual or family to (i) comprehend the medical facts, including the diagnosis, the probable course of the disorder, and the available management, (ii) appreciate the way heredity contributes to disorder, and the risk of recurrence in specified relatives, (iii) understand the options for dealing with the risk of recurrence, (iv) choose the course of action which seems appropriate to them in view of their risk and the family goals and in accordance with the decision, and (v) make the best possible adjustment to the disorder in the affected family member and/or the risk of recurrence of that disorder.

Presently, genetic counselling goes beyond mere presentations of risk facts and figures to the prevention and cure of disease, the relief of pain and the maintenance of health. For many disorders it is only possible to give precise recurrence risk conditions and also the order of risk, if exensive family studies are available.

A woman may be referred for genetic counseling if pregnant and undergoing prenatal testing or screening. Genetic counsellors educate the patient about their testing options and inform them of their results. If a prenatal screening or test is abnormal, the genetic counselor evaluates the risk of an affected pregnancy, educates the patient about these risks and informs the patient of their options.

A person may also undergo genetic counselling after the birth of a child with a genetic condition. In these instances, the genetic counselor explains the condition to the patient along with recurrence risks in future children. In all cases of a positive family history for a condition, the genetic counsellor can evaluate risks, recurrence and explain the condition itself.

Some of the genetic disorders that could be identified are Down's syndrome, cystic fibrosis, sickle cell disease, Tay-Sachs disease (a fatal disease affecting the central nervous system) and spina bifida. Some reputed hospitals offer genetic counseling as part of their maternity care programme.

Genetic counseling also involves:

- Educating the affected couple to understand the nature of the genetic disorder.
- Counseling and psychological support.
- Providing the necessary information on support groups and services to manage the genetic condition.

Ideally, it is best to seek genetic counseling before one become pregnant. It will be especially beneficial if the baby is at risk of inheriting genetic disorders.

The risk factors involved could be:

- If a standard prenatal screening test yields an abnormal result.
- Either parent or a close relative has an inherited disease or birth defect.
- Either parent already has children with birth defects or genetic disorders.
- If the women is over 35 years of age and wants to give birth to a baby.
- If someone have had miscarriages before.

REFERENCES

Butler J, et, al. Supportive nurse-midwife care is associated with a reduced incidence of cesarean section. American Jouran of Obstetrics and Gynecology 1993; 168:1407-13.

Capan P, et al. Nurse-managed clinics provide access and improved health care. Nurse practitioner 1993; 18:50-5.

Gabay M and Wolfe SM. Nurse-Midwifery, the Beneficial Alternative. Public Health Reports 1997; 112(5): 386-395.

Haire D and Elsberry C. Maternity care and outcomes in a high-risk service: the North Central Bronx Hospital experience. Birth 1991; 18:33-7.

Harvey S, et al. A randomized controlled trial of nurse-midwifery care. Birth 1996; 23:128-35

Hueston WJ, and Rudy M. A comparison of labor and delivery management between nurse-midwives and family physicians. Journal of Family Practice 1993; 375:449-54.

Murphy, PA and Fullerton, J. Outcomes of Intended Home Births in Nurse-Midwifery Practice: A Prospective Descriptive Study. Obstetrics & Gynecology 1998 92:3; 461-470.

Oakley D, et. al. Processes of care: comparisons of certified nurse-midwives and obstetricians. Journal of Nurse-Midwifery 1995; 40:399-409.

3

Pregnancy (Ante-natal)

A full-term pregnancy lasts approximately forty weeks, or nine calendar months, and is divided into three phases, called trimesters, of three months each. During each trimester, the pregnant woman experiences various physical and psychological changes.

NORMAL PREGNANCY

The earliest sign of pregnancy and the reason most pregnant women initially see a physician is missing a menstrual period. For sexually active women who are of reproductive age and have regular periods, missing a period for ≥ 1 wk is presumptive evidence of pregnancy.

Pregnancy is considered to last 266 days from the time of conception or 280 days from the first day of the last menstrual period if periods occur regularly every 28 days. Delivery date is estimated based on the last menstrual period. Delivery up to 2 wk earlier or later than the estimated date is normal.

SYMPTOMS AND SIGNS

Pregnancy may cause breasts to be engorged because of increased levels of estrogen (primarily) and progesterone-an extension of premenstrual breast engorgement. Nausea, occasionally with vomiting, may occur because of increased secretion of estrogen and the ? subunit of human chorionic gonadotropin (β-hCG) by syncytial cells of the placenta, beginning 10 days after fertilization. The corpus luteum in the ovary, stimulated by β-hCG, continues secreting large amounts of estrogen and progesterone to maintain the pregnancy. Many women become fatigued at this time, and a few women notice abdominal bloating very early. Women usually begin to feel foetal movement between 16 and 20 wk.

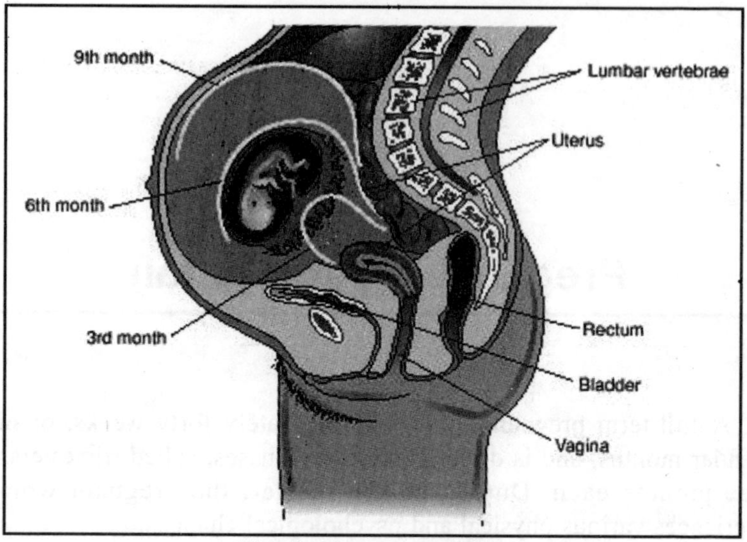

Fig. Symptoms and Signs

Pelvic examination findings include a softer cervix and an irregularly softened, enlarged uterus. The cervix usually becomes bluish to purple, probably because blood supply to the uterus is increased. Around 12 wk gestation, the uterus extends above the true pelvis into the abdomen; at 20 wk, it reaches the umbilicus; and by 36 wk, the upper pole almost reaches the xiphoid process.

DIAGNOSIS

Usually urine and occasionally blood tests are used to confirm or exclude pregnancy; results are usually accurate several days before a missed menstrual period and often as early as several days after conception. Levels of β-hCG, which correlate with gestational age in normal pregnancies, can be used to determine whether a foetus is growing normally. The best approach is to compare 2 serum β-hCG values, obtained 48 to 72 h apart and measured by the same laboratory. In a normal single pregnancy, β-hCG levels double about every 1.4 to 2.1 days during the first 60 days (7.5 wk), then begin to decrease between 10 and 18 wk. Regular doubling of the β-hCG level during the 1st trimester strongly suggests normal growth.

Other accepted signs of pregnancy include the following:

- Presence of a gestational sac in the uterus, seen with ultrasonography typically at about 4 to 5 wk and typically corresponding to a serum b-hCG level of about 1500 mIU/mL (a yolk sac can usually be seen in the gestational sac by 5 wk).

- Foetal heart motion, seen with real-time ultrasonography as early as 5 to 6 wk.
- Foetal heart sounds, heard with Doppler ultrasonography as early as 8 to 10 wk if the uterus is accessible abdominally.
- Foetal movements felt by the examining physician after 20 wk.

PHYSIOLOGICAL CHANGES DURING PREGNANCY

Pregnancy is associated with normal physiological changes that assist foetal survival as well as preparation for labour. It is important to know what 'normal' parametres of change are in order to diagnose and manage common medical problems of pregnancy such as hypertension, gestation diabetes, anaemia and hyperthyroidism.

REPRODUCTIVE SYSTEM

When a lady become pregnant, the lower part of her body is affected first and the part that undergoes the most significant changes is the uterus. It increases to 20 times its original weight, and 1, 000 times its initial capacity. The amount of its muscle, connective and elastic tissue, blood vessels, and nerves increases. Its shape changes from elongated to oval by the second month, to round by midgestation, then back through oval to elongated at term (the end of a normal nine-month pregnancy). The uterus softens beginning at the sixth week. It changes position as it increases in size, ascending into the abdomen by the fourth month and eventually reaching to the liver. It also becomes more contractile (the tendency to decrease in size), with irregular, painless Braxton Hicks contractions beginning in the first trimester. Lady may feel these contractions in the last weeks of pregnancy, when they are known as false labour.

Other parts of the reproductive system change along with the uterus. The cervix and vagina have an increased blood supply, which causes a darkening in colour apparent by the sixth week. The amount of elastic tissue increases to prepare the way for the stretching that will be required during delivery. Secretions increase, and a mucous plug develops in the cervix. The fallopian tubes, ovaries, and ligaments supporting the uterus all enlarge and elongate. The ovaries, of course, cease to ovulate.

During the fourth month, the uterus grows into the abdomen, causing the abdominal wall to expand to accommodate it. The connective and elastic tissues stretch and straighten, creating thinned areas called striae (stretch marks). While the red of the striae may fade, silver remnants usually remain after delivery. In 50 percent of women, striae develop in the third trimester. Late in pregnancy, the internal pressure from the large uterus may even cause the muscles of the abdominal wall to separate (diastasis).

Breasts undergo many changes during pregnancy to produce milk. In the first two months of pregnancy, the breasts may feel sore or full. They enlarge, and veins may become visible. Striae can develop. The nipples also increase in size and usually darken. By midpregnancy, colostrum (a thick, yellowish fluid) can be expressed, but milk is not produced until after delivery.

CARDIO VASCULAR SYSTEM

Progesterone decreases systemic vascular resistance reduces by about 20% early in pregnancy. Postural hypotension may result.

Diastolic and systolic blood pressure tend to fall during mid pregnancy and then return to normal by week 36.

Venous return in the inferior vena cava can be compromised in late pregnancy if a woman lies flat on her back - this is relieved by lying in the left lateral position.

Increased circulating angiotensin II encourages water and sodium retention leading to an increased plasma volume (to 50% by 30 weeks). This enables increased uterine blood flow to meet growing nutritional and oxygenation needs of the foetus. It also enables blood loss (average 500ml) at delivery to be met without physiological decompensation.

Advise women not to take up unaccustomed vigorous exercise in pregnancy as there is a risk of diversion of uterine blood flow to the skeletal muscles.

Blood flow to kidneys, skin and mucosa increases.

Cardiac output increases by 30-50% with 15% increase in heart rate and 25-30% increased stroke volume. Much of this adjustment occurs prior to 12 weeks gestation and so impaired cardiac function is likely to present problematically in early pregnancy or with the sudden increase in pre-load in the third stage of labour.

RESPIRATORY SYSTEM

Changes within the respiratory system are of great significance to the anaesthetist.

Respiratory Tract: Hormonal changes to the mucosal vasculature of the respiratory tract lead to capillary engorgement and swelling of the lining in the nose, oropharynx, larynx, and trachea. Symptoms of nasal congestion, voice change and upper respiratory tract infection may prevail throughout gestation. These symptoms can be exacerbated by fluid overload or oedema associated with pregnancy-induced hypertension (PIH) or pre-eclampsia.

Lung Volumes: Upward displacement by the gravid uterus causes a 4 cm elevation of the diaphragm, but total lung capacity decreases only slightly because of compensatory increases in the transverse and antero-posterior diametres of the chest, as well as flaring of the ribs. These changes are brought about by hormonal effects that loosen ligaments. Despite the upward displacement, the diaphragm moves with greater excursions during breathing in the pregnant than in the non-pregnant state. In fact, breathing is more diaphragmatic than thoracic during gestation, an advantage during supine positioning and high regional blockade.

From the middle of the second trimester, expiratory reserve volume, residual volume and functional residual volume are progressively decreased, by approximately 20% at term. Lung compliance is relatively unaffected, but chest wall compliance is reduced, especially in the lithotomy position.

Ventilation and Respiratory Gases: A progressive increase in minute ventilation starts soon after conception and peaks at 50% above normal levels around the second trimester. This increase is effected by a 40% rise in tidal volume and a 15% rise in respiratory rate (2-3 breaths/minute). Since dead space remains unchanged, alveolar ventilation is about 70% higher at the end of gestation.

Oxygen consumption increases gradually in response to the needs of the growing foetus, culminating in a rise of at least 20% at term. During labour, oxygen consumption is further increased (up to and over 60%) as a result of the exaggerated cardiac and respiratory work load.

URINARY SYSTEM

Glomerular filtration rate (GFR) increases by 50% early in pregnancy, increasing creatinine clearance. Serum creatinine and urea will fall by about 25%.

Increased GFR also increases filtered sodium. Aldosterone levels rise by 2-3 times to reabsorb the filtered sodium.

Increased GFR and impaired tubular reabsorption of glucose produce glucosuria in approximately 15% of normal pregnancies.

Proteinuria is abnormal in pregnancy.

The smooth muscle of the renal pelvis and ureter become relaxed and dilated, kidneys increase in length and ureters become longer, more curved and with an increase in residual urine volume. Bladder smooth muscle also relaxes, increasing capacity and risk of UTI. Approximately 5% of pregnant women have bacteriuria and there is a greater risk of developing pyelonephritis in pregnancy.

GASTROINTESTINAL SYSTEM

Mechanical Changes: The enlarging uterus causes a gradual cephalad displacement of stomach and intestines. At term the stomach has attained a vertical position rather than its normal horizontal one. These mechanical forces lead to increased intragastric pressures as well as a change in the angle of the gastroesophageal junction, which in turn tends toward greater oesophageal reflux.

Physiological Changes; The hormonal effects on the gastrointestinal tract are an issue of debate. Relaxation of the lower oesophageal sphincter has been described, but there have been differing views about the effect on motility of the gastrointestinal tract and the times at which it is most prominent.

Many believe that there is also retardation of gastrointestinal motility and gastric emptying, producing increased gastric volume with decreased pH, beginning as early as 8-10 weeks of gestation. Recent studies, however, have shed a different light on the subject. Measuring peak plasma concentrations of drugs absorbed exclusively in the duodenum in both non-pregnant and pregnant volunteers, at different times of gestation, it was shown that peak absorption occurred at the same interval in all women with the exception those in labour. This suggests that gastric emptying is delayed only at the time of delivery.

Pulmonary Aspiration: Pulmonary Aspiration of gastric contents can occur either following vomiting (active) or regurgitation (passive). Aspiration of solid material causes atelectasis, obstructive pneumonitis or lung abscess, while aspiration of acidic gastric contents results in chemical pneumonitis (Mendelson's syndrome). The most serious consequences follow aspiration of acidic materials containing particulate matter as may follow swallowing certain antacids such as magnesium trisilicate.

METABOLIC CHANGES

All metabolic functions are increased during pregnancy to provide for the demands of foetus, placenta and uterus as well as for the gravida's increased basal metabolic rate and oxygen consumption. Protein metabolism is enhanced to supply substrate for maternal and foetal growth. Fat metabolism increases as evidenced by elevation in all lipid fractions in the blood. Carbohydrate metabolism, however, demonstrates the most dramatic changes. Metabolically speaking, pregnant women live in a state of "accelerated starvation." First, nutritional demands of the growing foetus are met by the intake of glucose and, second, secretion of insulin in response to glucose is augmented. As early as 15 weeks of gestation, maternal blood glucose levels after an overnight fast are considerably lower than in the nongravid state.

Hypoglycaemia: Optimal blood glucose levels in pregnant women range between 4.4 to 5.5 mmol/1 (80 to 100mg/dl). In healthy non-pregnant individuals, signs of hypoglycaemia usually begin when the blood glucose level declines to approximately 2.2 mmol/1 (40mg/dl); in pregnant women, however, hypoglycaemia is defined as a concentration below 3.3 mmol/1 (60mg/dl). Hypoglycaemia initiates the release of glucagon, cortisol and, importantly, catecholamines. In the anaesthetised state, however, these compensatory mechanisms, particularly the release of epinephrine (adrenaline), are blocked. Autonomic derangements in the form of hypotension and tachycardia tend to ensue during high regional blockade or deep general anaesthesia, which may mask the symptoms and signs of hypoglycaemia.

RENAL PHYSIOLOGY

Renal plasma flow and glomerular filtration rate begin to increase progressively during the first trimester. At term, both are 50-60% higher than in the non-pregnant state. This parallels the increases in blood volume and cardiac output. The elevations in plasma flow and glomerular filtration result in an elevation in creatinine clearance. Blood urea and serum creatinine are reduced by 40%. The increase in glomerular filtration may overwhelm the ability of the renal tubules to reabsorb leading to glucose and protein losses in the urine. Thus, mild glycosuria (1-10 gm/day) and/or proteinuria (to 300 mg/day) can occur in normal pregnancy. There is also an increase in filtered sodium, but tubular absorption is increased by an increase in aldosterone secretion, via the renin-angiotensin mechanism. There is also a decrease in plasma osmolality. This is a measure of the osmotic activity of a substance in solution and is defined as the number of osmoles in a kilogram of solvent. In practice it indicates that the plasma concentrations of electrolytes, glucose and urea, fall if more water than sodium, for example, is retained. Over the whole period of gestation there is retention of 7.5L of water and 900 mmol of sodium.

After the 12th week of gestation, progesterone can induce dilation and atony of the renal calyses and ureters. With advancing gestation, the enlarging uterus can compress the ureters as they cross the pelvic brim and cause further dilatation by obstructing flow. These changes may contribute to the frequency of urinary tract infections during pregnancy.

SKELETAL CHANGES

- Increased ligamental laxity caused by increased levels of relaxin contribute to back pain and pubic symphysis dysfunction.
- Shift in posture with exaggerated lumbar lordosis.

SKIN CHANGES

- Increased oestrogen levels may cause hyperpigmentation of the umbilicus, nipples, abdominal midline (linea nigra) and face (chloasma).
- Hyperdynamic circulation and high levels of oestrogen may cause spider naevi and palmar erythema.
- Stria gravidarum ("stretch marks")

ENDOCRINE SYSTEM

Pituitary

- FSH/LH fall to low levels
- ACTH and melanocyte stimulating hormone increase
- Prolactin increases

Thyroid and Parathyroid

- Thyroxine binding globulin (TBG) concentrations rise due to increased oestrogen levels.
- T4 and T3 increase over first half of pregnancy but there is a normal to slightly decreased amount of free hormone due to increased TBG-binding.
- TSH production is stimulated, although in healthy individuals this is not usually significant. A large rise in TSH is likely to indicate iodine deficiency or subclinical hypothyroidism.

- Serum calcium levels decrease in pregnancy which stimulates an increase in parathyroid hormone (PTH).
- Cholecalciferol (vitamin D3) is converted to its active metabolite 1, 25-dihydroxycholecalciferol by placental 1α-hydroxylase.

Adrenal & Pancreas

- Cortisol levels increase in pregnancy which favours lipogenesis and fat storage.
- Insulin response also increases so blood sugar should remain normal or low.
- Peripheral insulin resistance may also develop over the course of pregnancy and gestational diabetes is thought to reflect a pronounced insulin resistance of this sort.

PSYCHOLOGICAL CHANGES

Psychological Changes in the First Trimester: Lady may not be able to see the changes that are happening during the first trimester, but they are significant. During this time, some new mothers might be filled with a feeling of anxiety about losing their new baby. These fears, though unfounded, are perfectly normal. Read about the many emotions that women experience during this critical period in foetal development.

Psychological Changes in the Second Trimester: Once the stress and anxiety of the first trimester have passed, the emotional changes of the second trimester begin. Though the feelings during this time will usually be less intense, they can be equally as troubling. Many mothers begin to feel self-conscious about the weight they are putting on to support their baby, and these feelings can lead to low self-esteem.

Psychological Changes in the Third Trimester: In the third trimester, women are anticipating childbirth and coping with significant physical changes. While fears of losing the baby have usually disappeared by this point, a new anxiety takes its place -- the fear of the baby's arrival. Also, worries about labour and birth are also common during the last three months of pregnancy.

DISCOMFORTS OF PREGNANCY

Symptoms of discomfort due to pregnancy vary from woman-to-woman. The following are some common discomforts. However, each mother-to-be may experience symptoms differently or not at all:

- Nausea and vomiting: About half of all pregnant women experience nausea and sometimes vomiting in the first trimester - also called morning sickness because symptoms are most severe in the morning. Some women may have nausea and vomiting throughout the pregnancy. The cause of morning sickness may be due to the changes in hormone levels during pregnancy.

  Morning sickness seems to be aggravated by stress, travelling, and certain foods high in protein and fat. To lessen the symptoms, eating small meals several times a day may help. A diet high in complex carbohydrates (such as whole wheat bread, pasta, bananas, and green, leafy vegetables) may also help reduce the severity of the nausea.

  If vomiting is severe, causing a woman to lose fluids and weight, it may indicate a condition called hyperemesis gravidarum. Hyperemesis can lead to dehydration and may require hospitalization for intravenous fluids and nutrition.

- Fatigue: As the body works overtime to provide a nourishing environment for the foetus, it is no wonder a pregnant woman often feels tired. In the first trimester, her blood volume and other fluids increase as her body adjusts to the pregnancy. Sometimes anaemia is the underlying cause of the fatigue. Anaemia is a reduction in the oxygen carried through the bloodstream by red blood cells. A simple blood test performed at the first prenatal visit will check for anaemia.

- Heartburn and indigestion: Heartburn and indigestion, caused by pressure on the intestines and stomach (which, in turn, pushes stomach contents back up into the esophagus), can be prevented or reduced by eating smaller meals throughout the day and by avoiding lying down shortly after eating.

- Bleeding gums: Gums may become more spongy as blood flow increases during pregnancy, causing them to bleed easily. A pregnant woman should continue to take care of her teeth and gums and go to the dentist for regular checkups. This symptom usually disappears after pregnancy.

- Pica: Pica is a rare craving to eat substances other than food, such as dirt, clay, or coal. The craving may indicate a nutritional deficiency.

- Swelling/fluid retention: Mild swelling is common during pregnancy but severe swelling that persists may indicate preeclampsia (abnormal condition marked by high blood pressure). Lying on the left side, elevating the legs, and wearing support hose and comfortable shoes may help to relieve the swelling.
- Skin changes: Due to fluctuations in hormone levels, including hormones that stimulate pigmentation of the skin, brown, blotchy patches may occur on the face, forehead, and/or cheeks. This is often called the mask of pregnancy, or chloasma, and often disappears soon after delivery. Pigmentation may also increase in the skin surrounding the nipples, called the areola. In addition, a dark line frequently appears down the middle of the abdomen.
- Stretch marks: Pinkish stretch marks may appear on the abdomen, breasts, thighs, or buttocks. Stretch marks are generally caused by a rapid increase in weight, and the marks usually fade after pregnancy.
- Constipation: Increased pressure from the pregnancy on the rectum and intestines can interfere with digestion and subsequent bowel movements. In addition, hormone changes may slow down the food being processed by the body. Increasing fluids, regular exercise, and increasing the fibre in diet are some of the ways to prevent constipation. Always check with physician before taking any medication for this condition.
- Backache: As a woman's weight increases, her balance changes, therefore, straining her back. Pelvic joints that begin to loosen in preparation for childbirth also contribute to this back strain. Proper posture and proper lifting techniques throughout the pregnancy can help reduce the strain on the back.
- Dizziness: Dizziness during pregnancy is a common symptom. To prevent injury from falling during episodes of dizziness, a pregnant woman should stand up slowly and hold on to the walls and other stable structures for support and balance.
- Headaches: Hormonal changes may be the cause of headaches during pregnancy, especially during the first trimester. Rest, proper nutrition, and adequate fluid intake may help alleviate headache symptoms. Always consult physician before taking any medication for this condition.

TESTS

The earliest pregnancy test was based on early pregnancy factor. This test can be performed within 48 hrs of fertilization but very costly. But at present there are lot of ways to detect pregnancy at an early stage. Tests are available to confirm pregnancy at home itself. Some of the confirmatory tests available now are:

- Home pregnancy tests.
- Quantitative serum analysis.
- Urine analysis
- Qualitative analysis.
- Sonograms.
- Physical examinations.

Basis for tests: Most chemical tests for pregnancy are based on the presence of beta subunit of HCG or human chorionic gonadotrophin in the blood or urine.HCG can be detected in urine or blood after implantation, which occurs 6-12 days after fertilization.

Trophoblast cells of the embryo which gets implanted in the uterine endometreium secretes this hormone which is later continued by placenta.

Quantitative blood analysis requires a minimum level of 1mIU/ml, of HCG to detect pregnancy when compared to urine test, qualitative test which requires a level of 20mIU/ml n and a level of 25 mIU/ml respectively. Thus the Quantitative blood analysis serves the best and is highly sensitive.

Home Pregnancy Test

Home pregnancy tests have become common nowadays. Though they are very much helpful and fairly accurate, their results always should be confirmed with a doctor.

- In pregnancy, the growing tissues of the new conception (early foetus) secrete a special hormone into body called 'Human Chorionic Gonadotrophin' (HCG). This enters blood as early as 10-12days following fertilisation. This can be traced from blood or urine by special tests. Home tests are done with urine.
- Depending upon the type and sensitivity of the test used, pregnancy can be detected as early as a day or two from the missed period.
- Technique for the usage of these tests will be included in the pack itself.

Usage: These kits are user friendly. First Urine should be collected in clean detergent free bottle. Preferably first morning sample is used as it contains more of HCG hormone levels. Urine is then taken in the dropper given with the kid. Only 2/3 drops of urine are added to the well where it is indicated. If there appears a pink line in the place indicated as tests and other pink in the control region then the tests is positive.(2 pink lines).If only one line appears in the test region then the test is negative, and if no lines appear then the test is invalid. Method of testing differs according to the brand.

It may happen that a test result comes negative although, in reality pregnant. This is more likely if:

- The cycles are irregular or are often delayed.
- The testing has been done very early in pregnancy. In such cases, if the test is repeated after one week, it may become positive. It is always advisable to confirm the pregnancy diagnosis by a qualified medical practitioner as all tests have their limitations.

Serum Beta HCG/Quantitative Blood Tests

This is the most sensitive test for pregnancy and detects the hormone even at earlier levels.

Urine Tests

This test is also based on the increased levels of HCG but less sensitive when compared to blood tests.

Sonography

Ultrasound scan can also be used for diagnosing pregnancy. Gestational sac can be visualized as early as four and half weeks of gestation (2½ weeks after ovulation).It is not necessary if the periods are regular and LMP (last menstrual period) is known. It is necessary if:

- Bleeding after missing a period.
- To ensure if the growth is proper.
- To rule out ectopic pregnancy.

FALSE POSITIVES AND NEGATIVES

False positives:

- In home pregnancy tests, there appear evaporation lines if the test is read after the specified reaction time independent of actual pregnancy.

- Women treated with HCG injection as part of infertility treatment, test positive irrespective of actual pregnancy.
- Some diseases like choriocarcinomas, IgA deficiencies, heterophilic antibodies, and even lung cancer also show elevated levels of HCG, giving false positive results.

False negatives:

The most common reasons for false negative result is when the testing is done very early. Quantative urine tests and the most sensitive urine tests can detect pregnancy as early as 6-12 days after implantation but the less ṣensitive home pregnancy tests require adequately elevated levels of hormone to detect it. Menstrution occurs after 14 days of ovulation and the likelihood of false negatives decreases once a menstrual period is late.

The accuracy of pregnancy tests is related to the day of ovulation not the day of intercourse. Because it is normal for the sperm to be waiting in the fallopian tube for 5 days. Once the egg is released fusion takes place leading to the formation of zygote. But it will take another 12 days for it to get implanted. Thus after implantation only there will be rise in HCG levels. Thus it takes approximately 17 days after intercourse .Any tests taken before this period will give negative results. Moreover it takes a few more days to reach adequate levels to be detected by less sensitive pregnancy tests.

OTHER PRENATAL TESTS

The various tests that are routinely done during pregnancy include:

- Blood group detection.

  To identify the blood group and Rh factors to prevent complications later.

- Blood tests for AIDS, hepatitis, rubella, VDRL

  Elisa tests is carried on to rule out any sexually transmitted diseases, specific blood tests to find out HbA2 (Thalassemia carriers), HBsAg (hepatitis B carriers.).VDRL to diagnose syphilis.

- Ultrasound/sonography to check for foetal heart beat and any abnormalities in foetal development.other conditions like spina-bifida and placental abnormalities can also be identified at an earlier stage.

- Urine test for albumin.

  Other tests may be required in special circumstances, particularly in high risk pregnancies. These include:

- Alpha-foetal protein (AFP) takes the measure of particular fetoprotein levels in the foetus and the mother's blood to rule out any developmental abnormalities of the foetus.
- Chorionic villus sampling (CVS) takes the measure of chorion covering the baby to detect any genetic abnormalities in the baby.
- Non-stress tests done to detect the response of the foetus to any external sound and tactile stimuli.
- Amniocentesis done with the fluid carefully taken from the amnion of the baby tested for any genetic abnormalities.

VIABILITY TESTS

Many pregnancy tests are used to study the viability of the pregnancy, series of quantative blood tests are taken to measure the gradual changes in the blood levels of HCG against a normal standard levels. Any abnormalities denote increased chances of miscarriages and ectopic pregnancy. Ultrasound can also be used for this purpose. The growth of the foetus is visually seen at regular intervals .Any abnormalities can be easily detected from the scan.

ANTE-NATAL CARE

Antenatal care (prenatal care), a series of checkups, at a hospitals and at a doctor's surgery, design to monitor the physical and mental health of a pregnant woman and the development of her baby. In addition, the expectant mother (and father) receive information and advice about pregnancy, labour, childbirth and care of the newborn infant.

The checks are generally done once a month up to 28 weeks of pregnancy, once a fortnight up to 36 weeks, and are carried out every week for the last month. At the first visit, personal details and family medical history are obtained, and also the date of the last menstrual period, state of health at this stage in pregnancy and the estimated date of delivery. All this information, along with examination and test results, is recorded on file and on a cooperation card. Many of the details are in an abbreviated form and can be explained by medical advisers. Ideally, the cooperation card should accompany the woman at all times in case of emergency.

Various routine tests are carried out including height and shoe size and weight. Les may be checked for varicose veins, ankles and hands may be looked at for the swelling and puffiness that results from oedema. The breasts are usually examined with the condition of the nipples being noted and the heart, lungs, eyes, hair, nails and teeth may be checked as a guide to general health.

Urine Tests may be carried out to detect urinary or kidney infections, or, if sugar, protein or ketones are present, to detect diabetes or kidney problems. Blood Pressure is monitored, and a Blood Test may be taken to disclose Rhesus Blood Group, Hemoglobin and Alpha-Fetoprotein level, and the presence of antibodies to German Measles or AIDS. Blood may be tested to detect Syphilis, Sickle-Cell Anaemia and Thalassaemia. The abdomen is examined to determine the size of the foetus, its position and the height of the top of the uterus (particularly valuable after the 32nd week).

Foetal heart beat is checked, and an internal examination is usually carried out to confirm the pregnancy and check that the cervix is closed. The size of the pelvis is assessed, and a Cervical Smear Test may be carried out. Several other tests are also utilized, some as routine and others to determine if there are specific problems with the foetus. Ultrasound scanning is now routine in all pregnancies to check the progress of the baby and is usually carried out at an early stage. It is also used in Amniocentesis testing, which may be done during the 14th-18th week of pregnancy. Other tests include Choronic Villus Sampling, Umbilical Vein Sampling and Fetoscopy. Together the routine and special tests all work to ensure the health of the mother and her baby.

OBJECTIVES

There is general acceptance that antenatal care should be provided for all pregnant women. Some obvious benefits of modern antenatal care are:

- Meeting consumer demand for health care during pregnancy.
- Screening, e.g., for congenital syphilis of foetal anomalies.
- Early detection of pregnancy problems, e.g., hypertension.
- Advice for pregnant women and preparation for delivery, including specific delivery plans.

The general objective of antenatal care is to ensure the best possible pregnancy outcomes for pregnant women and their unborn babies through optimal physical and psychological preparation before delivery. Two specific indices that reflect the status of antenatal care are the incidence of congenital syphilis in a population and the rate of unbooked deliveries presenting at maternity units.

ASSESSMENT

Obstetric care involves outpatient antenatal care, management of labour and delivery, and postpartum care. Although malpractices claims and research statistics in obstetrics usually reflect adverse outcomes in the labour and delivery process, antenatal care forms the firm groundwork from which obstetrics decisions are made. Antenatal care encompasses both the management of problems that arise during the pregnancy and the screening for factors that warrant further action. In the past, perinatal care focused primarily on improvements in foetal testing and advances in newborn care. Now the pregnant woman is recognized as part of a much wider social system that involves her family, community, cultural group, and society as a whole.

HISTORY AND PHYSICAL EXAMINATION

Pregnant women require routine prenatal care to help ensure their health and the health of the foetus. Also, evaluation is often required for symptoms and signs of illness. Common symptoms that are often pregnancy-related include vaginal bleeding, pelvic pain, vomiting, and lower-extremity edema.

Ideally, women who are planning to become pregnant should see a physician or nurse before conception, so that they can be counseled about pregnancy risks and ways to reduce them. The initial routine prenatal visit should occur between 6 and 8 wk gestation. Follow-up visits should occur at about 4-wk intervals until 28 wk, at 2-wk intervals from 28 to 36 wk, and weekly thereafter until delivery. Prenatal care includes screening for disorders, taking measures to reduce foetal and maternal risks, and counseling.

History

During the initial visit, a full medical history is obtained. It includes previous and current disorders and drug use (therapeutic, social, and illicit), presence of risk factors for complications of pregnancy, and obstetric history, with the outcome of all previous pregnancies, including maternal and foetal complications (e.g., gestational diabetes, preeclampsia, congenital malformations, stillbirth). Family history should include all chronic disorders in family members to identify possible hereditary disorders. During subsequent visits, queries focus on interim developments, particularly vaginal bleeding or fluid discharge, headache, changes in vision, edema of face or fingers, and changes in frequency or intensity of foetal movement.

Gravidity is the number of confirmed pregnancies; a pregnant woman is a gravida. Parity is the number of deliveries after 20 wk. Multifoetal pregnancy is counted as one in terms of gravidity and parity. Abortus is the number of pregnancy losses (abortions) before 20 wk regardless of cause (e.g., spontaneous, therapeutic, or elective abortion; ectopic pregnancy). Sum of parity and abortus equals gravidity. Parity is often recorded as 4 numbers: number of term deliveries (after 37 wk), number of premature deliveries (> 20 and < 37 wk), number of abortions, and number of living children. Thus, a woman who is pregnant and has had one term delivery, one set of twins born at 32 wk, and 2 abortions is gravida 5, para 1-1-2-3.

Physical Examination

A full general examination, including height and weight, is done first. In the initial obstetric examination, speculum and bimanual pelvic examination is done, noting the presence of lesions or discharge as well as colour and consistency of the cervix; also, foetal heart rate and, in patients presenting later in pregnancy, lie of the foetus are assessed. Pelvic capacity can be estimated clinically by evaluating various measurements with the middle finger during bimanual examination. If the distance from the underside of the pubic symphysis to the sacral promontory is > 11.5 cm, the pelvic inlet is almost certainly adequate. Normally, distance between the ischial spines is ? 9 cm, length of the sacrospinous ligaments is 4 to ? 5 cm, and the subpubic arch is ? 90°.

During subsequent visits, BP and weight assessment is important. Obstetric examination focuses on uterine size, fundal height (in cm above the symphysis pubis), foetal heart rate and activity, and maternal diet, weight gain, and overall well-being. Speculum and bimanual examination is usually not needed unless vaginal discharge or bleeding, leakage of fluid, or pain is present.

ANTENATAL EXAMINATION

At each visit the following examinations should be done.

- General:
  - Blood pressure
  - Body weight

- Abdominal:
  - — Fundal level
  - — Foetal lie
  - — Foetal presentation
  - — Foetal heart sounds (FHS)
- Record any new complaints
- Urine examination:
  - — By dipstick for protein, glucose and ketones
- Assessment of foetal well-being
  - — Foetal size through assessment of fundal level (FL)
  - — Foetal kick count: at least 10 movements every12 hours
  - — Foetal movements: absence precedes intrauterine foetal death (IUFD) by 48 hours
  - — Foetal heart sounds
  - — Ultrasound if it is available
  - — At 37 Weeks
  - — Assessment of foetal size, lie, presentation

PRESENTATION & POSITION OF THE FOETUS

The foetus' presentation and position affect how the foetus passes through the vagina. Most normal births involve a combination of vertex presentation with anterior position.

1. Presentation refers to how the foetus is situated in the uterus, while the part of foetus that is closest to the cervix is termed the presenting part. There are a few different types of presentation:

- Vertex or cephalic presentation . The most common and safest birth position where the baby's head is the presenting part.
- Transverse lie or shoulder presentation . Here a caesarean section is always needed.
- Breech, where the baby's buttocks presents first. Accounting for about 3 to 4% of all deliveries, the breech birth often involves a longer labour due to the fact that the buttocks does not as easily open the cervix as the head. Various types of breech exist. These include: complete breech is which the baby sits cross legged at the bottom of uterus; a frank breech, where the baby crosses its legs straight up with his feet near the face; and a footing breech, where one or both of the baby's

feet present first; very uncommon form is the knee breech where the baby's knee presents before the foot.

A breech presentation may not be discovered until after labour has begun, but where there are no other complications (such as a prolapsed cord) a vaginal birth is possible. However forceps or a vacuum extractor may be required. Where a breech presentation or transverse lie position is discovered during pregnancy, it may be possible to rotate the baby to an upright or vertex position using a procedure called external version.

Performed under the guidance of ultrasound, the physician manipulates the baby into a head-down position by applying gentle, but firm pressure to the baby's head and hip through abdomen. This procedure is generally most successful if it's performed at 36 weeks due to the fact that after 37 weeks less amniotic fluid makes it tougher to rotate the baby. However, there are risks, including inducing labour, producing pain in the abdomen, and although very rare, the risk of shearing the placenta from the uterine wall also exists.

2. The position of the baby refers to the direction that the foetus is facing. Most commonly the baby's position is anterior, where the back of the head is touching the abdomen wall. The less common posterior position is where the back of the baby's head is against the spine. However, most posterior babies rotate to an interior position before the second stage of labour .

   Where there is difficulty in delivery due to abnormal presentation and/or position, and the vaginal opening isn't stretching enough to let the baby emerge and a tear is likely, a doctor may perform an episiotomy .

DIAGNOSIS OF STAGE AND PHASE IN PREGNANCY

Symptoms and signs	Stage	Phase
Cervix not dilated	False pregnancy/ not in pregnancy	
Cervix dilated <4cm	First	Latent
Cervix dilated 4-9cm Rate of dilatation typically 1cm/hr or more Foetal descent begins	First	Active

Cervix fully dilated (10cm) Foetal descent continues No urge to push	Second	Early (non expulsive)
Cervix fully dilated (10cm) Presenting part of foetus reaches pelvic floor Woman has the urge to push	Second	Late expulsive

The third stage of pregnancys begins with the delivery of the baby and ends with the expulsion of the placenta.

The rate of dilatation of the cervix is the most exact measure of the progress of pregnancy. Cervical dilatation is usually estimated in centimetres, from 0 cm when the cervix is closed, to 10 cm at full dilatation. Assessment of cervical dilatation is not, however, as precise as one would like to believe. Personal experience has shown substantial variations in estimates of dilatation of different observers in the same situation, and even by the same observer on repeat examinations.

The recommended frequency of vaginal examinations to assess the progress of cervical dilatation varies greatly among units and in the literature. This variation illustrates the lack of consensus for the optimal timing of vaginal examinations in pregnancy. Like all assessments it seems most sensible that care should be individualized. The number and timing of vaginal examinations should be frequent enough to permit adequate assessment of progress and to detect any problems promptly.

ASSESSMENT OF ENGAGEMENT AND DESCENT OF THE FOETUS

The assessment of engagement and descent of the foetus can be done by measuring the fundal height, abdominal palpation and vaginal examination.

- Measuring the fundal height
- Abdominal palpation
- Vaginal examination

Measuring the Fundal Height and Abdominal Palpation

The examiner must ask and answer 6 questions:

1. Is the fundal height consistent with the estimation of maturity?
2. Is the lie longitudinal?
3. What is the presentation?

4. Is the cephalic presentation a vertex?
5. What is the position of the vertex?
6. Is the vertex engaged?

Is the Fundal Height Consistent with the Estimation of Maturity?

Many pregnant women have the distance from the lowest part of the uterus to the highest part of their uterus measured with a tape measure. Their caregiver may also feel and gently press the outside of the woman's pregnant uterus (abdominal palpation). This is to check the baby's size and position, the quantity of fluid around the baby and to diagnose multiple pregnancy. A Cochrane review found that there is too little evidence to show whether symphysis-fundal height measurement during pregnancy is more beneficial than abdominal palpation.

The height of the fundus in centimetres should equal approximately the weeks of gestation.

A tape measure is used to measure from the upper border of the symphysis pubis to the top of the fundus, generally along the midline of the abdomen. There are suggestions this has a dubious reliability but other studies indicate an acceptable degree of sensitivity.

Is the Lie Longitudinal?

- The lie is the relation of the long axis of the foetus to the mother
- Only a longitudinal lie is normal; transverse and oblique are not

What is the Presentation?

- The presenting part is the part of the foetus which occupies the lower pole of the uterus
- Only a cephalic presentation is normal after 32 weeks
- At 30 weeks, however, up to 25% of babies present by breech

Is the Cephalic Presentation a Vertex?

- This depends on the attitude of the foetus i.e. the relationship of its different parts to each other
- The normal attitude is full flexion, in full flexion every foetal joint is flexed

If the cephalic presentation is not a vertex it is a malpresentation.

What is the Position of the Vertex?

- It is conveniently expressed by referring to the position of one area of the presenting part, known as the denominator
- The denominator of the vertex is the occiput
- The position is the relationship of the presenting part to the mother's pelvis
- There are 8 recognised positions
  1. Direct Occipito Posterior (DOP) or Occipito Posterior (OP)
  2. Left Occipito Posterior (LOP)
  3. Left Occipito Anterior (LOA)
  4. Left Occipito Lateral (LOL) or Left Occipito Transverse (LOT)
  5. Right Occipito Posterior (ROP)
  6. Right Occipito Anterior (ROA)
  7. Right Occipito Lateral (ROL) or Right Occipito Transverse (ROT)
  8. Direct Occipito Anterior (DOA) or Occipito Anterior (OA)
- The lateral and anterior positions are regarded as normal
- Mostly the occiput posterior will rotate forward in pregnancy

Is the Vertex Engaged?

- Engagement means the descent of the bi-parietal diametre (this is the widest transverse diametre of the foetal skull) through the pelvic brim
- A convenient way to describe the amount of head above the brim is to identify the number of 'fifths' abdominally palpable
- When the head is engaged 2/5 or less will be felt abdominally
- When the head is fixed: 3/5 is palpable abdominally

Vaginal Examination

- If necessary, a vaginal examination may be used to assess descent by relating the level of the foetal presenting part to the ischial spines of the maternal pelvis
- Assessing descent of the foetal head by vaginal examination, 0 station is at the level of the ischial spine
- Moulding of the foetal head, an important observation in following the progress of pregnancy if cephalopelvic

disproportion is suspected, can also be determined by vaginal examination.

SCREENING AND ASSESSMENT OF HIGH RISK

The concept of risk in obstetrics can be examined at many levels. All problems that arise in pregnancy, whether common complaints or more hazardous diseases, convey some risk to the pregnancy, depending on how they are managed by the patient and her care provider. Risk assessment has received detailed attention in the past.

It has been shown that most women and infants suffering morbidity and mortality will come from a small segment of women with high-risk factors; by reassessing risk factors before pregnancy, during pregnancy, and again in labour, our ability to identify those at highest risk increases. Most of the emphasis for screening, risk assessment, and associated trials for therapeutic interventions have focused primarily on preclampsia and preterm birth prevention.

RISK APPROACH

There are few conditions encountered in the delivery of healthcare that lend themselves more perfectly to an integrative approach than pregnancy. The factors that create these circumstances are also factors that allow healthcare providers to use more integrative approaches with greater comfort when dealing with the pregnant patient. The following are the unique aspects of pregnancy:

1. Pregnancy is not a disease state.
2. Pregnancy is a significant life transition with little debate that all aspects of the individual are affected: mind, body, spirit and community.
3. Pregnancy is a condition that exemplifies the power of nature and the body's capacities.
4. Pregnancy is a condition that has benefited tremendously from the advances of modern medicine.
5. Pregnancy is a condition where the accepted goal of care is to be as minimally invasive as possible. (The same is not universally true of labour and delivery.)
6. Pregnancy is a condition where there is general recognition of the immediate need for and benefit of optimal health.

MODALITIES OF DIAGNOSIS; INVASIVE & NON-INVASIVE

The holy grail of prenatal diagnosis has been the identification of chromosome and single gene abnormalities through maternal blood sampling. This would allow safe accurate prenatal diagnosis, requiring much lower operator skills, and automation is potentially possible, making it cost-effective. In contrast, standard prenatal screening involves ultrasound and biochemical risk assessment followed by invasive prenatal diagnosis by chorionic villus sampling (CVS), amniocentesis or foetal blood sampling - all requiring clinical expertise to perform and a variable risk of foetal loss.

The most common call is consistently from parents wrestling with the decision about whether to have an invasive test such as chorionic villus sampling (CVS) or amniocentesis. Because both procedures carry a one per cent risk of miscarriage, parents agonise over whether to put their pregnancy at risk in order to have conclusive information on a genetic condition. If cffDNA testing were to provide risk-free but reliable diagnoses of aneuploidies and other genetic conditions it would prove extremely popular with many parents. For most parents the earlier reassurance that cffDNA testing would bring will be welcome. However, we must avoid making assumptions that an earlier diagnosis will necessarily be easier for parents to cope with. Making painful decisions about the future of what is most often a wanted pregnancy is difficult at any gestation. Furthermore, there is no evidence that earlier terminations for foetal abnormality have substantially less emotional impact on women and couples than those carried out later in the pregnancy.

Another concern from the parental perspective is the form cffDNA testing takes, being a simple blood test. Women are very accustomed to having blood taken in pregnancy and while holding out an arm for a needle to be inserted is not always pleasant, it is something with which every pregnant woman is familiar. The 'routine' nature of the procedure could mean that some women embark on it without considering the possible implications and so are particularly distressed if test results bring unexpected news about the pregnancy. This has implications for how pre-test counselling and consent issues are handled.

In fact there is a precedent for a non-invasive diagnostic tool in routine use in antenatal care, namely ultrasound scanning. Every time an ultrasound probe is placed on the abdomen of a pregnant woman there is the possibility that an abnormality will be detected. Although information provision to women about the purpose of antenatal ultrasound is improving, we cannot underestimate the profound impact on parents when the scan shows that there is something wrong. However well-informed a woman may be, such news will always come as a shock and generate considerable anxiety and distress. This will also be the case for a diagnosis made from cffDNA testing, even if it comes earlier in pregnancy.

ULTRASONIC

Obstetric ultrasonography has grown in popularity since it was introduced over four decades ago. It had proliferated and its use if not controlled, which suggests that ad hoc use is open to misuse and could be a drain on the limited human and economic resources available without corresponding improvement in foetal and maternal outcomes.

It is a fact that despite the amount of human and material resources available, the majority of the population are still living below the poverty line. Only 50 percent of the women receive antenatal care and if scarce resources are wasted on unnecessary equipment and the performance of scans by unskilled practitioners, technical, human and financial resources are wasted that could be used to increase access to the services and improve maternal and neonatal outcomes. Ultrasound can be a useful tool in the antenatal period when employed judiciously based on sound clinical judgement. It should not be used indiscriminately. It should be used by trained, accredited and regulated practitioners.

ANTENATAL PREPARATION

Antenatal care by a health professional can help pregnant women and their partners identify the need for any dietary or lifestyle changes and ways of sustaining those changes throughout the pregnancy and beyond the birth of the child. It also provides and opportunity to help the parents create the emotional foundations for the child's life; one of the most important elements of early parenting. Ultrasound examinations and population studies by psychologists and neurobiologists show that from about 10 weeks, an infant moves spontaneously, and by 15 weeks, movements may be felt as a reaction to the mother's laugh or cough, suggesting a response of self-protection or self-assertion.

Spectographic analysis of voice and cry sounds as early as 26 weeks show that the child has begun to adopt the mother's voice characteristics, and recognition of the mother's voice almost immediately after birth is often a remarkable observation of new, first time mothers. Another important goal of antenatal preparation is to establish a birth plan, one that empowers parents to make decisions on the place of birth and the choice of birth attendant or birth companion. This also includes securing access to any backup facility that may be required and the resources to access assistance. Antenatal preparation also provides an opportunity for parents to talk through their emotional needs in relation to parenting, which is especially important for pregnant adolescents and women with low self-esteem.

Antenatal preparation is also a time to rationalize the rituals of care, to act as a platform for the other types of care and empowerment, by providing an opportunity to establish a trusting relationship with a health professional and channels of communication that will help women develop the skills for life long decision-making. Parents can often be counseled about breastfeeding and how to access help with infant problems such as feeding, crying and sleep disruptions, which are typically the most problematic for parents, especially if it is their first child. The other major issue for which parents often seek guidance, is Sudden Infant Death Syndrome (SIDS). The prevalence of SIDS has shown a dramatic, worldwide reduction, which, to some extent, is directly related to guidance during antenatal care and major campaigns urging parents to place their infants in a supine, or back-lying position while sleeping.

Yet another important opportunity afforded by antenatal visits is the chance to discuss the diagnostic approach to the pregnancy. In some cases, tests such as ultrasound are offered indiscriminately, or to inform sex-selective abortions, especially in developing countries.

ANTENATAL COUNSELLING

When there is an anomaly in the unborn baby, there could be a lot of anxiety among parents. Obtaining more information from a specialist in this area, can relieve the anxieties and also provide answer to many questions. This step is called 'antenatal counselling'. It will help to plan the type of delivery, place of delivery (where treatment is available to the baby after birth), the type of tests required after birth. Also it helps to find out more about what is expected in the long run (prognosis) and whether the problem can occur again in the following children (familial incidence). Antenatal counseling comprises following procedure:

The first appointment needs to be earlier in pregnancy (prior to 12 weeks) than may have traditionally occurred and, because of the large volume of information needs in early pregnancy, two appointments may be required. At the first (and second) antenatal appointment:

- Give information, with an opportunity to discuss issues and ask questions; offer verbal information supported by written information (on topics such as diet and lifestyle considerations, pregnancy care services available, maternity benefits and sufficient information to enable informed decision making about screening tests).

- Identify women who may need additional care and plan pattern of care for the pregnancy.
- Check blood group and rhesus D (RhD) status.
- Offer screening for anaemia, red-cell alloantibodies, Hepatitis B virus, HIV, rubella susceptibility and syphilis.
- Offer screening for asymptomatic bacteriuria (ASB).
- Offering screening for Down's syndrome.
- Offer early ultrasound scan for gestational age assessment.
- Offer ultrasound screening for structural anomalies (20 weeks).
- Measure BMI and blood pressure (BP) and test urine for proteinuria.

After the first (and possibly second) appointment, for women who choose to have screening, the following test should be arranged before 16 weeks of gestation (except serum screening for Down's syndrome, which may occur up to 20 weeks of gestation):

- Blood tests (for checking blood group and RhD status and screening for anaemia, red-cell alloantibodies, hepatitis B virus, HIV, rubella susceptibility and syphilis).
- Urine tests (to check for proteinuria and screen for ASB).
- Ultrasound scan
- Serum screening at 14 to 20 weeks.

16 Weeks

The next appointment should be scheduled at 16 weeks to:

- Review, discuss and record the results of all screening tests undertaken; reassess planned pattern of care for the pregnancy and identify women who need additional care
- Investigate a haemoglobin level of less than 11g/dl and consider iron supplementation if indicated
- Measure BP and test urine for proteinuria
- Give information, with an opportunity to discuss issues and ask questions; offer verbal information supported by antenatal classes and written information.

18-20 Weeks

At 18-20 weeks, if the woman chooses, an ultrasound scan should be performed for the

detection of structural anomalies. For a woman whose placenta is found to extend across the internal cervical os at this time, another scan at 36 weeks should be offered and the results of this scan reviewed at the 36-week appointment.

25 Weeks

At 25 weeks of gestation, another appointment should be scheduled for nulliparous women. At this appointment:

- Measure and plot symphysis-fundal height.
- Measure BP and test urine for proteinuria.
- Give information, with an opportunity to discuss issues and ask questions; offer verbal information supported by antenatal classes and written information.

28 Weeks

The next appointment for all pregnant women should occur at 28 weeks. At this appointment:

- Offer a second screening for anaemia and atypical red-cell alloantibodies.
- Investigate a haemoglobin level of less than 10.5 g/dl and consider iron supplementation, if indicated.
- Offer anti-D to rhesus-negative women.
- Measure BP and test urine for proteinuria.
- Measure and plot symphysis-fundal height.
- Give information, with an opportunity to discuss issues and ask questions; offer verbal information supported by antenatal classes and written information.

31 Weeks

Nulliparous women should have an appointment scheduled at 31 weeks to:

- Measure BP and test urine for proteinuria.
- Measure and plot symphysis-fundal height.

- Give information, with an opportunity to discuss issues and ask questions; offer verbal information supported by antenatal classes and written information.
- Review, discuss and record the results of screening tests undertaken at 28 weeks; reassess planned pattern of care for the pregnancy and identify women who need additional care

34 Weeks

At 34 weeks, all pregnant women should be seen in order to:

- Offer a second dose of anti-D to rhesus-negative women.
- Measure BP and test urine for proteinuria.
- Measure and plot symphysis-fundal height.
- Give information, with an opportunity to discuss issues and ask questions; offer verbal information supported by antenatal classes and written information.
- Review, discuss and record the results of screening tests undertaken at 28 weeks; reassess planned pattern of care for the pregnancy and identify women who need additional care.

36 Weeks

At 36 weeks, all pregnant women should be seen again to:

- Measure BP and test urine for proteinuria.
- Measure and plot symphysis-fundal height.
- Check position of baby.
- For women whose babies are in the breech presentation, offer external cephalic version (ECV).
- Review ultrasound scan report if placenta extended over the internal cervical os at previous scan.
- Give information, with an opportunity to discuss issues and ask questions; offer verbal information supported by antenatal classes and written information.

38 Weeks

Another appointment at 38 weeks will allow for:

- Measurement BP and urine testing for proteinuria.
- Measurement and plotting of symphysis-fundal height.
- Information giving, with an opportunity to discuss issues and ask questions; verbal information supported by antenatal classes and written information.

40 Weeks

For nulliparous women, an appointment at 40 weeks should be scheduled to:

- Measure BP and test urine for proteinuria.
- Measure and plot symphysis-fundal height.
- Give information, with an opportunity to discuss issues and ask questions.

41 Weeks

For women who have not given birth by 41 weeks:

- A membrane sweep should be offered.
- Induction of labour should be offered.
- BP should be measured and urine tested for proteinuria.
- Symphysis-fundal height should be measured and plotted.
- Information should be given, with an opportunity to discuss issues and ask questions; verbal information supported by written information.

General

Throughout the entire antenatal period, healthcare providers should remain alert to signs or symptoms of conditions which affect the health of the mother and foetus, such as domestic violence, pre-eclampsia and diabetes.

ANTENATAL EXERCISES

Circulatory Exercises

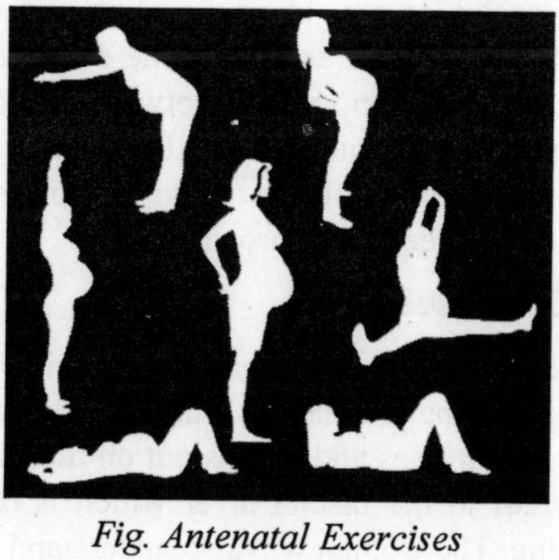

Fig. Antenatal Exercises

Circulatory exercises should be frequently, particularly in the morning and late evening. They should be performed in a half-lying or sitting position with the legs elevated and are intended to maintain and improve the circulation. Vigorous movements of the feet will assist venous return and minimize varicosities, swelling of the ankles and cramp.

Foot Exercises

Sit or lie at an angle of 45 degrees (half-lying) with the back against a wedge and pillows, the legs supported and the knees straight. Bend and stretch the ankles briskly at least 12 times, emphasizing dorsiflexion rather than plantar flexion to avoid cramp. Keeping the knees and hips still, circle both ankles in as large a circle as possible at least 12 times in each direction.

Leg Tightening

Sit or lie (half-lying) in same position as above. Pull both feet upwards at the ankle and press the back of the knees down onto the support. Hold this position for a count of 5, breathing normally, then relax. Repeat 10 times.

A pregnant woman should be advised to avoid prolonged standing, and sitting or lying with her legs crossed. She should be encouraged to sit with her feet raised on a low stool. If oedema is present, she could lie at an angle of 45 degrees with her legs raised a little higher than her hips.

Its is important to retain a wide angle at the groin in order to prevent compression, which could cause circulatory stasis. A pillow under the bottom of the mattress will elevate her feet when sleeping. Sitting instead of standing must be encouraged whilst doing household chores such as ironing, peeling vegetables etc. The woman should be reminded that walking will aid her circulation especially the deep venous blood flow. She should be wear good supporting footwear and avoid high heels, which might cause injury through instability. If a woman has always worn high heels then she should not wear completely flat shoes but something with a lower heel and a broader base.

Pelvic Floor Exercises

Pelvic floor exercises should receive top priority in any programme of physical exercise during pregnancy. Muscles toned antenatally will be able to cope with the stresses and strains put on them by pregnancy and to give extra support to the fascial layer which is relaxing under the influence of relaxing. The woman will also understand how to re-educate them after delivery to help to prevent any long-term urinary problems or prolapse. Pelvic floor exercises should be taught, even late in pregnancy. Healthy, exercise muscles stretch and recoil more conveniently which can facilitate delivery. It has been observed that pelvic floor muscles are stronger post-natally in women who exercised during pregnancy than in those who did not and that antenatal pelvic floor exercises reduced the risk of postpartum stress incontinence in primigravidae. It has also been highlighted that the pelvic floor muscles play a part in maintaining the stability of the pelvis.

Abdominal Exercises

Because of their attachment to the linea alba, exercises involving the oblique abdominal, for example, twisting or knee rolling, should be avoided during later pregnancy to avoid the risk of tearing the linea alba and causing diastasis of the rectus muscles. However, it is very important to exercise the deep abdominal muscles during pregnancy. Transverus abdominis has been found to be the core stability muscle and needs to work as efficiently as possible to help maintain the integrity of the pelvis. It has been shown that the transverses abdominis is much more important than rectus abdominis in preventing postural and back problems and so should be the main muscle to exercise during pregnancy and postpartum. It has a high proportion of slow twitch type I fibres which respond to a gentle not maximal contraction. The transverses exercise can be performed in any position, for example, sitting, standing, high-kneeling, prone-kneeling or side-lying. Kneeling on all fours is usually a comfortable position to start to learn the exercise, which should then be practiced in any functional position during the day.

Transversus Exercise

Keeping spine in the mid position, breathe in then gently draw in the lower abdominal muscles on the outward breath and hold the contraction for up to 10 seconds whilst continuing to breathe normally, then relax slowly. Repeat 10 times.

Transversus and Pelvic Floor Exercise

The actions of both the transverses and the pelvic floor muscles will be enhanced by combining the two exercises. This may be done by working transverses then bringing in a pelvic floor contraction or vice versa. It is important to use this combined contraction to protect the spine and pelvic joints when performing functional activities such as moving and handling objects, changing positions, unavoidable standing.

As pregnancy progresses, the pelvic tilt alters putting a strain on the ligaments and joints of the lower back and pelvis which may lead to pain and discomfort. Pelvic tilting is a useful exercise to relieve back pain and discomfort. Pelvic tilting is a useful exercise to relieve back pain and stiffness, and promote good posture. Performed more quickly, the exercise helps to relieve backache in labour.

Pelvic Tilting

Lie at an angle of 45 degrees (half-lying) supported by a wedge and pillows, with knees bent and the feet flat on the surface.

Pull in the abdominal muscles, tighten the muscles of the buttocks and press the small of the back down onto support. Hold the position for a count of 5, breathing normally, then relax. Repeat up to 10 times.

The exercise may be performed more rhythmically (pelvic rocking) to help relieve any tension and postural backache whenever the need arises. Once mastered in this position, pelvic tilting or rocking can be encouraged in several positions, for example sitting, reverse sitting astride a chair, side-lying, standing, supported kneeling and prone kneeling.

DIET

Poor diet affects the health of socially disadvantaged people from the cradle to the grave. The social and economic reasons are complex, but the potential for health gain through improved diet is enormous. A poor diet in pregnancy together with other contributing risk factors and limits placental function and foetal growth.

It has been suggested that low birth weight perpetuates the intergenerational cycle of poor health by programming children toward the potential of adult diseases including hypertension, diabetes, obesity, and coronary heart disease. People in lower socio-economic groups may have a diet high in cheap energy foods including, meat products, full cream milk, fats, sugars, preserves and potatoes with very little intake of vegetables, fruit, and wholewheat bread. Such a diet is lower in essential nutrients such as calcium, iron, magnesium, folate, and vitamin C than that of the higher socio-economic groups. In terms of the protective role of antioxidants and other dietary factors there is scope for considerable health gain if a diet rich in vegetables, fruit, unrefined cereal, fish, and small quantities of quality vegetable oils could be more accessible to poor people. However healthy lifestyle choices are not always accessible and/or affordable to people on low incomes or who live in areas where, for example, shops do not offer fresh fruit and vegetables. However, it is important that health professionals discourage the over reliance on food stuff to supply their recommended daily requirement of folic acid as dietary supplementation is still required to protect against neural tube defects. It is now generally accepted that increased folate intake before and during pregnancy reduces the occurrence and recurrence of neural tube defects, namely spina bifida, anencephaly and encephalocoele. It is recommended that women take 400 g of folic acid daily prior to conception and during the first trimester of pregnancy. Simply delivering a healthy eating message and providing supporting information in the form of a leaflet does not complete the health education process.

A diet low in folate around the time of conception not only predisposes to neural tube defects but also to lower birth weight and a shorter pregnancy. In conclusion the dietary advice should focus on a well-balanced and varied diet with an emphasis on complex carbohydrates and protein, and with adequate daily folate (0.5mg, or 5mg if high NTD risk), iron (15mg), calcium (1200mg) and fluids (2-3L). Foods likely to be contaminated with listeria should be avoided e.g., raw meat, raw seafood, soft cheeses. Many first trimester women can minimise nausea by frequent small meals rich in B group vitamins and low in spice and fat. Severe caloric restriction can result in reduced foetal growth, so as a general policy weight reduction is best deferred to post-natally.

SUBSTANCE USE

Tobacco, alcohol and drugs can have harmful effects on anyone's health. When a pregnant or nursing woman uses these substances, her baby also is exposed to them, for all substances cross the placenta through the umbilical cord and enter into the baby's bloodstream.

While pregnant, it is best to eat well, stay healthy and avoid ingesting anything that might be harmful to the mother's or baby's health.

Street Drugs

A pregnant woman who uses drugs like cocaine, crack, heroin and methadone may have a baby born addicted to the substances she took during her pregnancy. Cocaine is one of the most harmful drugs to unborn babies. Cocaine can cause a woman to miscarry and may cause preterm birth, bleeding, foetal death and foetal strokes, which can lead to brain damage and death. After birth, a baby who has been exposed to cocaine prenatally goes through withdrawal, signs of which include jitters and irritability. These babies are hard to comfort and are often unable to respond to their mothers. Cocaine use during pregnancy also may be linked to an increased risk of sudden infant death syndrome, or SIDS.

Amphetamines or "speed" also are harmful to unborn babies. One study showed that the fetuses of mothers who used speed during pregnancy had decreased weight, length and head size. Another study showed that these babies had more strokes, or bleeding into their brains.

Marijuana

Marijuana can affect foetal and infant development and may cause miscarriage. Although the effects of marijuana on an unborn baby are still unknown, studies have indicated that prenatal marijuana use is linked to premature births, small birth size, difficult or long labour and an increase in newborn jitteriness.

Marijuana smoked by a pregnant woman remains in the baby's fat cells for seven to 30 days. Smoking marijuana can affect the amount of oxygen and nutrients the baby receives, which may affect growth. Marijuana is never safe during pregnancy and it can harm the baby at any stage. In addition, marijuana can have long-term effects on infants and children, such as having trouble paying attention or learning to read.

Alcohol

Drinking alcohol can increase the risk of miscarriage, stillbirth, newborn death and foetal alcohol syndrome (FAS). Babies with FAS have low birth weight, heart defects, facial defects, learning problems and mental retardation. Since it is not known if there is a safe level of alcohol during pregnancy, the best advice is not to drink at all. Even one drink a day has been shown to have effects on the growing foetus. The best time to stop drinking alcohol is before conceiving. If pregnancy is unplanned, lady should stop drinking as soon as she suspect she is pregnant.

Tobacco

Women who smoke during pregnancy are more likely to have babies who are too small. Smoking also increases the risk of miscarriage, preterm labour, stillbirth and newborn death. Babies born weighing less than 5 pounds may have more health problems early in life and learning problems later in school.

Prescription Drugs

Some prescribed medications may be harmful to unborn or nursing baby. If lady is taking any prescribed drugs, tell health care provider as soon as possible so that medications can be changed or adjusted as needed.

Over-the-Counter Medicines and Vitamins

Avoid over-the-counter medicines such as antacids, laxatives, sleeping pills, cold medications and pain relievers. While some are safe for pregnant women, many are not. This applies to large doses of over-the-counter vitamin preparations as well, for taking large doses of extra vitamins can be harmful to baby.

Caffeine

Caffeine is present in coffee, tea, cola drinks and some medications. For at least 10 years, there has been controversy over whether caffeine is harmful during pregnancy. Some studies suggest caffeine is harmful, pointing to an increased risk of miscarriage, early delivery or lower birth weight. Other studies have shown that women who consume a moderate amount of caffeine do not experience these problems. Because results are conflicting, no one knows the true risk. We recommend drinking as little caffeine as possible.

EDUCATION FOR CHILD-BIRTH

Childbirth education is a significant vehicle of health promotion for women, infants, and families. The birth event often has been the focus of medicine and nursing. Early childbirth classes were focused entirely on developing and practicing techniques for use in managing pain and facilitating the progress of labour. More recent developments in perinatal education have broadened the focus to incorporate family adaptation to the pregnancy and parental roles for the newborn.

Childbirth education can contribute significantly to the promotion of healthy lifestyles. People who take prenatal classes receive extensive information about nutritional and fluid needs during pregnancy, exercise suited to lifestyle and preferences, smoking cessation, stress management, dangerous medications and street drugs, ways to foster healthy relationships, and the importance of avoiding alcohol. Expectant parents who begin classes as early as the first trimester can initiate health-promoting behaviours sooner and improve their chances of giving birth to a full-term, adequately nourished infant who experiences minimal foetal stress.

The prevention of preterm birth is currently a major focus of many health-oriented organizations and programs. Lifestyle and environmental factors that increase the risk of preterm labour and birth include receiving late or no prenatal care, smoking, drinking alcohol, using illegal drugs, being exposed to diethylstilbestrol, experiencing domestic violence (including physical, sexual, or emotional abuse).

PREVENTION FROM RADIATION

It is important to prevent radiation during the pregnancy. Clinical diagnosis is unreliable and, if not confirmed by appropriate investigation, will lead to unnecessary treatment in some cases. Suggestive symptoms of chest pain or breathlessness must be investigated. The diagnosis is often made clinically as a result of swelling, calf pain or tenderness. It should be confirmed non-invasively by duplex ultrasound scanning of the leg veins and Doppler ultrasonography. If the diagnosis is still in doubt, further investigative procedures undertaken should be designed to minimize exposure of the foetus to radiation, especially in the first trimester. Limited venography may be performed with abdominal shielding, though a negative result does not exclude an iliac vein thrombosis. A clinical diagnosis of pulmonary embolism may be made on a history of dyspnoea, chest pain, cough or haemoptysis. Oxygen saturation and arterial gases may help. A chest X-ray is sometimes required to exclude other conditions which may present with similar signs and symptoms, such as pneumonia. The diagnosis is confirmed by the use of perfusion scanning. This may be performed antenatally as the procedure exposes the foetus to only to only a very low dose of radiation.

Immediate treatment involves intravenous heparinisation of the patient. In the antenatal period, this can then be converted to a subcutaneous form of heparin, rather than warfarin.

PSYCHOSOCIAL AND CULTURAL ASPECTS OF PREGNANCY

Pregnancy is a unique developmental transition resulting in a woman being no longer responsible just for herself but also for another. Because of the enormous physical and mental changes that must occur in the transition, it is a time of particular vulnerability, both physically and mentally. Mental health is influenced by multiple factors from the woman's earlier life and own development, current relationships and support, and the cultural context in which the pregnancy occurs.

Different theoretical models influence the understanding of both motherhood and mental illness in the perinatal period; the medical model emphasizes the role of hormones, sleep deprivation, and early influences on biologic responses to stress; feminist theories look at the influence of the medicalization of childbirth reinforcing feminine helplessness as a cause of difficulties, while attachment and interpersonal theories emphasize the importance of changing relationships at this time of development change. Theorists in evolutionary psychology emphasize the role of depression as a response to inadequate support, in order to ensure their partner, in particular, increases his investment in the child. These theories all provide valid views and are not necessarily at odds with one another. How the mother adapts to these changes as she prepares for motherhood will depend on multiple factors. This will include her own theoretical perspective, biology, personality, background, general health, current supports, and whether this child was planned and wanted.

ADJUSTMENT TO PREGNANCY

Even if a pregnancy is well-planned and long-anticipated, the realities of adjusting to the impending changes can be daunting. On an emotional level, things may seem unstable and out of control and the emotional upheaval can make a person feel anxious and vulnerable. Here are some suggestions for working through coping with some of this upheaval and helping to adjust to the pregnancy process:

The physical changes that pregnancy brings can be challenging enough, but the hormonal shifts and mood swings can make a woman feel really off-balance. It may help to understand that all of the upheaval is absolutely normal. Bursting into tears, seemingly irrational responses, feeling overwhelmed, depressed, crabby and elated - are all very typical feelings during the early weeks of pregnancy. For some women, the emotional ups and downs continue throughout pregnancy, while for others it just seems to be in the beginning weeks that the hormones are temporarily imbalanced. Time and understanding may take care of the bulk of these feelings, but if patient feel overwhelmingly depressed or anxious, try talking to a trusted partner, friend, family member or physician. It may also help to see a trained or professional counselor, or join a support group of other expectant mothers.

The impending lifestyle change can be one of the issues that creates the most reluctance for expectant mothers. There may be pressure from outside sources to start or stop working, move to a different apartment or house, or make other major life changes - in addition to the major life change of becoming a parent. A few ladies may have preconceived ideas about what it means to be a mother and fear that she will not be able to meet those expectations.

Regardless of whether the pregnancy was planned or unplanned, or what other difficult realities and situations surround the conception and preparation for the new addition, making the adjustment to the impending life changes is an important part of the pregnancy process. The women should take the time to identify concerns, issues and fears and talk them through - seeking help if necessary and remember that even though she is becoming a parent.

SINGLE PARENT

The structure of families have changed over the past 20 years single-parent families have become even more common than the so-called "nuclear family" consisting of a mother, father and children. Today we see all sorts of single parent families; headed by mothers, headed by fathers, headed by a grandparent raising their grandchildren. Life in a single parent household - though common - can be quite stressful for the adult and the children. Members may unrealistically expect that the family can function like a two-parent family, and may feel that something is wrong when it can not. The single parent may feel overwhelmed by the responsibility of juggling caring for the children, maintaining a job and keeping up with the bills and household chores. And typically, the family's finances and resources are drastically reduced following the parents' breakup.

Single parent families deal with many other pressures and potential problem areas that the nuclear family does not have to face. Some of these are:

- Visitation and custody problems;
- The effects of continuing conflict between the parents;
- Less opportunity for parents and children to spend time together;
- Effects of the breakup on children's school performance and peer relations;
- Disruptions of extended family relationships;
- Problems caused by the parents' dating and entering new relationships.

The single parent can help family members face these difficulties by talking with each other about their feelings and working together to tackle problems. Support from friends, other family members and the church or synagogue can help too.

TEENAGE PREGNANCY

Attempting to understand the phenomenon of adolescent pregnancy and to provide adequate care for pregnant adolescents requires an understanding of cognitive and psychosocial development of adolescents.

Although age ranges are often assigned to the developmental tasks for early, middle, and late adolescence, the chronologic age does not always correspond to the level of maturity. Additionally and individual adolescent may be functioning at one level cognitively and at another level psychosocially.

Early adolescence is characterized by turmoil stemming from the physical changes of puberty, loss of body control, and an intense preoccupation with physical appearance. Adjusting to their new body image makes early adolescents self-conscious and raises their concerns about being normal and appearing acceptable. Psychosexual development may correspond with undifferentiated exploratory sexual behaviour with members of the same or opposite sex.

Middle adolescence focuses on self-identification and self-realization. Girls show more interest in developing intense, loving relationships with boys. Boys are more interested in the pleasure of sexual activity than in the maintenance of loving relationships. Both genders exhibit behaviour that is more defiant, narcissitic, and self-reliant. With narcissism comes a sense of personal omnipotence and personal fables, which are stories about one's own uniqueness and invulnerability. For boys, this may be a sense of immortality that fosters risk taking behaviour; for girls, it may be a belief that she cannot become pregnant so she does not need to use contraception.

REFERENCES

Midwifery Perspectives Vienna Midwifery Seminar College of Midwifery Southern Health Board June 2002

Home Birth in Ireland: A review. ICM Triennial Conference Midwives for the Family and the World Vienna April 2002*

Home Birth in Ireland 1993 - 1997.A review of community midwifery practice Rhona O'Connell Mary Cronin Health Services Research Group March 2002

Challenges to Midwifery Practice Cork/Kerry Nurse Education Seminar February 2001.

Authoritative Knowledge in Childbirth. Midwives Association of Ireland, AGM November 1998.

4

Intra-natal Period

In general intranatal period is the whole period when a women conceive and till she gives birth to a baby, or any thing occurring chiefly with reference to the child during the act of birth. As far as possible all women should have institutional deliveries and delivery by a Skilled Birth Attendant (doctor, nurse, LHV and ANM). Institutional delivery -is one which occurs in a hospital, Government or private where facilities and care for provision of safe delivery exists. Families of women insisting on delivery at home must ensure that she is taken to the nearest FRU/CHC/ PHC if and when complications arise. In an institutional delivery, an ANM/ LHV/Staff Nurse/

MO (PHC) must be engaged for the birth. If these functionaries are not available a trained dai/TBA who has adequate experience should be engaged. The family should be prepared for any kind of emergency and a vehicle for transportation in such a case should also be arranged. After delivery, in case the placenta is not delivered completely within 30 minutes, the woman must be rushed to the nearest FRU/District Hospital for manual removal of placenta & treatment.

PHYSIOLOGY OF LABOUR, MECHANISM OF LABOUR

NORMAL LABOUR

Emanuel Friedman in his elegant treatise on labour (1978) stated correctly that "the clinical features of uterine contractions namely frequency, intensity, and duration cannot be relied upon as measures of progression in labour nor as indices of normality. Except for cervical dilatation and foetal decent, none of the clinical features of the parturient patient appears to be useful in assessing labour progression." Friedman sought to select criteria that would limit normal labour and thus be able to identify significant abnormalities of labour. These limits, admittedly arbitrary, appear to be logical and clinically useful. The graphic representation of labour plotting descent and dilatation against time has become known as the Friedman curve. It, or a modification of it, is used extensively to evaluate labouring patients.

Labour has been divided functionally into a preparatory division (including latent and acceleration phases of the dilatation curve), a dilatational division comprising only the linear phase of maximum slope of dilatation, and a pelvic division encompassing the linear phase of maximum descent.

FUNCTIONAL CLASSIFICATION OF LABOUR

Principal Clinical Features on the Functional Divisions of Labour

Characteristic	Preparatory Division	Dilatational Division	Pelvic Division
Functions	Contractions coordinated, polarized, oriented; cervix prepared	Cervix actively dilated	Pelvis negotiated; mechanisms of labour; foetal descent; delivery
Interval	Latent and acceleration phases	Phase of maximum slope	Deceleration phase and second stage
Measurement	Elapsed duration	Linear rate of dilatation	Linear rate of descent
Diagnosable disorders	Prolonged latent phase	Protracted dilatation; protracted descent	Prolonged deceleration; secondary arrest of dilatation; arrest of descent; failure of descent

ABNORMAL LABOUR

Dystocia (literally difficult labour) is characterized by abnormally slow progress in labour. It is the consequence of four distinct abnormalities that may exist singly or in combination. Uterine forces that are not sufficiently strong or appropriately coordinated to efface and dilate the cervix. Forces generated by voluntary muscles during the second stage of labour that are inadequate to overcome the normal resistance of the bony birth canal and maternal soft parts. Faulty presentation or abnormal development of the foetus of such character that the foetus cannot be extruded through the birth canal.

Abnormalities of the birth canal that form an obstacle to the descent of the foetus.

Labour Disorders	
Pattern	**Diagnostic Criterion**
Prolonged latent phase	Nulliparas 20 hr or more Multiparas 14 hr or more
Protracted active phase dilatation	Nulliparas 1.2 cm/hr or less
Protracted descent	Nulliparas 1 cm/hr or less Multiparas 2 cm/hr or less
Prolonged deceleration phase	Nulliparas 3 hr or more Multiparas 1 hr or more
Secondary arrest of dilatation	Arrest 2 hr or more
Arrest of descent	Arrest 1 hr or more
Failure of descent	No descent in deceleration phase of second stage

Etiologic factors that appear to be responsible for the development of prolonged latent phase disorders in multiparas most often include excessive sedation administered during the course of the latent phase and poor prelabor soft-tissue preparation. In addition, false labour and myometrial dysfunction are found but can be diagnosed only retrospectively.

Arrest disorder: Secondary arrest of dilatation pattern with documented cessation of progression in the active phase. Prolonged deceleration phase pattern with deceleration phase duration greater than normal limits. Failure of descent in the deceleration phase and second stage. Arrest of descent characterized by halted advancement of foetal station in the second stage.

These four abnormalities are similar in etiology, response to treatment, and prognosis, being readily differentiated from the normal dilatation and descent curves (broken lines).

Etiology of arrest disorders are as follows. The striking association with cephalopelvic disproportion makes these disorders especially ominous; whenever encountered, arrest patterns should signal the likelihood that a bony impediment exists. Other factors very often occur in combination with each other and with disproportion as well.

Immediately after incising the uterus and foetal membranes, the operators fingers are insinuated between the symphysis pubis and the foetal head until the posterior surface is reached. The head is carefully lifted anteriorly and, as necessary, superiorly to bring it from beneath the symphysis forward through the uterine and abdominal incisions.

MECHANISM OF LABOUR

The definition or clinical diagnosis of labour is a retrospective one. There is no laboratory test that gives a "labour titer" or an x-ray procedure that can define the difference between the labouring and non-labouring patient. Realizing these limitations, the patient is diagnosed as being in labour when a combination of conditions exist. Perhaps a good working definition may be stated as follows: When in the presence of perceived uterine contractions, there is progressive cervical dilation and descent of the presenting part which leads to the eventual expulsion of the products of conception, the patient is in labour.

The "mechanism of labour" refers to the sequencing of events related to posturing and positioning that allows the baby to find the "easiest way out." For the most part the foetus is a passive respondent in the process of labour, while the mother provides the uterine forces and structural configuration of the passageway through which the passenger must travel. For a normal mechanism of labour to occur, both the foetal and maternal factors must be harmonious. An understanding of these factors is essential for the obstetrician to appropriately intervene if the mechanism deviates from the normal. The following definitions must be mastered to be able to discuss and understand the mechanism of labour:

1. Attitude. This refers to the posturing of the joints and relation of foetal parts to one another. The normal foetal attitude when labour begins is with all joints in flexion.
2. Lie. This refers to the longitudinal axis of the foetus in relation to the mother's longitudinal axis; i.e., transverse, oblique, or longitudinal (parallel).
3. Presentation. This describes that part on the foetus lying over the inlet of the pelvis or at the cervical os.
4. Point of Reference or Direction. This is an arbitrary point on the presenting part used to orient it to the maternal pelvis [usually occiput, mentum (chin) or sacrum].
5. Position. This describes the relation of the point of reference to one of the eight octanes of the pelvic inlet (e.g., LOT: the occiput is transverse and to the left).

6. Engagement. This occurs when the biparietal diametre is at or below the inlet of the true pelvis.
7. Station. This references the presenting part to the level of the ischial spines measured in plus or minus centimetres.

The single most important determinant to the mechanism of labour is probably pelvic configuration. The classic work of Caldwell and Maloy is reviewed in the text and should be understood. Their classification of the pelvis into four major types (gynecoid, android, anthropoid, and platypelloid) helps the student understand the possible difficulties that may arise in a labouring patient. A quote that should be remembered is: "No two pelves are exactly the same, just as no two faces are the same. For each pelvis there is an optimum mechanism that may be wholly different from the so-called normal mechanism described."

An important principle is that most pelves are not purely defined but occur in nature as mixed types. Regardless of the shape, the baby will be delivered if size and positioning remain compatible. The narrowest part of the foetus attempts to align itself with the narrowest pelvic dimension (e.g., biparietal to interspinous diametres) which means the occiput generally tends to rotate to the "most ample portion of the pelvis."

The mechanical steps the baby undergoes can be arbitrarily divided, and clinically they are usually broken down into six or eight steps for ease of discussion. It must be understood, however, that these are arbitrary distinctions in a natural continuum.

The following six divisions of labour are easy to use:

1. Flexion and Engagement. This occurs at various times before the forces of labour begin.
2. Descent. This occurs as a result of active forces of labour.
3. Internal Rotation. This occurs as a result of impingement of the presenting part on the bony and soft tissues of the pelvis.
4. Extension. This is the mechanism by which the head normally negotiates the pelvic curve.
5. External Rotation(Restitution). This is the spontaneous realignment of the head with the shoulders.
6. Expulsion. This is anterior and then posterior shoulders, followed by trunk and lower extremities in rapid succession.

Abnormal mechanisms of labour do occur, and the operator must be able to recognize these early and intervene when appropriate. The above mechanisms of labour should be come "second nature" to the practitioner and indeed does become such by careful observation. Those patients who have undeliverable or uncorrectable problems should be unhesitatingly delivered by the abdominal route because inappropriate operative vaginal intervention may lead to damage to both mother and foetus. Some of the undeliverable situations include persistent mentum posterior, persistent brow presentation, some types of breech presentations, and shoulder presentation.

MANAGEMENT OF LABOUR

The stages of labour are often thought to be a mystery. In all honesty it is a mystery in many ways. Each woman will have a different labour and yet many parts are the same.

During labour, the first and generally longest stage of birth at 12 to 24 hours, the contractions of the uterine muscles will cause the cervix to efface (shortening or thinning of the cervix; 0-100% thinned out) and dilate (the opening of the cervix; expressed in centimetres). Another term used to indicate progress in labour is the baby's station or the location of the baby's presenting part, in relation to certain bones in the pelvis. This indicates how much the baby has advanced or moved through the pelvis and is usually expressed in centilitres above (minus) and below (plus) the level of a certain point on the pelvis.

All these changes serve to gradually move the foetus through the cervix and vagina (or birth canal) and out of the body.

Labour is the first stage of birth and the longest, usually being anywhere between (for a first pregnancy; in subsequent pregnancies labour is generally much shorter). Assessing the start of labour is one of the most important aspects of the management of labour.

SIGNS AND SYMPTOMS

- Painful contractions with a certain regularity.
- Effacement and/or dilatation of the cervix.
- Leakage of amniotic fluid.
- Bloody discharge or "bloody show" (a small amount of blood mixed with mucus from the cervix) often serves as a clue that labour is about to begin.
- Rupture of the membranes or the woman's water breaking is a clear sign that something irreversible has occurred. Indeed,

about 80 to 90% of women whose membranes have ruptured go into labour spontaneously within 24 hours.

- However, it should be noted that contractions may be felt long before labour actually starts, and cervical dilatation may be present weeks before the end of pregnancy.

Upon admittance to the hospital, an examination of the baby's station, presentation, position (forward/backward) and foetal heartbeat as well as the mother's weight, blood pressure, pulse, heart and breathing rates, temperature, effacement and contraction strength, duration, and frequency all are noted to see how far along labour is. Often the membranes are also checked to see if they have ruptured.

The heart rate of mother and foetus is checked about every 15 minutes as 30 to 50% of babies who develop problems or die during delivery do so without warning. Enemas and pubic shaving, were once standard procedure but, according to the World Health Organization, have long been considered unnecessary and should not be undertaken except at the woman's request. The WHO also states that dilation of the cervix is the most accurate indication of the progress of labour.

The first stage of birth is often divided into three categories: early, active, and transition. A summary of each of these stages is found in the table below:

	Length	Dilation	Contractions
Early Labour	2 - 9 hours	0 - 4 centimetres	30 to 60 seconds long Start at 20 - 30 minutes apart and slow but gradually become more frequent and stronger; 5 minutes apart by the end of this phase.
Active Labour	The rest of labour, usually shorter than Early phase	4 - 8 centimetres	45 to 60 seconds apart and stronger, peak sooner. Contractions become more and more intense once water breaks.
Transition Phase	10 - 90 minutes	8 -10 centimetres	60 to 90 seconds long. These contractions, which peak suddenly and peak more than once, can be as close as 1 and 1.5 to 2 minutes apart. May feel as if the contractions are right on top of each other.

The transition phase is the sign that labour is almost over and the woman and baby are moving into the second stage of birth delivery.

THE LABOUR ROOM

There are three stages of labour. The first stage occurs from the time true labour begins until the cervix is completely dilated and effaced. During the second stage the baby is delivered. The third stage follows the birth of the baby through the birth of the placenta.

Testing During Labour and Delivery

- Pelvic Exam - The most important test performed during labour is the pelvic exam used to determine the progression of labour.
- Foetal monitoring - Foetal monitoring is used to detect the baby's heart rate and response to uterine contractions.

THE FIRST STAGE

The first stage of labour is the longest. There are three phases within the first stage. At the end of the first stage, the cervix is dilated to 10 centimetres. In mothers having their first child, this stage usually lasts 12 to 16 hours. For women having second or subsequent children, the first stage lasts around 6-7 hours.

1. Early Labour: During the early or latent phase, the cervix dilates to 4 centimetres. The duration of the first phase is the longest, averaging around 8 hours. Contractions may be irregular, progressing to rhythmic and methodical. The pain felt at this early stage may be similar to menstrual pain: aching, fullness, cramping and backache. Walking is usually more comfortable than sitting. Most women spend these hours at home, or they may be checked at the hospital and sent home until labour becomes more active.
2. Active Labour: Active labour is marked by regular contractions that become longer, stronger and closer together over time. Most providers recommend that lady go to the hospital when contractions are five minutes apart, lasting more then 60 seconds for at least an hour. Measure contractions from the start of one contraction to the beginning of the next.
3. Transition: Transition is the most difficult phase of labour. It is the shortest, lasting from 30 minutes to two hours. The pain may be intense, as the cervix stretches and the baby descends into the birth canal

SECOND STAGE

The second stage labour lasts anywhere from one contraction to up to two hours. The labour nurse or physician will tell when it is time to push. It is important that not to push until instructed. When "crowning" occurs, within the next few pushes, the baby is born. Fluid will be removed from the baby's mouth and nose with a bulb syringe. The baby will take its first breath, and may begin to cry. Immediately after birth, the baby is still connected to the placenta by the umbilical cord. The cord is clamped and cut.

THIRD STAGE

The third stage of labour refers to the period following the completed delivery of the newborn until the completed delivery of the placenta. Relatively little thought or teaching seems to be devoted to the third stage of labour compared with that given to the first and second stages. A leading North American obstetrics text devotes only 4 of more than 1500 pages to the third stage of labour but significantly more to the complications that may arise immediately following delivery. One respected author states: "This indeed is the unforgiving stage of labour, and in it there lurks more unheralded treachery than in both the other stages combined. The normal case can, within a minute, become abnormal and successful delivery can turn swiftly to disaster."

Another interesting aspect of the third stage is the marked discrepancy in what is believed to be its appropriate and optimal conduct. A clear division exists between authorities who advocate the physiological approach and those who advocate the active approach to management. While management strategies are often controversial, for disagreement to persist when fairly compelling evidence supports one of the two approaches is somewhat unusual.

The third stage of labour commences with the completed delivery of the foetus and ends with the completed delivery of the placenta and its attached membranes. The clinician immediately recognizes that from a practical perspective, the risk of complications continues for some period after delivery of the placenta. For this reason, many authorities have advocated a so-called fourth stage of labour, which begins with the delivery of the placenta and lasts for an arbitrary period afterward. The most commonly chosen duration is 1 hour; however, periods as long as 4 hours have been suggested. The length of the third stage itself is usually 5-15 minutes. The absolute time limit for delivery of the placenta, without evidence of significant bleeding, remains unclear. Periods ranging from 30-60 minutes have been suggested.

Signs of Placental Separation

Traditionally, 4 signs of placental separation are taught.

1. The most reliable sign is the lengthening of the umbilical cord as the placenta separates and is pushed into the lower uterine segment by progressive uterine retraction. Placing a clamp on the cord near the perineum makes it easier to appreciate this lengthening. Never place traction on the cord without countertraction on the uterus above the symphysis; otherwise, one may mistake cord lengthening due to impending prolapse or inversion for that of uncomplicated placental separation.
2. The uterus takes on a more globular shape and becomes firmer. This occurs as the placenta descends into the lower segment and the body of the uterus continues to retract. This change may be clinically difficult to appreciate.
3. The uterus rises in the abdomen. The descent of the placenta into the lower segment, and finally into the vagina, displaces the uterus upward.
4. A gush of blood occurs. The retroplacental clot is able to escape as the placenta descends to the lower uterine segment. The retroplacental clot usually forms centrally and escapes following complete separation; however, if the blood can find a path to escape, it may do so before complete separation and thus is not a reliable indicator of complete separation. This occurrence is sometimes associated with increased bleeding and a prolonged third stage, with the delivery of the leading edge of the placenta and maternal surface first (Matthews Duncan method), rather than the cord insertion and foetal surface, which is more common (Schultze method).

Commence preparations for the third stage of labour well before delivery of the baby. In the antepartum period, discuss with the patient and her partner their preferences for the delivery process with an open dialogue regarding any risk factors present and what implications they might have for the woman. Thoroughly discuss any concerns or variations from accepted practice.

Physiological Versus Active Management

The controversy surrounding third-stage management exists between authorities who advocate the physiological, or expectant, approach and those who advocate the active approach.

FOURTH STAGE

The delivery of the placenta does not mark the end of risk for bleeding; on the contrary, the uterus may have a tendency to relax slightly following placental delivery, and this is the point at which problems most commonly begin. The prophylactic use of a uterotonic helps ensure that the uterus continues to contract and retract, but the obstetrician must remain vigilant. Nearly every clinician can recount an episode of being briefly distracted at this point only to have his or her attention abruptly reclaimed by a cascade of blood.

Following delivery of the placenta, palpate the abdomen to assess and monitor uterine tone and size. At this point, uterine massage is reasonable, especially if concern exists regarding uterine tone. Uterine massage can be uncomfortable; therefore, explain the rationale to the patient. If intravenous access is in place, a continuous infusion of oxytocin for a period following delivery is reasonable. If ongoing concerns exist regarding uterine tone, then start an oxytocin infusion or administer a longer-acting agent. Encourage early breastfeeding to promote endogenous oxytocin release.

Once good, sustained uterine tone has been established, the presence of any bleeding from the lower genital tract can be assessed. If bleeding is minimal, assess the placenta for completeness. (First, manage any significant lower genital tract bleeding.) Assessment of the placenta before repair of an episiotomy or any lacerations is advised in order to avoid disrupting these repairs if uterine exploration or instrumentation is necessary.

Examine the foetal side for any evidence of vessels coursing to the edge of the placenta and into the membranes. Such vessels suggest the presence of a succenturiate placental lobe. If the vessels are torn and the lobe is not present, it is quite likely retained and may subsequently lead to bleeding or infection. If this is the case, turn the placenta over and lay it on a flat surface to examine the maternal side, with special attention to any defect suggestive of a missing, retained cotyledon. Note other abnormalities of the placenta, and consider whether pathological examination is warranted. Cultures of the placenta seem to be of little value in the diagnosis or management of foetal or uterine infection.

The lower genital tract is examined using adequate lighting and appropriate positioning and analgesia. Any episiotomy or lacerations are repaired. During this time, note any ongoing blood loss from the upper vagina, and, if present, reassess uterine tone and size. Closely observe the patient for blood loss over the next hour, with skilled assessment of uterine tone and size at least every 15 minutes. The duration of close observation and the presence and/or length of any uterotonic administration depends on the risk factors present and the clinical course.

REFERENCES

Arditti, Rita. Women as Objects: Science and Sexual Politics. Science for the People, Sept. 1974.

Arms, Suzanne. Immaculate Deception. 1975. One of the classics that helped change the practices of birthing in the USA.

Courter, Gay. The Midwife. Houghton Mifflin Co. 1981. A novel about the roots of midwifery from Prussia to the United States.

Davis, Elizabeth. Heart and Hands. 2nd. Edition. Celestial Arts, 1992. A Midwife's guide to pregnancy, childbirth and the art and science of midwifery.

Donnison, Jean. Midwives and Medical Men: A History of Inter-Professional Rivalries and Women's Rights. Schocken books, 1977.

Edwards, Margot and Waldorf, Mary. Reclaiming Birth: History and Heroines of American Childbirth Reform. The Crossing Press, 1984

Ehrenreich, Barbara and English, Derdre. Witches, Midwives and Nurses: A History of Women Healers. The Feminist Press, 1973.

Gordon, Linda. Woman's Body, Woman's Right: A Social History of Birth Control in America. New York: Grossman, 1977.

Graham, Harvey. Eternal Eve, the History of Gynaecology and Obstetrics. Doubleday & Company, 1951.

Kitzinger, Sheila. The Midwife Challenge. Pandora, 1991. Describes midwifery worldwide from a historical perspective.

5

Post-natal Period

Postnatal is the period beginning immediately after the birth of a child and extending for about six weeks. The period is sometimes incorrectly called the postpartum period, which refers to the mother and, less commonly, puerperium. Biologically, it is the time after birth, a time in which the mother's body, including hormone levels and uterus size, return to prepregnancy conditions. Lochia is post-partum vaginal discharge, containing blood, mucus, and placental tissue. During the first stages of this period, the newborn also starts his/her adaptation to extrauterine life, the most significant physiological transition until death.

A woman who is delivering in a hospital may leave the hospital as soon as she is medically stable and chooses to leave, which can be as early as a few hours postpartum, though the average for spontaneous vaginal delivery (SVD) is 1-2 days, and the average caesarean section postnatal stay is 3-4 days. During this time the mother is monitored for bleeding, bowel and bladder function, and baby care. The infant's health is also monitored.

PHYSICAL

The mother is assessed for tears, and is sutured if necessary. Also, she may suffer from constipation or hemorrhoids, both of which would be managed. The bladder is also assessed for infection, retention and any problems in the muscles. The major focus of postpartum care is ensuring that the woman is healthy and capable of taking care of her newborn, equipped with all the information she needs about breastfeeding, reproductive health and contraception, and the imminent life adjustment. Some medical conditions may occur postnatally, such as Sheehan Syndrome and peripartum cardiomyopathy. In some cases, this adjustment is not made easily, and hormonal disturbances may lead to postnatal depression or even puerperal psychosis.

PSYCHOLOGICAL

Postnatal depression is common, with approximately 30% of women suffering from it, potentially as early as 24 hours postpartum. It is usually limited in duration, lasting 36 to 48 hours. Apart from empathy and support from caregivers and family, treatment is not required. Approximately 10-20% of women will suffer the symptoms of major depression, and should be treated accordingly. Postpartum depression may be the response to the hormonal changes and life adjustment the woman goes through immediately after childbirth. Postnatal Psychosis (also known as puerperal psychosis), is a more severe form of mental illness than postpartum depression. Care provided by a postpartum doula will support the mother, assist with breastfeeding and baby care which enhances her confidence, helping to lessen her chances of developing postpartum depression or other postpartum mood disorders.

NORMAL PUERPERIUM, PHYSIOLOGY DURATION

The puerperium is defined as the period from birth to the first 6 weeks postpartum. Multiple anatomic and physiologic changes occur during this time, and there is the potential for significant complications such as infection or haemorrhage.

PHYSIOLOGY

Involutional Changes: The uterus usually undergoes complete involution by 6 weeks postpartum, going from a weight of 1, 000 g to a weight of 100 g or less. The endometrium begins to regenerate early in the postpartum period, essentially completing the regeneration by the third week. The last part of the uterus to return to normal is the placental attachment site, which may take up to 6 weeks to regenerate. The sloughed tissue becomes part of the lochia. Initially, the lochia contains blood mixed with decidua and is called the lochia rubra. By the 3rd or 4th day, the lochia becomes pale and watery, although it is still tinged with blood; at this stage, it is termed the lochia serosa. After the 10th day, the lochia becomes yellowish-white (the lochia alba). The vagina, which is dusky, engorged, spacious, and smooth after delivery, diminishes in size and regains its normal ragouted, pink appearance by approximately 3 weeks postpartum.

Anatomically, the dilatation of the calyces, renal pelvis, and ureters that is characteristic of pregnancy may persist as long as 8 weeks postpartum. Functionally, the increased renal plasma flow, glomerular filtration rate, and creatinine clearance rate associated with pregnancy return to normal by 6 weeks after delivery.

The changes in the cardiovascular system that occurred during pregnancy (ie, increase in heart rate, cardiac output, and blood volume) generally return to baseline by approximately 6 weeks postpartum. Peripheral vascular resistance also returns to the prepregnancy level by this time. Most of these parametres return to normal puerperium, lactation, breast-feeding, breast feeding, breast-feeding, postpartum, postpartum depression, postpartum haemorrhage, uterine infection, mastitis, episiotomy infection within the first 2 weeks postpartum.

OVULATION AND MENSTRUATION

After delivery, ovulation occurs at an average of 10 weeks but may occur as early as 27 days after delivery in non-lactating women. In women who breast-feed for at least 3 months, the average time to ovulation is 17 weeks. In non-lactating women, the mean time to menstruation is 6-8 weeks after delivery, and 70% menstruate by 12 weeks after delivery. In lactating women, the return to menstruation is more gradual, so that one half to three fourths have menstruated by 36 weeks. For obvious reasons, lactation is not an ideal or necessarily effective method of birth control.

LACTATION

Breast-feeding should be encouraged for several reasons. First and foremost, breast milk is the ideal source of nutrients for the neonate. Breast milk also provides some degree of immunologic protection for the neonate. Nursing is contraindicated in patients with certain viral infections such as CMV, hepatitis B, and HIV infection.

The breast and nipples of a woman who is nursing her infant require little attention in the puerperium other than attention to cleanliness and fissures. Some parturients may request lactation suppression during the postpartum period. Lactation is suppressed in 60-70% of women who wear a fight brassiere and avoid stimulation of the nipples. Althoughbreast engorgement may occasionally cause a temperature elevation of short duration, any rise in temperature during the puerperium might be a sign of infection.

Lactogenesis

One distinguishing characteristic of mammals is their capacity to nourish their young with secretions from the mammary glands. On the basis of studies in animals, lactogenesis can be arbitrarily divided into two stages. During the first stage, which occurs during the third trimester of pregnancy, the lobular-alveolar complex is stimulated to differentiate such that there are increases in synthesis of enzymes necessary for the production of milk components. These special constituents of human milk include major proteins such as a-lactalbumin, [3-1actoglobulin, and casein, as well as triglycerides and lactose. The second stage is characterized by secretion of colostrum, followed by significant milk secretion approximately 5 days after delivery.

In concert with cortisol, insulin, estrogen, progesterone, and placental lactogen, prolactin stimulates growth and development of the milk-secreting apparatus of the mammary gland. Prolactin is the principal hormone that stimulates lactogenesis, and levels increase progressively throughout pregnancy from a mean of less than 20 ng/mL in a nonpregnant woman to an average of 250-300 ng/mL during the third trimester. Prolactin exerts its principal action by binding to specific membrane receptors on mammary tissue to stimulate gene transcription of messenger RNA and subsequent synthesis of lactose, casein, milk fat, and a-lactalbumin.

During pregnancy, the high estrogen levels produced by the foetal-placental unit stimulate an increase in circulating puerperium, lactation, breast-feeding, breast feeding, breastfeeding, postpartum, postpartum depression, postpartum haemorrhage, uterine infection, mastitis, episiotomy infection prolactin; however, the high estrogen-progesterone levels also suppress the number of available prolactin-binding sites in mammary tissue so that lactogenesis is delayed until placental separation leads to a rapid decline in these steroid levels. After delivery, prolactin concentrations remain elevated and increase further during suckling. Because higher prolactin levels lead to more prolactin-binding sites, prolactin can induce an up-regulation of its own receptors, thereby further increasing its biologic activity.

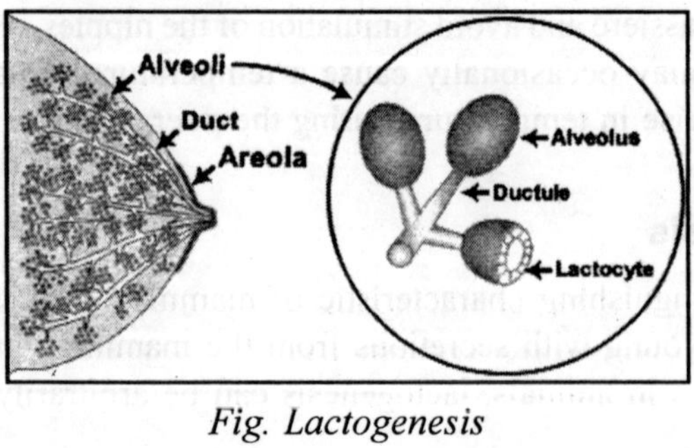

Fig. Lactogenesis

Although both human placental lactogen and growth hormone are structurally similar to prolactin and have intrinsic lactotrophic properties, their role in lactogenesis in humans is unclear. During pregnancy, growth hormone is suppressed to very low levels, whereas placental production of human placental lactogen is parallel to the increase in placental growth during the second half of pregnancy. In animal models, human placental lactogen can mimic the biologic action of prolactin by binding to the prolactin receptor. Because levels of human placental lactogen decline rapidly and become undetectable 24 hours after delivery, a role for human placental lactogen in the maintenance of lactation is unlikely.

In mammary tissues, cortisol induces the development of the rough endoplasmic reticulum and Golgi membranes that are necessary for increased synthesis of milk proteins. Thus, cortisol appears to be essential for prolactin stimulation of casein production.

During pregnancy, estrogens promote ductal development while progesterone stimulates lobular-alveolar maturation of the mammary gland. In addition, the high levels of estrogens present during pregnancy augment the release of prolactin from the pituitary gland, and the high levels of progesterone act to suppress lactogenesis by reducing the ability of prolactin to up-regulate its own receptors. Progesterone also exerts other anti-lactogenic effects by reducing estrogen binding to mammary tissue.

Thyroid hormones appear to play a permissive role in lactogenesis because administration of T4 augments mammary development and milk production.

POSTNATAL ASSESSMENT AND MANAGEMENT

On admission to the postnatal ward, the midwife makes the woman comfortable and responds to her immediate needs. A complete report on the woman and her baby is received from the midwife transferring the woman from labour ward to the postnatal ward. Any complications, such as postpartum haemorrhage, perineal tears, or a depressed emotional state should be reported on, as well as the relevant interventions. The postnatal midwife needs to know how the baby is doing in the case where he does not accompany the mother to the ward.

OBSERVATIONS

On admission to the postnatal ward the temperature, pulse, blood pressure, uterine contraction and blood loss are assessed. Check the last Hb level as it may decrease after the intrapartum and postpartum blood loss. The frequency of observations is guided by the condition of the patient.

GENERAL ASSESSMENT

Enquire whether the woman is experiencing pain or discomfort. Ask specifically about her emotional state, lochia, micturition, defaecation, breastfeeding and infant care, mobilization, exercise, sleep and diet. Examine the perineum for signs of infection. Educate the woman about vulval and perineal hygiene.

ASSESSMENT AND MANAGEMENT OF SPECIFIC HEALTH PROBLEMS

Uterine Atomy

Uterine atony accounts for 80 to 90% of postpartum haemorrhage in the first 24 hours of the postnatal period. It occurs when the uterus does not contract effectively after childbirth and bleeding persists from the placental site. The midwife should educate the woman to look out for the following signs:

- The uterus is not palpable as a hard mass.
- Vaginal bleeding persists.
- Full bladder (a full bladder will prevent the uterus from contracting).

Educate the woman on simple methods to assist micturition such as a nearby running tap. Should this fail then she should seek appropriate assistance. The cause of retention of urine, such as a painful episotomy site or vulval haematoma, should be established and the condition managed.

The midwife should be on the alert for the following instances where there is an increased susceptibility to develop an atonic uterus.

- Multiparous women.
- Overdistension of the uterus during pregnancy (multiple pregnancy, large baby, polyhydramnios).
- History of PPH with previous delivery.
- Prolonged labour.
- Preciptous labour and delivery.
- Oxytoxin induction during labour.

Health education should be given to the woman to encourage regular checks that the uterine contraction is sustained, that vaginal bleeding is average, and that the bladder is emptied regularly. Rubbing up the uterine funds should be demonstrated to the woman and she should be encouraged to report odd or abnormal findings promptly.

Abnormal findings must be documented and reported to the doctor immediately. Exploration of the uterus under general anaesthesia and removal of the retained placental products may be necessary. If an antibiotic is prescribed, the midwife should advise on the significance of compliance and importance of completing the prescribed course of antibiotics.

Subinvolution

Subinvolution is a term used to describe a uterus that remains large and fails to reduce in size and mass. It may result from retained placental fragments, infection and myoma. Appropriate health education is essential and subinvolution should be suspected if the following are evident:

- The lochia fails to progress from rubra to serosa.
- The woman gives a history of excessive bleeding.
- The uterus is tender to palpation (which suggests endometritis).
- There is leucorrhoea and back pain.
- There is an accompanying infection.
- An enlarged uterus is palpated.

PROMOTING PHYSICAL AND EMOTIONAL WELL-BEING

The postnatal period is the final transition, a time of major life change and of potential stress as a woman becomes a mother and a couple become a family.

The following points should be kept in mind:

- Temperature: Usually elevated to 38°C during the first 24 hours post-delivery. It may increase beyond 38°C after 24 hours. If it persists beyond 48 hours it suggests infection and calls for action. Exclude other causes and/or symptoms such as pain in the calf, foul odour of lochia, infection or dehydration.
- Pulse: Ranges between 50 to 90 bpm. Tachycardia may result following haemorrhage, or a difficult labour and birth.
- Blood pressure: An elevated BP may suggest pre-eclampsia, chronic hypertension, renal disease, or anxiety. A drop in BP may be normal for the mother, or it may indicate postpartum haemorrhage.

- Respiration: This should remain within normal range of 16 to 24 breaths per minute.

Assessment of the psychological wellbeing of the woman post-delivery does not always receive the vigilant monitoring that it deserves. Midwives must be able to implement preventive measures; differentiate one condition from the other; identify the early signs and symptoms of each condition; and report promptly to the doctor when warning signs of puerperal depression or psychosis set in. Education about the psychological care and support must be emphasized during antenatal parenting must be emphasized during antenatal parenting sessions which couples participate in jointly.

LACTATION MANAGEMENT

Optimally, a woman is able to put her infant to breast immediately following birth, but for some mothers this is not an option and the breastfeeding relationship is delayed. For some the delay lasts only minutes; for others, it may be hours, days, or weeks. Many mothers experience little to no difficulty when putting their infants to the breasts to feed, but some mothers confront difficulties, which may require them to seek the assistance of a lactation consultant for successful management and continuation of the breastfeeding relationship.

Whether the obstacle is caused by the mother's or the infant's health, the age of the new mother, lifestyle, returning to work or school, lack of support, or any other special circumstance, she can be assisted to a successful and rewarding relationship by support, encouragement, and counseling techniques that include current breastfeeding information. The establishment and maintenance of breastfeeding should be one of the major goals of good postpartum care. Human breast milk is the optimal food for newborn infants. Through the ages the human species has been dependent on it for its reproduction, animal milk being used only as an emergency measure if no human milk was available, usually with disastrous consequences.

Breastfeeding is a primary health care strategy, improving the health of mothers and infants and children as well as lowering the risk of several chronic diseases of adults. Its benefits are well documented. Lack of knowledge of lactation management among health care providers has been a significant contributing factor in the failure to reach breastfeeding rates. An important reason for this lack of knowledge is that many schools of medicine, nursing and nutrition have not integrated lactation management education into their curricula.

The peripartum hospital experience should include adequate support, instruction, and care to ensure the successful initiation of breastfeeding. Such management is part of a continuum of care and education that begins during the prenatal period, promotes breastfeeding as the optimal method of infant feeding, and includes information about maternal and infant benefits.

IMMUNIZATION

Immunizations starts already in the postnatal period. Policies in countries may vary. Immunizing the mother is an important way of preventing a disease or a malformation in the newborns. If this was done for this birth, the opportunity in the perinatal period should not be missed for the next pregnancy.

THE TARGET DISEASES

Tuberculosis

Tuberculosis caused an estimated 2.6 million deaths worldwide in 1996. The pandemic of HIV infection and an increase in multi drug-resistant Mycobacterium tuberculosis have profoundly worsened the public health burden of the disease. BCG is the most widely used vaccine in the world. The efficacy in preventing pulmonary TB varies widely in the world, but BCG immunization at birth will reduce the morbidity and mortality from tuberculous meningitis and disseminated disease among children. In some countries where the risk of tuberculosis is low, and where the tuberculin reaction is used for case finding, BCG immunization is only used for individuals at increased risk. Generally, the BCG should continue to be given as soon after birth as possible in all populations at high risk of tuberculosis infection.

Diphtheria

Diphtheria is a threat especially in temperate climates. Immunization is by diphtheria toxoid, an inactivated preparation of diphtheria toxin. It does not prevent the infection, but prevents the systemic manifestations. The immunization is recommended for children in all countries at 6, 10 and 14 weeks after birth.

Tetanus

Tetanus is caused by a potent neurotoxin produced by Clostridium tetani, growing in necrosed tissues in dirty wounds and in the umbilical cord affecting neonates if delivery has not been clean. Immunization is by tetanus toxoid (TT), an inactivated preparation of the toxin. All children should receive TT immunization at 6, 10 and 14 weeks.

Women (pregnant or non-pregnant) of childbearing age who have not previously been immunized with TT in their infancy or adolescence should be immunized, both to protect themselves and to protect their newborns against neonatal tetanus.

A five-dose schedule is recommended for the previously unprotected woman as follows:

- TT1 at first contact or as early as possible in pregnancy.
- TT2 at least 4 weeks after TT1.
- TT3 at least 6 months after TT2.
- The two last doses are given after at least one year, or during a subsequent pregnancy.

Pertussis

Pertussis (whooping cough) is a respiratory infection caused by Bordetella pertussis. Many of the symptoms are caused by toxins. Immunization takes place by injection of vaccines containing pertussis bacteria killed by chemicals or heat, or by acellular vaccines recently introduced in some industrialized countries, containing pertussis antigens. It is recommended for children at 6, 10 and 14 weeks.

Poliomyelitis

Poliomyelitis is a viral infection spread via the faecal-oral route, and also via the pharyngeal route. The risk of paralysis among infants is approximately 1 in 200 infections among infants <1 year old, and 1 in 100 infections among children aged 1-14 years. Immunization is possible by injection of the inactivated vaccine, or by oral administration of a vaccine composed of attenuated polio viruses. All infants should be vaccinated with oral poliomyelitis vaccine (OPV) according to the following schedule:

- OPV 0 at birth or as late as 2 weeks after birth
- OPV 1 at 6 weeks
- OPV 2 at 10 weeks
- OPV 3 at 14 weeks.

Measles

Measles is an acute viral infection, transmitted by close respiratory contact. Deaths occur primarily through secondary infections of the respiratory and/or gastrointestinal tract. The immunization by attenuated virus preparations is recommended at 9 months of age, well after the postnatal period.

Hepatitis B

Hepatitis B is caused by a virus, transmitted through contact with blood and by sexual intercourse. Perinatal (vertical) transmission from mother to infant takes place during delivery. Child to child transmission is also common during childhood. Many infected infants become hepatitis B virus (HBV) carriers, some may develop serious liver disease. Immunization with vaccine containing the hepatitis B surface antigen (HBsAg) is recommended for all infants as soon as possible after birth, with a second dose at 6 weeks and a third dose at 14 weeks. In Africa, where perinatal infection is less common, immunization can begin later, the three doses can be given then at 6, 10 and 14 weeks, together with other vaccines. Immunization of health workers is also recommended.

Passive Immunization Post Partum against Rhesus-sensitization

One of the most effective immunological interventions post partum is the Rh-prophylaxis in Rh-negative women who did not produce anti Rh-D antibodies during pregnancy, and who gave birth to a Rh-positive infant. They receive anti Rh-D 200 μg within 24 hours or at the latest 72 hours post partum. This eliminates foetal Rh-D positive erythrocytes that have reached the maternal circulation during labour and delivery, and prevents Rh-sensitization of the mother in a high percentage. The implementation of Rh-prophylaxis requires an elaborate organization and is not universally available. Where the possibility exists, all pregnant women are screened for Rh-D, and if they are Rh-negative, Rh-D antibodies are determined at 32 weeks of pregnancy. After birth Rh-D of infants of Rh-negative mothers is determined, and anti Rh-D should be available if the infant is Rh-D positive.

Postpartum Rubella Vaccination

The postpartum period is an appropriate time for immunization against rubella, because pregnancy is a relative contraindication to rubella immunization, and the probability of pregnancy occurring within 30 days of delivery is extremely small. It has been shown to be effective. If during pregnancy a rubella test has been done and has shown the woman to be non-immune to rubella, immunization can be offered in the early puerperium. Thus congenital malformations due to rubella in subsequent pregnancies may be prevented.

THE IMMUNIZATION SCHEDULE IN THE PRENATAL AND POSTNATAL PERIOD

The following schedule is recommended during pregnancy and postnatally:

- If in a country most women of childbearing age have not been immunized with tetanus toxoid (TT) in their infancy or before pregnancy, it is recommended that they receive the first dose (TT1) at first contact during pregnancy, and TT2 at least 4 weeks after TT1. TT3 should be given at least 6 months after TT2. The two remaining doses should be given after subsequent intervals of one year minimum. If pregnant women have documentation of prior receipt of tetanus-toxoid-containing vaccines in early childhood or school-age, they may receive a booster dose during pregnancy.
- Soon after birth BCG is recommended in all populations at high risk of tuberculosis infection. The starting dose of oral poliomyelitis vaccine (OPV 0) is also recommended soon after birth, and the first dose of hepatitis B vaccine (HB 1) in those countries where perinatal transmission is frequent.
- At the age of 6 weeks the first dose of the combined vaccines against diphtheria, pertussis and tetanus (DPT 1) is given as well as the OPV 1 dose, and the HB 2 dose. In countries with a low perinatal transmission rate of hepatitis B, the HB 1 dose may be given at this age.
- At 10 weeks DPT 2 and OPV 2 are given, and HB 2 in countries with a low transmission rate.
- At 14 weeks DPT 3 and OPV 3 are given, and HB 3 in all countries.

FAMILY DYNAMICS AFTER CHILDBIRTH

Family roles govern the perceived expectations and responsibilities placed on children by parents and siblings. Children's perception of their place in the family constellation influences how they feel about themselves, and how they interact with others. Components of family structure during formative years that reflect emotional and affiliative ties are implicated in the psychological status, coping and relating styles of mature individuals.

Although many genetic and environmental factors contribute to differences between siblings, some differences in behaviour of siblings have been attributed to the effects of birth order, an individual's rank by age among siblings. The place of the individual within the family, the first social structure encountered, has been suggested as a contributing factor in shaping human personalities, and influencing interactions in subsequent social structures.

Although the view that birth order is the sole predictor of development across the lifespan has never been widely accepted, an individual's birth order is a possible influence on relationships with parents and siblings, which may affect personality formation and social behaviour across the lifespan. Socialisation differences experienced by individuals due to their ordinal position of birth may result in overt personality and behaviour differences. In the absence of siblings, first borns tend to be socialised by adults, whereas later borns are exposed to the socialising influences of older siblings. Adults socialised as first borns, are sometimes theorised to be more achievement oriented, while their younger siblings are often believed to be more successful in social endeavours, experience greater enjoyment during risk taking behaviour and be more independent of authority. It is acknowledged that such characterisations are general and imprecise at best.

STRESS

Ability to negotiate and cope with stressors, the stimuli or experiences that increase risk of personal, social or cognitive difficulties, has been associated with children's development, emotional adjustment and physical wellbeing. There are great individual differences in children's vulnerability or resilience when confronted with stress. Age, health status, temperament, heredity, cognitive appraisal of stressors and locus of control are some of the factors implicated in this variation. Adaptation to distinct stressors is a unique trajectory for each individual. Resiliency could also be viewed as a dynamic process since it may be situation specific to an extent. Inability to handle stress effectively in childhood has been associated with adjustment problems, anxiety disorders, antisocial behaviour, hyper- vigilance and psychosomatic illness. Protective factors against stress include personality factors such as flexibility and sociability.

Relationships with others outside the family, including peers, teachers and community involvement, can also act as buffers and assist a child in dealing with stressors. Yet it is the bond between siblings, and parents and children, that have been implicated as key determinants of resiliency to stress in childhood. Compatibility between the individual's characteristics and those of the family, and parental expectations have also been associated with individual coping styles. Greater compatibility may result in greater resiliency when confronted with stressful situations.

Although successful coping is reliant on many individual and environmental factors, personal characteristics, such as locus of control and competency are associated with greater resiliency and more adaptive coping styles. These individual determinants of coping style may override family factors with either a positive or negative outcome. They may also be determined in part by family interactions. It has been suggested that the first born personality exhibits greater resiliency. It could be suggested that the archetypal experiences of first born individuals may foster greater locus of control, providing the individuals with greater confidence in their ability to negotiate stressful stimuli. Causative inferences concerning these factors must be undertaken cautiously, if at all, since a variety of influences shape individual response to stress, most of which are difficult to control in empirical investigations.

FAMILY WELFARE SERVICES; METHODS, COUNSELLING

The coverage of several key services is poor, especially in the most of the postnatal care cases in many areas. Better access to good quality services is a precondition for improving quality and client orientation. This is because quality care depends not only on the contact between client and provider taking place, but also on it being frequent enough to establish a relationship of trust and confidence and to sustain changes in health behaviour, once initiated.

Postnatal depression is a common and potentially serious health problem, with adverse consequences not only for the mother's mental health and functioning, but also for the psychological health of the partner and, significantly, for the cognitive and social development of the infant. The prevalence of major depressive disorder in the weeks following delivery approximates to one in ten mothers, with symptoms typically enduring for 2-6 months. As is the case for all depressive disorders, the combination of a high prevalence rate, extended duration of symptoms and a marked adverse effect on health status means that postnatal depression imposes a considerable clinical, social and economic burden at the population level, which is further exacerbated by low levels of case recognition, treatment and public awareness. Research into treatments that might reduce the burden of postnatal depression remains modest, although controlled studies suggest that both pharmacological and psychological interventions can have a discernible impact on clinical outcome.

It was within this context that a health services research component was incorporated into a cross-cultural study of postnatal depression. The main intent of the health services research was to complement the work on diagnosis and the assessment of motherhood experience by developing and applying qualitative and quantitative research tools for assessing the availability of and access to appropriate care, as well as the actual uptake of services by mothers with postnatal depression.

RECORDS AND REPORTS

The essential record keeping tool is the antenatal card. This gives essential information on personal details, history, examination, and special investigations and pregnancy progress. The card must be retained by the woman throughout her pregnancy and brought to clinic or hospital for any antenatal attendance and at delivery. Continuity of antenatal care is more easily assured by this practice. Records that must be kept at the antenatal clinic are pregnant women's names, dates of attendance, results of blood tests and copies of any ultrasound reports. High and special risk groups may require hospital files to be opened.

REFERENCES

Boston Women's Health Book Collective. The New Our Bodies, Ourselves. New York: Simon and Schuster, 1992. Conrad, Peter and Kern, Rochelle, eds. The Sociology of Health and Illness: Critical Perspectives. 2nd Ed. New York: St. Martin's Press, 1986.

Courter, Gay. The Midwife . Houghton Mifflin Co. 1981. A novel about the roots of midwifery from Prussia to the United States.

Courter, Gay. The Midwife's Advice . Penguin. 1992. Paperback 1994. A sequel to The Midwife. A novel about the relationships of women, birthing and family planning in the United States.

Davis, Elizabeth. Heart and Hands. 2nd. Edition . Celestial Arts, 1987. A Midwife's guide to pregnancy, childbirth and the art and science of midwifery.

Donnison, Jean. Midwives and Medical Men: A History of Inter-Professional Rivalries and Women's Rights Schocken books, 1977.

Edwards, Margot and Waldorf , Mary. Reclaiming Birth: History and Heroines of American Childbirth Reform The Crossing Press, 1984

Ehrenreich, Barbara and English, Derdre. Witches, Midwives and Nurses: A History of Women Healers The Feminist Press, 1973.

Gaskin, Ina May. Spiritual Midwifery The Farm 1978. A classic. Contains many birth stories as well as more technical information for parents and midwives. Revised in 1980 and 1990.

6

Normal Neonates

A neonate is simply a newborn baby. Hence neonatal intensive care unit, NICU. We generally define the neonatal period as being the first month of life. A human infant less than a month old is a new born or a neonate. The term "newborn" includes premature infants, postmature infants and full term newborns. Upon reaching the age of one or beginning to walk, infants are referred to as "toddlers" (generally 12-36 months).

NORMAL NEONATE

In medical terms a baby born and until the four weeks of birth is called a neonate. A normal neonate is that newborn baby which has took birth without any caesarian operation and is of appropriate weight according to the birth chart of pediatrics.

PHYSIOLOGICAL ADAPTATION

The First Few Hours

Immediately at delivery, the neonate's respiratory effort, heart rate, colour, tone, and reflex irritability should be assessed; all are key components of the Apgar score assigned at 1 and 5 min after birth. Apgar scores between 8 and 10 indicate the neonate is making a smooth transition to extrauterine life; scores ? 7 at 5 min (particularly if sustained beyond 10 min) are linked to higher neonatal morbidity and mortality rates. Many normal neonates have cyanosis 1 min after birth that clears by 5 min. Cyanosis that does not clear may indicate congenital cardiopulmonary anomalies or CNS depression.

In addition to Apgar scoring, neonates should be evaluated for gross deformities (e.g., clubfoot, polydactyly) and other important abnormalities such as heart murmurs. The evaluation should ideally be performed under a radiant warmer with the family close by.

Preventive interventions include administration into both eyes of an antimicrobial agent (e.g., 1% silver nitrate solution 2 drops, 0.5% erythromycin 1 cm ribbon) to prevent gonococcal and chlamydial ophthalmia, and administration of vitamin K 1 mg IM to prevent hemorrhagic disease of the newborn.

Subsequently, the neonate is bathed, wrapped, and brought to the family. The head should be covered with a cap to prevent heat loss. Rooming-in and early breastfeeding should be encouraged so the family can get to know the baby and can receive guidance from staff during the hospital stay. Breastfeeding is more likely to be successful when the family is given frequent and adequate support.

The First Few Days

Physical examination: The neonate should undergo a thorough physical examination within 24 hour. Performing the examination alongside the mother and family members allows the family to ask questions and the clinician to point out physical findings and provide anticipatory guidance.

Basic measurements include length, weight, and head circumference. Length is measured from crown to heel; normal values are based on gestational age and should be plotted on a standard growth chart. When gestational age is uncertain or when the infant seems large or small for age, the gestational age can be precisely determined using physical and neuromuscular findings. These methods are typically accurate to ± 2 wk.

Many clinicians begin with examination of the heart and lungs when the infant is quiet. The examiner should identify the location where the heart sounds are loudest (to exclude dextrocardia). Normal heart rate is 100 to 160 beats/min. The rhythm should be regular, although an irregular rhythm from premature atrial or ventricular contractions is not uncommon. A murmur heard in the 1st 24 hour is most commonly caused by a patent ductus arteriosus. Daily heart examination confirms the disappearance of this murmur, usually within 3 days. Femoral pulses are sought and compared with brachial pulses. A weak or delayed femoral pulse suggests aortic coarctation or other left ventricular outflow tract obstruction. Central cyanosis suggests congenital heart disease, pulmonary disease, or sepsis.

The respiratory system is evaluated by counting respirations over a full minute because breathing in neonates is irregular; normal rate is 40 to 60 breaths/min. The chest wall should be examined for symmetry, and lung sounds should be equal throughout. Grunting, nasal flaring, and retractions are signs of respiratory distress.

After cardiac and pulmonary evaluation, a systematic head to toe examination is performed. In a vertex delivery, the head is commonly molded with overriding of the cranial bones at the sutures and some swelling and ecchymosis of the scalp (caput succedaneum). In a breech delivery, the head has less molding, with swelling and ecchymosis occurring in the presenting part (i.e., buttocks, genitals, or feet). The fontanelles vary in diametre from a fingertip breadth to several centimetres. A large anterior fontanelle may be a sign of hypothyroidism. Also common is a cephalohematoma, an accumulation of blood between the periosteum and the bone that produces a swelling that does not cross suture lines. It may occur over one or both parietal bones and occasionally over the occiput. Cephalohematomas usually are not evident until soft-tissue edema subsides; they gradually disappear over several months.

The eyes may be easier to examine the day after birth because the birth process causes swelling around the eyelids. Eyes should be examined for presence of the red reflex; absence occurs with glaucoma, cataracts, and retinoblastoma. Subconjunctival haemorrhages are common and caused by forces exerted during delivery.

Low-set ears may indicate genetic anomalies, including trisomy 21. The external auditory canal should be examined. Clinicians should look for external ear pits or tags, which are sometimes associated with hearing loss and kidney abnormalities.

The clinician should inspect and palpate the palate to detect a posterior palate defect. Some neonates are born with an epulis, a benign hamartoma of the gum, which if large enough can cause feeding difficulties and may obstruct the infant's airway. These lesions can be removed without recurrence. Neonates can also be born with primary or natal teeth. Natal teeth do not have roots and may need to be removed because they may fall out and be aspirated. Inclusion cysts called Epstein's pearls may occur on the roof of the mouth.

When examining the neck, the clinician must lift the chin to look for abnormalities such as cystic hygromas, goiters, or branchial arch remnants. Torticollis can be caused by a sternocleidomastoid hematoma from birth trauma.

The abdomen should be round and symmetric. A scaphoid abdomen may indicate a diaphragmatic hernia, through which intestines have migrated to the chest cavity in utero, sometimes causing pulmonary hypoplasia and postnatal respiratory distress. An asymmetric abdomen suggests an abdominal mass. Splenomegaly suggests congenital infection or hemolytic anaemia. The kidneys may be palpable with deep palpation, the left more easily than the right. Large kidneys may be due to obstruction, tumor, or cystic disease. The liver is normally palpable 1 to 2 cm below the costal margin. An umbilical hernia, due to a weakness of the umbilical ring musculature, is common but rarely significant.

In boys, the penis should be examined for hypospadias or epispadias. In term boys, testes should be present in the scrotum. Scrotal swelling may signify hydrocele, inguinal hernia, or, more rarely, testicular torsion. With hydrocele, the scrotum transilluminates. Torsion, a surgical emergency, causes ecchymosis and firmness. In term girls, the labia are prominent. Mucoid vaginal and serosanguineous secretions (pseudomenses) are normal; they result from exposure to maternal hormones in utero and withdrawal at birth. A small tag of hymenal tissue at the posterior fourchette, believed to be due to maternal hormonal stimulation, is sometimes present but disappears over a few weeks. Ambiguous genitals (intersex) may be a consequence of several uncommon conditions (e.g., congenital adrenal hyperplasia; 5α-reductase deficiency; Klinefelter's, Turner's, or Swyer syndrome); referral to an endocrinologist is indicated for evaluation and a discussion with the family about the benefits and risks of immediate vs delayed gender assignment.

Orthopedic examination focuses on detection of hip dysplasia. Risk factors for dysplasia include female sex, breech position in utero, twin gestation, and family history. The condition is assessed by using the Barlow or Ortolani maneuver. In the Ortolani maneuver, the neonate is placed on his back with his feet facing the examiner. With an index finger on the greater trochanter and a thumb on the lesser trochanter, the examiner first fully flexes the legs at the knees and hips, then fully abducts the legs while exerting pressure upward and inward until the knees touch the examining table. A palpable clunk of the femoral head with abduction signifies movement of an already dislocated femoral head into the acetabulum and constitutes a positive test for hip dysplasia.

The maneuver may be falsely negative in infants > 3 months because of tighter hip muscles and ligaments. If the examination is equivocal or the infant is high risk (e.g., girls who were in the breech position), hip ultrasonography should be done at 4 to 6 wk; some experts recommend screening ultrasonography at 4 to 6 week for all infants with risk factors.

The neurologic examination includes an evaluation of the neonate's tone, level of alertness, movement of extremities, and reflexes. Typically, neonatal reflexes, including the Moro, suck, and rooting reflexes, are elicited. The Moro reflex, the neonate's response to startle, is elicited by pulling the arms slightly off the bed and releasing suddenly. In response, the neonate extends the arms with fingers extended, flexes the hips, and cries. The rooting reflex is elicited by stroking the neonate's cheek or lateral lip, which prompts the infant to turn the head toward the touch and open the mouth. The suck reflex can be elicited by using a pacifier or gloved finger. These reflexes are present for several months after birth and are markers of a normal peripheral nervous system.

A neonate's skin is usually ruddy; cyanosis of fingers and toes is common in the 1st few hours. Vernix caseosa covers most neonates > 24 week gestation. Dryness and peeling often develop within days, especially at wrist and ankle creases. Petechiae may occur in areas experiencing trauma during delivery, such as the face, in a delivery where the face is the presenting part; however, neonates with diffuse petechiae should be evaluated for thrombocytopenia. Many neonates have erythema toxicum, a benign rash with an erythematous base and a white or yellow papule. This rash, which usually appears 24 hour after birth, is scattered over the body and can last for up to 2 week.

INITIAL AND DAILY ASSESSMENT

The practical nurse has a unique opportunity of closely observing and providing care for the newborn infant after delivery. Because of the newborn infant's helplessness, his needs must be met initially by nursing personnel. Many nursing assessments and evaluations are conducted for the well-being of the infant. Nursing care does not stop with the newborn infant. Interaction with the parents is also important in the development of a family unit.

CARE OF THE NEWBORN IN THE DELIVERY ROOM

There are several needs of a newborn infant that require close attention. Establishing and maintaining respirations are the two needs that must be met immediately.

Establishing and Maintaining the Newborn's Airway

The physician suctions the infant before it is completely born with a bulb syringe or a DeLee trap. A DeLee trap is used if meconium was present in the amniotic fluid. The infant's mouth is suctioned first and then his nose. Once the infant is delivered, his head is held slightly downward to promote drainage of mucus and fluid. The infant's face is wiped thoroughly clean. If the infant doesn't breathe spontaneously, he should be stimulated to cry by slapping his heels, lightly tapping the buttocks, and/or rubbing his back gently. The infant is then positioned with his head slightly down when placed in the radiant warmer. The bulb syringe is used to remove mucus from his mouth and nose.

Common Characteristics of Newborn Respirations

- Nose breathers. Sleeps with mouth closed, does not have to interrupt feedings to breathe.
- Irregular rate.
- Usually abdominal or diaphragmatic in character.
- Ranges from 40 to 60 breathers per minute.
- Breathing is quiet and shallow.
- Easily altered by external stimuli.
- Periods of apnea less than 15 seconds is normal.
- Acrocyanosis may occur during periods of crying. Acrocyanosis refers to cyanotic look of the baby's hands and feet when he is crying. When the baby stops crying, his hands and feet get pink again.

Signs and Symptoms of Newborn Respiratory Distress

- Increased rate or difficulty breathing-growing and seesaw breathing. In normal respirations, the infant's chest and abdomen rise. With seesaw respirations, the infant's chest wall retracts and his abdomen rises with inspirations.
- Sternal or subcostal retractions.
- Nasal flaring.
- Excessive mucus, drooling.
- Cyanosis.

Maintaining Body Temperature

- Dry the infant thoroughly immediately after delivery. The infant is extremely vulnerable to heat loss because his body surface area is great in relation to his weight and he has relatively little subcutaneous weight. Heat loss after delivery is increased by the cool delivery room and the infant's wet skin.
- Place the infant in a radiant heat warmer.
- Place a stockinette cap on the infant's head to prevent heat loss through the head.

- Wrap the infant snugly in a warm blanket.
- Place the infant closely to the mother's skin. Skin-to-skin contact with the mother will help prevent heat loss.

Identify the Infant After Delivery

- The infant must be properly identified before leaving the delivery room. An identification (ID) band is placed on the infant's wrist and leg. An identical band matching the infant's band is placed on the mother's wrist.
- The infant's footprints or palm prints placed next to the mother's thumb print is rarely done in most facilities. Each facility has its own instant identification method.

Establish Parent-Infant Bonding Process

- Parent-infant bonding is the initial step in the process of attraction and response between the newborn and the parents. This paves the way for development of love and affiliation that forms a strong family unit.
- This process should begin as soon after delivery as possible. In the delivery room as soon as the infant is dry and identified, he should be given to the parents. The infant is more alert during the first hours (approximately four) after birth than in the immediate subsequent hours.

APGAR SCORING OF THE NEWBORN

SIGN	0	1	2	1 min	5 min
Heart Rate	Absent	Less Than 100	Over 100	2	2
Respiratory Effort	Absent	Slow, Irregular	Good Cry	1	2
Muscle Tone	Limp	Some Flexion	Active Motion	1	2
Reflex Irritability	No Response	Grimace	Cry	1	2
Color	Pale	Body Pink, Extr. Blue	All Pink	1	2
TOTAL SCORE				6	10

Fig. APGAR Scoring

The initial APGAR scoring is performed in the delivery room by the physician. APGAR scoring is a method of evaluating the condition of the newborn at one minute and at five minutes after delivery.

Purpose

The APGAR scoring chart is used to evaluate the conditions of the baby at birth, determine the need for resuscitation, evaluate the effectiveness of resuscitative efforts, and to identify neonates at risk for morbidity and mortality.

Objective Signs Used for Evaluation

1. Heart rate.
2. Respiratory effort.
3. Muscle tone.
4. Reflex irritability.
5. Colour.

Scoring

1. Evaluations at each of the five categories are initially done at one minute after birth.
2. Each item has a maximum score of two and a minimum score of zero.
3. The final APGAR score is the sum total of the five items, with a maximum score of ten. The higher the final APGAR score, the better condition of the infant.
4. Evaluations at one minute quickly indicate the neonate's initial adaptation to extrauterine life and whether or not resuscitation is necessary.
5. The five-minute score gives a more accurate picture of the neonate's overall status, including obvious neurologic impairment or impending death.

PROCEDURE FOR ADMISSION TO THE NURSERY

a. Carry out the hospital policy for gowning and the three-minute scrub. If lady is already wearing scrubs, it is not necessary to gown. If the initial scrub has already been completed when coming on duty, a one-minute scrub is acceptable.

b. Receive the infant from the transporter. Take the infant from the transporter or the transporter's arms. Verify the ID bracelet on the infant's arm and leg with the delivery room personnel. Make sure the information is accurate (i.e., mother's name, sex of the infant, date and time of birth, and doctor's name).

Take the report from the delivery room person. The report concerns pertinent information of the mother's labour and of the newborn's birth.

c. Remove the delivery room blanket from the infant.

d. Weigh the infant. Place a protective paper cover over the scale first and make sure the scale is balanced. Place the infant on the scale. Document the infant's weight on the:

   1. Delivery room record.
   2. Instant data card.

e. Place the infant in an open warmer for the remainder of the admission procedures to maintain adequate temperature.

   1. Measure the infant.
      a. Length (from top of head to the heel with the leg fully extended).
      b. Head circumference - repeat after molding and caput succedaneum are resolved.
      c. Chest circumference (at the nipple line).
      d. Abdominal circumference.
   2. Record measurements in inches and centimetres.
   3. Document the information in the appropriate areas on the delivery room record, and the instant data card.
   4. Take infant's vital signs and document on the delivery room record.
      a. Temperature-only the first one is done rectally, the remainder are axillary.
      b. Heart rate and respirations-count a full minute because of the irregularities in rhythm.

f. Aspirate fluids.

   1. Aspirate the infant's mouth and nose gently with a bulb syringe.
   2. Insert a number 5 French catheter into the baby's nares to check for patency.
   3. Insert a number 8 French catheter in the baby's mouth down into the stomach and gently aspirate stomach contents.
   4. Record the colour and amount of aspirate on the delivery record sheet.

g. Evaluate the infant's physical condition.

1. Note the infant's cry, colour, and activity for signs of respiratory distress throughout the assessment.
2. Do a complete head-to-toe assessment, looking for any gross abnormalities on his hands, feet, palate, spine, and so forth.
3. Document if the infant voids or passes meconium.
4. Document presence of reflexes (dealt with more extensively in the typical newborn).
   a. Moro.
   b. Sucking.
   c. Grasping.
5. Count the number of vessels in the cord and document.
6. Assess head for molding, caput succedaneum, or cephalhematoma and document in appropriate records.
7. Observe and record any birthmarks.

h. Place the infant on his side to promote drainage of mucus. Note that he is supported by a pillow to his backside.

i. Provide for infant's safety while in open warmer.

j. Place the infant in an isolette if his temperature is below 98°F rectally. If the infant's temperature is above 98°F rectally, place him in an open crib.

NOTE: Step "j" is done after the initial assessment and procedures are completed.

Administration of Vitamin K

Vitamin K is given as a prophylaxis for hemorrhagic disease. It is administered intramuscular (IM) in the vastus lateralis.

Eye Prophylaxis for the Newborn

This procedure is required by law in all states as prophylaxis against gonorrhea. The medications used are as follows:

a. Erythromycin Ophthalmic Ointment. This has become the drug of choice and is received in a sterile syringe from the pharmacy. It is injected into each eye from the inner to outer canthus immediately after birth. It does not appear to cause much eye irritation.

b. 1% Silver Nitrate Solution. Two drops are applied in each eye in the conjunctival sac, not the cornea. The infant eyes may or may not be irrigated after instillation, depending on local policy.

The infant may get profuse discharge and chemical conjunctivitis for a few days with no residual damage. One percent silver nitrate solution is no longer recommended for use.

Initial Bath

a. The amount of time required for the initial bath is determined by local policy. If the infant's temperature is greater than 98°F rectally, the bath may be done after all admission procedures are done. Otherwise, wait until the infant's temperature has stabilized above 98°F.

b. The procedure for actually completing the bath is also determined by local policy. Allow the parent to participate if possible. Remove as much of the vernix as possible. Some may not come off during the first bath because it is so "sticky."

Cord Care for the Newborn Infant

a. Inspect the cord frequently for signs of bleeding immediately after it has been cut.

b. Apply triple dye (refer to local policy) to the cord after the infant has had his bath and has been determined to be stable. The dye prevents infection and helps the cord to dry.

c. Swab the cord with alcohol at least three times per day (refer to local policy). The alcohol aids in drying.

d. Observe for cord detachment. The cord detaches in ten to fourteen days. The cord dries faster when left uncovered. Have the parents roll the infant's diaper down some in front initially so the cord is not covered.

e. Observe for signs of infection and report findings immediately. The signs of infection are purulent drainage, redness, and possible swelling (more than usual).

Bonding Process

a. Bonding should be initiated in the delivery room.

b. The significant other should be allowed to participate in as much of the care as possible during the admission process to develop the bond between him and the infant.

c. Transport the infant back to the mother as soon as local policy allows to take advantage of the alert state newborns have during those first few hours after birth.

1. This is considered a critical time for both individuals to interact and get to know one another.
2. It is an excellent time to establish breast-feeding while the infant is awake.
3. Approximately the first four hours after delivery, the infant returns to a sleep state or less alert state.

ESSENTIAL OF THE NEWBORN CARE; THERMAL CONTROL

A complete inspection of the newborn infant is performed within 24 hours after delivery. The goal is to compile a complete record of the newborn that will act as a database for subsequent assessment and care.

a. Assemble necessary equipment.
   i. Pediatric stethoscope.
   ii. Penlight.
   iii. Tape measure.
   iv. Rectal thermometre.
   v. Infant scale.
b. Wash hands for a full three minutes.
c. Approach and identify the infant.
d. Provide for a warm, well-lighted, draft-free area, keeping the infant undressed for as short a time as possible.
e. Place the infant on a flat, protected surface.
f. Take the infant's temperature. The infant's temperature is taken rectally only on admission. Subsequent temperatures are to be taken by the axillary method.
g. Determine the infant's apical heart rate. Count for a full minute.
h. Determine the infant's respiratory rate. Count for a full minute. Note any signs of respiratory distress (retractions, grunting, nasal flaring) rate over 60 bpm, or periods of apnea. Auscultate the infant's lungs.
i. Balance the scale.
j. Weigh the naked infant. Most newborns weigh between six to nine pounds (2, 700 and 4, 000 grams). Record the weight in pounds and ounces, as well as in grams.
k. Measure the infant's length from top of the head to the heel with the leg fully extended and record measurements.

l. Measure the infant's head circumference and record measurements. The normal head circumference is 13 to 14 inches (33 to 35 cm). Cranial molding from a vaginal delivery may affect this measurement. The measurement should be repeated on the second and third day after delivery.

m. Measure the infant's chest circumference at the nipple line and record the measurement.

n. Observe the general contour of the infant's head. Gently palpate the sutures and fontanelles. The anterior fontanelle is approximately two inches long and is gem/diamond shaped. The posterior fontanelle is smaller than the anterior fontanelle. Normally, the fontanelle feels soft and is either flat or slightly indented. The anterior fontanelle usually bulges when the infant cries, coughs, or vomits.

o. Observe the general appearance of the infant's neck. The infant's neck is usually short, thick, and covered with folds of tissue. The infant should be able to move his neck from side to side, from flexion to extension, and can hold his head in the midline position.

- Observe the infant's eyes for symmetry of size and shape. Note the infant's eye movements. Strabismus caused by poor neuromuscular control is normal. An infant older than ten days should look in the direction in which mother turn. Note the colour of the infant's eyes.
- Inspect the infant's ears for structure, shape, and position. The ears should be firm with wee-formed cartilage. Tops of the auricles should be parallel to the outer canthus of the eye.

p. Inspect the infant's nose for patency.

q. Inspect the infant's mouth for cleft palate by gently depressing his tongue when he cries. Check the mucous membranes. Observe the soft and hard palate. Make sure they are in tact.

r. Inspect the infant's skin and nails. Observe for jaundice, birthmarks, milia, petechiae, and lanugo. Observe the infant's hands and feet for normal creases. Observe the colour of the infant's nail beds; they should be pink. Acrocyanosis may be present up to 24 degrees, especially when the infant is crying.

s. Inspect the size, shape, and symmetry of the infant's chest. Normally, an infant's chest is circular or barrel-shaped. The breast tissue of both male and female infants may be slightly engorged during the first few days of life.

t. Palpate the infant's peripheral pulses (femoral, brachial, and radial).

u. Inspect the size and shape of the infant's abdomen. The abdomen should be cylindrical in shape. Sunken or distended abdomen should be reported. Check the umbilical cord for the number of vessels.

v. Auscultate the infant's abdomen for bowel sounds. Bowel sounds should be present within one to two hours after birth.

w. Observe for excessive drooling, coughing, gagging, or cyanosis during feeding.

x. Place the infant on his abdomen and observe his spine for curves, masses, or abnormal openings.

y. Inspect the male infant's genitalia. The penis should be checked for location of the urinary meatus. The scrotum may appear edematous and proportionately large.

z. Inspect the female infant's genitalia. The labia majora may appear edematous and cover the clitoris and the labia minora.

aa. Observe the infant's spontaneous or involuntary movements for symmetry, spasticity, or rigidity. Gently straighten his arm or leg. Release it and observe whether it returns to its normal position. If the extremity remains limp, the infant may be hypotonic. If the extremity is difficult to straighten and rapidly flexes when released, he may be hypertonic.

bb. Dress the infant carefully and return him to his bassinet.

cc. Record all significant nursing observations in the infants' health record. Report observations to the Charge Nurse.

Phenylketonuria Test

A phenylketonuria (PKU) test is done to check for rising levels of phenylalanine. Phenylalanine is a naturally occurring amino acid essential to growth. After milk or formula (both contain phenylalanine) feedings begin, levels rise due to a deficiency of the liver enzyme that converts phenylalanine to tyrosine. Due to this metabolic deficiency, poisons build up in the bloodstream and cause mental retardation. If the infant is found to have rising levels of phenylalanine, many protein foods can be withheld from the diet and synthetic foods substituted. The following steps are performed to collect a blood specimen for a PKU test on the newborn infant.

a. Ensure that the infant has been on milk or formula feeding for three full days. Four days are preferred.
b. Explain to the parents the purpose of the test
c. Perform a heel stick to obtain needed specimen.
d. Place one drop of blood on each of the three circles on the filter paper or in accordance with local policy.
e. Label and transport the specimen to the laboratory.
f. Notify the parents of follow-up care of the infant, if the infant is discharged prior to his third or fourth day of life. This test must be done.

GOALS OF NEWBORN NURSING CARE

a. To continue appraisal of the newborn throughout his hospital stay.
    1. Observe and record the infant's vital signs.
    2. Monitor weight loss or gain (daily by some local policy).
    3. Monitor bowel and bladder function.
    4. Monitor activity and sleep patterns.
    5. Monitor interactions and bonding with parents.
c. To provide safeguards against infection (that is, handwashing).
d. To initiate feedings.
e. To provide guidance and health instruction to parents.

BREASTFEEDING, PREVENTION OF INFECTIONS

Signs of hunger are demonstrated by the infant searching for food, sucking motions, and crying. The mother may begin to breast-feed at this time if she had planned to breast-feed, her condition is stable, and she desires to feed the infant.

a. Preparation of the Nipples. Preparation of the nipples should begin during pregnancy.
    1. Roll nipples. The mother should roll her nipples with her thumb and forefinger two to three times each day.
    2. Massage breast.
        - Place hand over the other above the breast.
        - Gently, but firmly, exert pressure evenly with the thumbs across the top and fingers underneath the breast.

— Come together with the heel of the hand on each side and release at the areola, being careful not to touch the areola and nipple.

— Gently lift the breast from beneath and drop lightly.

3. Roughen nipples with a towel.

b. Initiation of Breast-feeding.

1. Initial feeding is usually with one ounce of sterile water to determine if the newborn can swallow. The mother should begin feeding with five minutes of actual sucking time on each breast and increase feeding time after the baby has fed three consecutive times without difficulty. Each feeding should be initiated by alternating the breasts. The baby may receive glucose water after feeding until the milk comes in the breast.

2. The advantages of breast-feeding are as follows:

   a. Colostrum contains less fat and sugar and more protein and salts than breast milk. It also contains large amounts of antibodies and vitamins and acts as a laxative to help expel meconium.

   NOTE: Colostrum is the thin yellowish fluid secreted for the first several days after birth.

   b. Colostrum comes before the milk in the mother's breast.

   c. Protein is more digestible than cow's milk.

   d. The fat that is present is rich in essential fatty acids needed for brain growth.

   e. Colostrum contains lactose, which favors the development of bacteria in the intestines that serves as a protective function during infancy.

   f. The calcium-to-phosphorous ratio is ideal for the absorption of calcium needed for bone growth.

   g. It appears less likely to produce an obese child, promotes better tooth and jaw alignment, and protects against allergy development during infancy.

   h. Breast-feeding is convenient and eliminates formula preparation.

   i. Breast-feeding is economical.

c. Contraindications.

1. Nipple or breast lesions may appear (depending on the type).

2. If the mother becomes pregnant, the milk will usually start to dry up.
3. Maternal illness.
4. Need of mother to return to work (although excellent battery operated breast pumps are now available and very inexpensive).
5. Inability of the mother to psychologically adjust.
6. A woman with cardiac or established renal disease may be discouraged from nursing.
7. Infections.

d. Common Breast-Feeding Problems.

1. Delayed milk production. This is usually the earliest of breast-feeding problems. It occurs if the baby is not breast-fed within a short time after birth or not fed frequently enough.
2. Sore breasts.
   a. The mother should let the baby breast-feed initially for ten to thirty minutes every two to three hours and gradually increase the amount of time. If her breasts are not empty after feeding, have the mother to express the milk into a bottle and refrigerate for later feedings.
   b. Improper position may cause soreness. Advise the mother that the infant should have a portion of the areola, in addition to the nipple in his mouth. Just chewing or sucking on the nipple may cause breast soreness.
3. Engorgement. This normally occurs on or about the third postpartum day. It results from an increase of milk into the milk ducts combined with increased blood and lymph supply to the breast. The breast becomes hard and painful. It is usually more common in the first-time breast-feeding mother. Engorgement can be prevented by:
   a. Manual expression of milk if the breasts are full but the infant is not ready to nurse, or if the infant can't get hold of the nipple because the skin is too tight.
   b. Wearing a supportive bra.
   c. Frequent nursing, if not too painful.
   d. Warm compresses applied to the sore breasts.
   NOTE: The thumb and forefinger are placed on opposite sides of the breast just behind the areola. The lactiferous

sinuses (ampulla A) are compressed, and milk is forced out.

4. Leaking breasts.
   a. This is a common annoyance. A conditioned response will occur in the mother when she sees or hears a baby that causes the milk to let down.
   b. The mother should fold her arms across her breasts and press them firmly against her chest wall. This will stop the leaking. Advise her to place absorbent pads in her bras.
5. Maternal anxiety. This will decrease milk production.
   a. An infant reacting to maternal anxiety will usually act in one of two ways.
   1. He will suck, stop, cry, suck, stop, cry, and then may regurgitate.
   2. He will suck, stop, cry, refuse to nurse, and continue to cry.
   b. Teach the mother relaxation techniques. Tell her to feed her baby in a quiet area.
6. Sore, cracked, or fissured nipples.
   i. Causes.
   a. Infant not having the nipple and areola properly in the mouth.
   b. "Friction" of the baby's gums on the nipple.
   c. Infant being allowed to suck on an empty breast.
   d. Washing the nipples with soap, which is drying.
   e. Failure to break suction before removing the infant from the breast.
   ii. Nursing interventions. Teach the mother proper nursing techniques and proper breast care.
7. Breast infection.
   a. Most often caused by the causative organism, Staphylococcus areus.
   b. Entry is gained through a cracked or fissured nipple.
   c. The infection is usually interstitial and not intraductal, so the infection will not harm the baby.
   d. Nursing interventions. Instruct the mother on proper breast care. If breast soreness is present, have the mother to express milk into a bottle to feed to her baby.

Bubbling the Newborn

a. Methods used to bubble the baby are baby placed on shoulders, baby held upright leaning slightly forward, and baby held across the lap. Rub or gently pat his back until air is expelled.

b. When no belch follows feeding, position the baby on his right side or abdomen.

NOTE: Hiccupping is common.

c. The baby should be bubbled frequently.

1. Bottle-feeding-every 1/2 ounce initially.
2. Breast-feeding-between each breast.

d. Always be sure to support the head.

IMMUNIZATION

Immunization of neonates carries three inherent questions (i) Is the neonatal immune system mature enough to elicit an immune response, and if not, how early can immunization be carried out? (ii) If an immune response is not elicited, will tolerance be induced? (iii) Can offspring of immune mothers be immunized against an antigen despite high levels of passively transferred maternal antibodies to that antigen?

Maternal and neonatal immunization is an increasingly promising strategy given the threat of antibiotic resistance. In developing countries, however, issues of vaccine cost, availability, delivery, and efficacy in the field are major barriers to the use of vaccines established as safe and effective.

A variety of neonatal immunization strategies have already proven successful. For example, the bacillus Calmette-Guerin (BCG) vaccine - a live attenuated where TB is a common and potentially lethal disease. A meta-analysis of BCG studies involving newborns and infants concluded and infants concluded that the vaccine was effective for up to 10 years after infant vaccination, and that it reduced the risk of infection, on average, by more than 50 percent. Likewise, hepatitis B vaccination of newborns has been shown effective in preventing neonatal infections and their sequelae.

Tuberculosis (TB) has been a significant public health problem all over the world and it has been recognized as a global emergency by WHO in 1993. In 1995, out of the total TB cases notified in the world, South-East Asia region accounted for 42% of cases. The highest number of TB patients were found in the Indian sub-continent with estimated incidence rates of more than 100/million population. In India, 1.5% of the population suffers from radiologically active TB, out of which 0.4% are infectious. Five lakh people die each year due to the disease. About 20 to 25 lakh cases are added annually to the pool.

TB has been classified as one of the six vaccine preventable diseases by WHO and BCG vaccination has been made a part of the National Immunization Program in India and abroad. BCG induced protection is essentially elicited through the generation of appropriate cell mediated immunity (CMI). Eight controlled trials of BCG vaccination conducted all over the world have shown the protective efficacy of BCG to be 0-80%. Particularly, BCG vaccination has been shown to reduce the incidence of disseminated TB and tubercular meningitis (TBM) in vaccinated children. The protective efficacy of the vaccine against these two forms of tuberculosis is 70-80%.

The success of any immunization program is judged by the development of immunity against the disease for which vaccination has been done, that is reflected by reduction in the incidence and eventual control/eradication of the disease from the community. It is important to note that vaccination is a process of administration of an antigen into the body, whereas, immunization refers to the development of active immunity, be it cell mediated, humoral or both against the antigen administered in the body which in turn prevents the development of disease by the same organism. It is, therefore, not the BCG vaccination coverage of the child population which is important, but the development of immunity against acquiring tuberculosis by the population in general and by children in particular.

MINOR DISORDERS OF NEWBORN AND ITS MANAGEMENT

A dysmorphic feature in a newborn is an abnormality of shape, size, or structure. Each finding traditionally is classified as minor or major. Among normal newborns, more than 13% have at least one minor anomaly, whereas only 1% have two or more minor anomalies.

Low birth weight is one of the most serious challenges in maternal and child health, in both developing and developed countries. The proportion of infants with low birth weight, both preterm and small for gestational age, ranges from 2-3% in some developed countries to 25-30% in many areas of developing countries. It seems to be a fair indicator of status of development in any community. Low birth weight is the main contributing factor in perinatal and infant mortality and morbidity. Half of all perinatal and one third of all infant deaths are due to low birth weight. Further prematurity contributes to mental and physical handicaps particularly in those who have not received expert neonatal care.

Although in 30-50% of cases the cause of low birth weight is unknown, but in developing countries maternal malnutrition and anaemia are additional important causes. In maternal and foetal causes majority of them are either preventable or manageable. Intervention programmes directed to pregnant women in avoiding a low birth weight neonate is easier, cost effective and efficient than treating the low birth weight babies. Proper nutritional programmes, identifying high risk pregnancy, treating anaemia in pregnancy, proper spacing of pregnancies, health education and socio-economic development measures are some of the recommended remedies to avert a low birth weight neonate delivery. Further studies are in progress to identify reasons for placental insufficiency syndrome.

The present study has shown a proportion of P&LBW neonates as 12.7% (150/1178) of live births, of these 150 P&LBW neonates 12% (18) died and 88% (132) could be saved. The low mortality rate in our study perhaps refers to better socioeconomic clientele of Shaikh Zayed Hospital. Low mortality till the time of discharge from hospital was due to either efficient management or higher proportion (almost 50%) of neonates falling in the gestational age of 36-38 weeks .As many infants born between 35 - 37 weeks of gestation will not need any special care at birth and will be able to stay with their moms in a regular newborn nursery1 .Neonates born with very low gestational age and birth weights of under 1.5 kg had very high mortality which indicates that neonatology unit needs to be upgraded in terms of equipment, techniques and manpower. The congenital anomaly detected among the P & LBW neonates is 7.3%, which compares well with similar rates in many countries. According to literature the frequency of inherited and congenital anomaly varies from 1-10% of live births if all minor defects are included. The congenital anomaly distribution by gravidity, birth weight, gestational age and maternal age did not show any significant association.

Current knowledge and proper monitoring of pregnant mothers during the antenatal period can identify and manage many known risk factors leading to SGA. These include placental development, renal diseases, hypertension, diabetes mellitus, bronchial asthma, anaemia, smoking etc., just to mention a few. This data on the probability of survival of infants in high risk pregnancy can be of great value in guiding management. This information can help both clinical staff and parents to decide if and when to intervene a pregnancy.

BIRTH INJURY DISORDERS

Birth injury is damage sustained during the birthing process, usually occurring during transit through the birth canal. A difficult delivery, with the risk of injury to the foetus, may occur if the birth canal is too small or the foetus is too large (as sometimes occurs when the mother has diabetes). Injury is also more likely if the foetus is lying in an abnormal position before birth. Overall, the rate of birth injuries is much lower now than in previous decades. Many newborns experience minor injuries from the birthing process, with swelling or bruising only in certain areas.

Head Injury: In most births, the head is the first part to enter the birth canal and experiences much of the pressure during the delivery. Swelling and bruising are not serious and resolve within a few days. Cephalohematoma is a bleeding injury in which a soft lump forms over the surface of one of the skull bones but below its thick fibrous covering. A cephalohematoma does not need treatment and disappears over weeks to months. Very rarely, one of the bones of the skull may fracture. Unless the fracture forms an indentation (depressed fracture), it heals rapidly without treatment.

Nerve Injury: Rarely, nerve injuries may occur. Pressure to the facial nerves caused by forceps can result in weakness of the muscles on one side of the face. This injury is evident when the newborn cries and the face appears asymmetric. No treatment is needed, and the newborn usually recovers within a few weeks.

Injuries to the spinal cord due to overstretching during delivery are extremely rare. These injuries can result in paralysis below where the injury occurred. Damage to the spinal cord is often permanent.

Bone Injury: Rarely, bones may be broken (fractured) during a difficult delivery. A fracture of the collarbone is most common. Fractures of bones in the newborn are splinted and almost always heal completely and rapidly.

ANAEMIA

Anaemia is a disorder in which there are too few red blood cells in the blood. Normally, the newborn's bone marrow does not produce new red blood cells between birth and 3 or 4 weeks of age. Anaemia can occur when red blood cells are broken down too rapidly, too much blood is lost, or more than one of these processes occurs at the same time.

Any process that leads to red blood cell destruction, if sufficiently severe, results in anaemia and high levels of bilirubin (hyperbilirubinemia). Hemolytic disease of the newborn may cause the newborn's red blood cells to be destroyed rapidly. The red blood cells may also be rapidly destroyed if the newborn has a hereditary abnormality of the red blood cells. An example is hereditary spherocytosis, in which the red blood cells appear small and spherical in shape when viewed under a microscope.

Infections acquired before birth, such as toxoplasmosis, rubella, cytomegalovirus, herpes simplex, or syphilis, may also rapidly destroy red blood cells, as can bacterial infections of the newborn acquired during or following birth.

Another cause of anaemia is blood loss. Blood loss can occur in many ways, for example, if there is a large transfusion of the foetal blood across the placenta and into the mother's circulation (foetal-maternal transfusion) or if too much blood gets trapped in the placenta at delivery, when the umbilical cord is clamped. The placenta may separate from the uterine wall before delivery (placental abruption), leading to haemorrhage of the foetal blood. Rarely, anaemia may result from a failure of the foetal bone marrow to produce red blood cells. One example of this is a genetic disorder called Fanconi's anaemia. Another rare example is that due to exposure of the mother and foetus to certain drugs used during pregnancy.

Symptoms and Treatment

A newborn who has suddenly lost a large amount of blood during labour or delivery may appear pale and have a rapid heart rate and low blood pressure, along with rapid, shallow breathing. Milder anaemia may result in lethargy, poor feeding, or no symptoms. When the anaemia is a result of rapid breakdown of red blood cells, there is also increased production of bilirubin, and the newborn's skin and the whites of the eyes appear yellow (jaundice).

A newborn who has rapidly lost a large amount of blood, often during labour and delivery, is treated with intravenous fluids followed by a blood transfusion. Very severe anaemia caused by hemolytic disease may also require a blood transfusion, but the anaemia is more often treated with an exchange blood transfusion, in which part of the newborn's blood is gradually removed and replaced with equal volumes of fresh donor blood. The exchange transfusion also removes bilirubin in the circulation and thus treats the hyperbilirubinemia.

APNEA OF PREMATURITY

Apnea of prematurity is a pause in breathing that lasts for more than 20 seconds. Apnea of prematurity commonly occurs in newborns who are born before 34 weeks of pregnancy, increasing in frequency and severity among the most prematurely born. In these newborns, the part of the brain that controls breathing (respiratory centre) has not matured fully. As a result, the newborns may have repeated episodes of normal breathing alternating with brief pauses in breathing. In very tiny premature newborns, apnea can be caused by temporary obstruction of the pharynx due to low muscle tone or a bending forward of the neck; this is called obstructive apnea. Over time, as the respiratory centre matures, episodes of apnea become less frequent, and by the time the newborn approaches term, they no longer occur.

Symptoms and Diagnosis

Premature newborns are routinely attached to a monitor that sounds an alarm if the newborn stops breathing for a prolonged time or if the heart rate slows. Depending on the length of the episodes, stoppage of breathing may decrease the oxygen levels in the blood, which results in a bluish discolouration of the skin (cyanosis). Low levels of oxygen in the blood may slow the heart rate (bradycardia).

Apnea can sometimes be a sign of a disorder, such as infection of the blood (sepsis), low blood sugar (hypoglycemia), or a low body temperature (hypothermia). Therefore, the doctor evaluates the newborn to rule out these disorders when there is a sudden or unexpected increase in frequency of episodes.

Treatment

Treatment of apnea depends on the cause. Apnea caused by obstruction of the pharynx may be decreased by keeping the newborn lying on his back or side with his head in the midline position. If episodes of apnea become frequent, and especially if the newborn has cyanosis, the newborn may be treated with a drug that stimulates the respiratory centre, such as caffeine or aminophylline. If these treatments fail to prevent frequent and severe episodes of apnea, the premature newborn may need treatment with continuous positive airway pressure (CPAP) or a ventilator.

Virtually all premature newborns stop having episodes of apnea several weeks before they reach term. Although a few infants are discharged from the hospital and placed on home monitors before they have completely outgrown their episodes of apnea, this practice is not standard or generally accepted. An association between apnea in the premature newborn and the risk for sudden infant death syndrome (SIDS), which usually occurs months after birth, has not been proven. Likewise, there is no proof that discharging an infant home on an apnea monitor decreases the risk of SIDS.

BRONCHOPULMONARY DYSPLASIA (BPD)

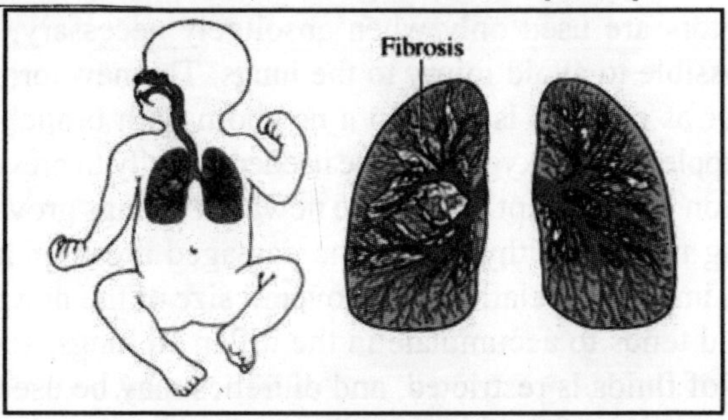

Fig. Bronchopulmonary Dysplasia

Bronchopulmonary dysplasia (chronic lung disease) is a disorder due to repetitive lung injury. Bronchopulmonary dysplasia occurs most often in premature newborns who had severe lung disease at birth, such as respiratory distress syndrome, particularly in those who needed treatment with a ventilator for more than a few weeks after birth. The delicate tissues of the lungs can become injured when the air sacs are over-stretched by the ventilation or by high oxygen levels. As a result, the lungs become inflamed and additional fluid accumulates within the lungs. Full-term newborns who have lung disease (such as pneumonia) occasionally develop bronchopulmonary dysplasia.

Symptoms and Diagnosis

Affected newborns usually breathe rapidly and may have respiratory distress, with drawing in of the lower chest while breathing in and low levels of oxygen in the blood, causing a bluish discolouration of the skin (cyanosis). Some newborns with severe cases exhale air from the lungs slowly and develop "air trapping, " in which the chest appears to be over-expanded. Although a few newborns with very severe bronchopulmonary dysplasia die even after months of care, most newborns survive. Over several years, the lung injury heals. However, later these children are at increased risk of developing asthma and viral pneumonia, such as that caused during winter months by respiratory syncytial virus (RSV).

The diagnosis of bronchopulmonary dysplasia is made in the premature newborn who has received ventilation for a prolonged time and who has signs of respiratory distress and a prolonged need for supplemental oxygen. Measurement of low levels of oxygen in the blood and results of a chest x-ray support the diagnosis.

Prevention and Treatment

Ventilators are used only when absolutely necessary, and then as gently as possible to avoid injury to the lungs. The newborn is taken off the ventilator as early as is safe. In a newborn with bronchopulmonary dysplasia, supplemental oxygen may be needed initially to prevent cyanosis. Good nutrition is important to help the newborn's lungs grow and to keep the new lung tissue healthy. Thus, the damaged areas of lung become less and less important relative to the overall size of the newborn's lungs. Because fluid tends to accumulate in the inflamed lungs, sometimes the daily intake of fluids is restricted, and diuretics may be used to increase the rate of excretion of fluid in the urine.

After discharge from the hospital, newborns with bronchopulmonary dysplasia should not be exposed to cigarette smoke or fumes from a space heater or wood-burning stove. They should be protected from exposure to people who have upper respiratory tract infections. In certain cases, doctors can give them partial immunity to RSV infection by administering doses of a specific antibody to that virus. This antibody must be injected monthly during the fall and winter.

HYPERBILIRUBINEMIA

Hyperbilirubinemia is an abnormally high level of bilirubin in the blood. Aging red blood cells are removed by the spleen, and the hemoglobin from these red blood cells is broken down and recycled. The heme portion of the hemoglobin molecule is converted into a yellow pigment called bilirubin, which is carried in the blood to the liver where it is chemically modified and then excreted in the bile into the newborn's digestive tract. It is removed from the body when the newborn passes stools. Bilirubin in the stools of newborns gives them their yellow colour.

In most newborns, the level of bilirubin in the blood increases in the first days after birth, causing the newborn's skin and the whites of the eyes to appear yellow (jaundice). If feedings are delayed for any reason, as occurs when newborns are sick or have a digestive tract problem, blood levels of bilirubin can become high. Also, breastfed newborns tend to have somewhat higher blood levels of bilirubin during the first week or two.

Hyperbilirubinemia may also occur when a newborn has a serious medical disorder, such as infection in the blood (sepsis). It may also be caused by hemolysis (rapid breakdown of red blood cells), as occurs with Rh incompatibility or ABO incompatibility.

In the large majority of cases, elevated levels of bilirubin in the blood are not serious. However, very high bilirubin levels can produce brain damage (kernicterus). Very premature and critically ill newborns are at higher risk for developing kernicterus. In almost all cases, moderately elevated blood levels of bilirubin due to breastfeeding are not of concern. However, newborns who are slightly premature and are breastfeeding, especially if discharged early from the hospital, must be monitored closely for hyperbilirubinemia because they can develop kernicterus if the bilirubin level becomes very high.

Symptoms and Diagnosis

Newborns with hyperbilirubinemia have a yellow colour to their skin and the whites of their eyes (jaundice). It may be more difficult to recognize jaundice in dark-skinned newborns. Jaundice usually first appears on the newborn's face and then, as the bilirubin level increases, progresses downward to involve the chest, abdomen, and finally the legs and feet. Newborns with hyperbilirubinemia who are showing symptoms of kernicterus may become lethargic and feed poorly; these newborns should be examined immediately by a doctor. The later stages of kernicterus involve irritability, muscle stiffening or seizures, and a fever.

It is important that a doctor assess the degree of jaundice in all newborns during the first days of life. Some newborns have developed dangerously high levels of bilirubin after being discharged from the hospital on the first day after birth before their blood level of bilirubin had risen. Therefore, it is very important that newborns discharged early be examined at home by a visiting nurse or in the doctor's office within a few days after discharge to assess their bilirubin levels. This is especially true for newborns born a few weeks prematurely and those breastfeeding.

A doctor first examines the newborn under good lighting and then measures the level of jaundice by holding a specialized piece of equipment (bilirubinometre) against the newborn's skin or by testing a small sample of blood.

Treatment

Mild hyperbilirubinemia does not require special treatment. Offering frequent feedings accelerates the passage of stools, thus reducing the reabsorption of bilirubin from the intestinal contents and lowering the bilirubin level. Moderate hyperbilirubinemia can be treated with phototherapy, in which the newborn is placed without clothes under fluorescent bilirubin lights.

The light exposure alters the composition of the bilirubin in the newborn's skin, changing it to a form that is more readily excreted by the liver and kidneys. The newborn's eyes are shielded with a blindfold. Newborns can also be treated at home by having them lie on a fibre-optic "bilirubin blanket, " which exposes their skin to bright light. These newborns need to have their blood levels of bilirubin tested repeatedly until they decrease.

Rarely, it may be necessary for a mother to change from breastfeeding to formula feeding temporarily to ensure that the newborn is obtaining adequate volumes with each feeding. The mother should resume breastfeeding as soon as the bilirubin levels start to decrease. Moderate hyperbilirubinemia sometimes continues for weeks in infants who are breastfed, a normal phenomenon that poses no problems for the infant and that does not usually require withholding of breastfeeding.

If the newborn's blood level of bilirubin approaches a dangerous level, it can be lowered rapidly by performing an exchange blood transfusion. In this procedure, a sterile catheter is placed into the umbilical vein located in the cut surface of the umbilical cord. The newborn's bilirubin-containing blood is removed and replaced with equal volumes of fresh blood.

LARGE FOR GESTATIONAL AGE (LGA)

A newborn, whether delivered preterm, term, or postterm, whose weight is above that of 90% of babies of the same gestational age at birth (above the 90th percentile) is considered large for gestational age. Some newborns are large for gestational age because of genetic factors, such as having large parents. Another cause is diabetes in the mother.

If the mother has diabetes during pregnancy, a large amount of glucose (sugar) crosses the placenta and results in high levels of glucose in the foetus's blood, with the release of increased amounts of insulin.

The result is accelerated growth of the foetus, including almost all organs with the exception of the brain, which grows normally. Vaginal delivery of a very large-for-gestational-age foetus may be problematic, increasing the risk of injury. Therefore, such a foetus may have to be delivered by caesarean section.

The large-for-gestational-age newborn born to a diabetic mother typically has a florid (reddish) complexion and appears obese and sometimes lethargic. Large-for-gestational-age newborns born to mothers who do not have diabetes are large, but not reddish or lethargic. After birth, when the supply of glucose from the placenta stops, the continuing rapid production of insulin leads to low levels of glucose (hypoglycemia). Often hypoglycemia produces no symptoms. Sometimes, the newborn is listless, limp, or jittery. Despite their large size, newborns of diabetic mothers often do not feed well for the first few days. Occasionally, newborns born to diabetic mothers have an abnormally high red blood cell count. As the red blood cells are broken down, bilirubin is formed, and these newborns tend to have high bilirubin levels, resulting in jaundice.

Large-for-gestational-age newborns born prematurely to diabetic mothers are also more likely to have immature lungs and to develop respiratory distress syndrome, even when born only a few weeks before full term. They also have a higher rate of birth defects than other newborns.

Testing the amniotic fluid in mothers with diabetes before delivery can be performed to determine lung maturity and the likelihood of the newborn developing respiratory distress syndrome after birth. If labour appears imminent, a corticosteroid may be given to increase lung maturity. To treat hypoglycemia in the newborn, intravenous glucose or frequent feedings by mouth or by tube into the stomach are often needed. Treatment of other complications, such as respiratory distress syndrome, is needed. Large-for-gestational-age newborns born to diabetic mothers are likely to be significantly overweight later in childhood and as adults, which puts them at risk for type 2 diabetes.

MECONIUM ASPIRATION SYNDROME

Meconium aspiration syndrome is respiratory distress in a newborn who has breathed (aspirated) meconium into the lungs before or around the time of birth. Meconium is the dark green fecal material that is produced in the intestines before birth. Normally, meconium is expelled after birth when a newborn starts to feed. However, in response to stress, such as an inadequate blood oxygen level, the foetus may pass meconium into the amniotic fluid. The same stress causes the foetus to take forceful gasps, so that the meconium-containing amniotic fluid may be breathed into the lungs. After delivery, the aspirated meconium may block the airways leading to portions of the newborn's lungs, which may cause them to collapse. Alternatively, when some airways are only partially blocked, air may be able to reach the parts of the lung beyond the block but may be prevented from being breathed out. Thus, the involved lung may become over-expanded. Progressive over-expansion of a portion of the lung can eventually result in rupture and then collapse of the lung. Air may then accumulate within the chest cavity around the lung (pneumothorax). Meconium breathed into the lungs may also cause inflammation of the lungs (pneumonitis).

Meconium aspiration syndrome is often most severe in postmature newborns because the meconium is very concentrated in a smaller amount of amniotic fluid and it causes more irritation than in a term newborn. Newborns with meconium aspiration syndrome are also at increased risk for developing persistent pulmonary hypertension. An affected newborn suffers from respiratory distress, in which he breathes rapidly, draws in his lower chest wall while breathing in, and grunts during breathing out. The newborn's skin may be bluish (cyanotic) if the blood levels of oxygen are reduced.

A doctor makes the diagnosis based on the observation of thick meconium in the amniotic fluid at the time of birth, respiratory distress in the newborn, and abnormal chest x-ray results. At delivery, if the newborn is covered with meconium, the newborn's mouth, nose, and throat are immediately suctioned to remove any meconium. If the newborn is lethargic or unresponsive, a tube may need to be passed into the windpipe to suction as much meconium as possible from the respiratory tract.

The newborn is treated with oxygen and placed on a ventilator if necessary. If the newborn needs intubation, then repeated suctioning is performed to try to remove more of the meconium. A newborn on a ventilator is observed closely for serious complications, such as pneumothorax or persistent pulmonary hypertension. Most newborns with meconium aspiration syndrome survive. However, if the disorder is severe and especially if it leads to persistent pulmonary hypertension, it can be fatal.

NECROTIZING ENTEROCOLITIS

Necrotizing enterocolitis is injury to the inner surface of the intestine. Necrotizing enterocolitis usually occurs in premature newborns. The cause is not understood. Diminished blood flow to the intestine in a sick premature newborn may result in injury to the inner layers of the intestine, allowing bacteria that normally exist within the intestine to invade the damaged intestinal wall. If the injury progresses through the entire thickness of the bowel wall and the intestinal wall perforates, intestinal contents leak into the abdominal cavity and cause peritonitis. Necrotizing enterocolitis can also lead to infection of the blood (sepsis). In the most severe cases, necrotizing enterocolitis can be fatal.

Newborns with necrotizing enterocolitis may develop swelling of the abdomen. They may vomit bile-stained intestinal fluid, and blood may be visible in the stools. These newborns soon appear very sick and lethargic and have low body temperature and repeated pauses of breathing (apnea spells). The diagnosis of necrotizing enterocolitis is confirmed by abdominal x-rays. Blood samples are taken for blood cultures to identify the bacteria responsible for the infection.

Prevention, Treatment, and Prognosis

Feeding the premature newborn breast milk rather than formula appears to provide some protection. In tiny or sick premature newborns, the risk may also be reduced by delaying feedings for several days and then increasing the amount of feedings slowly. Feedings are stopped if necrotizing enterocolitis is suspected. A suction tube is passed into the newborn's stomach to remove pressure from swallowed air and formula, thereby decompressing the intestine. Intravenous fluids are given to maintain hydration, and antibiotics are begun after blood cultures have been obtained.

About 70% of newborns with necrotizing enterocolitis do not need surgery. If the intestine perforates, then surgery is needed. Surgery may also be needed if the condition progressively worsens despite treatment. In the tiniest and sickest newborns, "peritoneal drains" are placed into the abdominal cavity on each side of the lower abdomen. The drains allow stool and peritoneal fluid to drain from the abdominal cavity and, along with antibiotics, may allow symptoms to improve. The condition of many newborns treated with drains stabilizes, so that an operation can be performed more safely at a later time. In some cases, the newborns recover completely without needing additional surgery.

Larger infants need surgery in which portions of the bowel are removed and the ends of the healthy bowel are brought out to the skin surface to create a temporary opening for the excretion of bodily wastes (ostomy). Intensive medical treatment and surgery when needed have improved the prognosis for newborns with necrotizing enterocolitis. More than two thirds of such newborns survive.

PERSISTENT PULMONARY HYPERTENSION

Persistent pulmonary hypertension is a serious disorder in which the newborn's arteries to the lungs remain constricted after delivery, thus limiting the amount of blood flow to the lungs and therefore the amount of oxygen in the bloodstream.

Normally, the blood vessels to the lungs are tightly constricted during foetal life. The lungs do not need much blood flow before birth because the placenta eliminates carbon dioxide and transports oxygen to the foetus. Immediately after birth, the umbilical cord is cut and the newborn's lungs must take over the role of oxygenating the blood and removing carbon dioxide. To achieve this, it is necessary not only that the fluid filling the air sacs be replaced by air, but that the arteries bringing blood to the lungs widen (dilate) so that an adequate amount of blood flows through the lungs. In response to severe respiratory distress, or as a consequence of certain drugs taken by the mother before delivery (such as large doses of aspirin), the blood vessels to the lungs may not dilate as they normally should. As a result, there is insufficient blood flow to the lungs and not enough oxygen reaches the blood.

Persistent pulmonary hypertension is more common in newborns who are term or postterm and in newborns whose mothers were regular users of aspirin or indomethacin during pregnancy. In many newborns, the respiratory distress that initiates persistent pulmonary hypertension results from other lung diseases, such as meconium aspiration syndrome or pneumonia, but persistent pulmonary hypertension can also develop in newborns with no other lung disorder.

Symptoms and Diagnosis

Sometimes persistent pulmonary hypertension is present from birth; other times, it develops over the first day or two. Breathing is usually rapid, and there may be severe respiratory distress if the newborn has an underlying lung disease. The most prominent feature is a bluish discolouration of the skin (cyanosis) due to low blood oxygen levels. Sometimes low blood pressure (hypotension) leads to symptoms such as weak pulses and a pale, grayish hue to the skin.

A doctor may suspect persistent pulmonary hypertension if the mother used aspirin or indomethacin during pregnancy or had a stressful delivery, or if the newborn has severe respiratory distress and measurement of oxygen levels is unexpectedly low. A chest x-ray is performed, but definitive diagnosis requires an echocardiogram.

Treatment

Treatment involves placing the newborn in an environment with 100% oxygen to breathe. Alternatively, a ventilator providing 100% oxygen may be needed. A high percentage of oxygen in the blood helps open the arteries going to the lungs.

To make the blood slightly alkaline, which may also open these arteries, the newborn is often given intravenous sodium bicarbonate. In more severe cases, a very small concentration of the gas nitric oxide may be added to the oxygen that the newborn is breathing. Inhaled nitric oxide opens the arteries in the newborn's lungs and reduces pulmonary hypertension. This treatment may be needed over several days. If all other treatments fail, extracorporeal membrane oxygenation (ECMO) can be used. In this procedure, blood from the newborn is circulated through a machine that adds oxygen and removes carbon dioxide and then returns the blood to the newborn. ECMO has been lifesaving, allowing many newborns to survive until the pulmonary hypertension resolves.

PNEUMOTHORAX

Pneumothorax is a collection of air within the chest cavity surrounding a lung that develops when air leaks out of the lung. Pneumothorax most often occurs in a newborn with stiff lungs, such as a newborn with respiratory distress syndrome or meconium aspiration syndrome. Occasionally, it occurs as a complication from the use of continuous positive airway pressure (CPAP) or a ventilator. If the pneumothorax is under pressure, it can result in collapse of the lung and in difficulty breathing. Also, if under pressure, the pneumothorax can compress the veins bringing blood to the heart. As a result, less blood fills the chambers of the heart, the output of the heart decreases, and the newborn's blood pressure decreases.

Air that leaks from the lungs into the soft tissues in front of the heart is called pneumomediastinum. Unlike pneumothorax, this condition usually does not affect breathing.

Diagnosis and Treatment

Pneumothorax is suspected when a newborn with underlying lung disease, or a newborn on continuous positive airway pressure (CPAP) or a ventilator, develops worsening respiratory distress or a drop in blood pressure. When examining the newborn, a doctor notices a diminished sound of air entering and leaving the lung on the side of the pneumothorax. In premature newborns, a fibre-optic light may be used to light up the affected side of the newborn's chest while in a darkened room (positive transillumination); this procedure is used to look for air in the pleural cavity. A chest x-ray provides a definitive diagnosis.

No treatment is needed in newborns who do not have symptoms. A term newborn with mild symptoms may be placed in an oxygen hood. However, if the newborn's breathing is labored, and particularly if the circulation of blood is impaired, the air must be rapidly removed from the pleural cavity, which can be done using a needle and syringe. If the newborn is in significant distress, is receiving CPAP, or is on a ventilator, a doctor may need to place a chest tube to continuously suction and remove air from the chest cavity. The tube can usually be removed after several days. A pneumomediastinum can be seen on an x-ray; no treatment is needed.

POLYCYTHEMIA

Polycythemia is an abnormally high concentration of red blood cells. A markedly increased concentration of red blood cells may result in the blood being too thick, which slows the flow of blood through small blood vessels and interferes with the delivery of oxygen to tissues. A newborn who is born postmaturely or whose mother has severe high blood pressure, smokes, or lives at a high altitude is more likely to have polycythemia. Polycythemia may also result if the newborn receives too much blood from the placenta at birth, as may occur if the newborn is held below the level of the placenta for a period of time before the umbilical cord is clamped.

The newborn with polycythemia may have a ruddy or dusky colour. Most such newborns do not have other symptoms. However, the newborn may be sluggish, feed poorly, have rapid heart and respiratory rates, and, rarely, may have seizures. If the newborn has such symptoms and a blood test indicates too many red blood cells (high hematocrit), a partial exchange blood transfusion is performed, in which the newborn's blood is removed and replaced with equal volumes of albumin solution or saline, thus diluting the remaining red blood cells and correcting the polycythemia.

POSTMATURITY

A postmature newborn is a newborn delivered after more than 42 weeks in the uterus. Postmature (postterm) delivery is much less common than premature (preterm) delivery. The reason for a pregnancy to continue beyond term is usually unknown. Reduced function of the placenta is the greatest risk to fetuses who go beyond term. Near the end of a term pregnancy, the placenta begins to shrink. As it shrinks, the placenta becomes less able to provide adequate nutrients to the foetus. To compensate, the foetus begins to use its own fat and carbohydrates to provide energy. As a result, its growth rate slows, and occasionally its weight may decrease. If the placenta shrinks sufficiently, it may not provide adequate oxygen to the foetus, particularly during labour. A lack of adequate oxygen may result in foetal distress and, in extreme cases, may result in injury to the foetal brain and other organs. Foetal distress may cause the foetus to pass stools (meconium) into the amniotic fluid. The foetus may also take deep, gasping breaths triggered by the distress and thereby inhale the meconium-containing amniotic fluid into the lungs before or during birth. As a result, the newborn may have difficulty breathing after delivery (meconium aspiration syndrome).

Symptoms

A postmature newborn has dry, peeling, loose skin and may appear emaciated, especially if the function of the placenta was severely reduced. The newborn often appears alert. The skin and nail beds may be stained green if meconium was present in the amniotic fluid. A postmature newborn is prone to developing low blood sugar levels (hypoglycemia) after delivery, especially if oxygen levels were low during labour.

Treatment

The postmature newborn who experienced low oxygen levels and foetal distress may need resuscitation at birth. If meconium has been breathed into the lungs, a ventilator may be needed. Intravenous glucose solutions or frequent breast milk or formula feedings are given to prevent hypoglycemia. If these problems do not occur, the major goal is to provide good nutrition so that the newborn can catch up to the weight that is appropriate for him.

PREMATURITY

A premature newborn is a newborn delivered before 37 weeks in the uterus; such a newborn has underdeveloped organs. About 8% of newborns are born prematurely (preterm). Many of these newborns are born just a few weeks early and do not experience problems related to their prematurity. However, the more prematurely newborns are born, the more they are prone to a number of serious and even life-threatening complications. Very premature birth is the single most common cause of death in the newborn. Also, newborns born very prematurely are at high risk for chronic problems, especially delayed development and learning disorders. Such disorders occur because the internal organs have not had time to develop adequately before birth.

The reason for a premature birth cannot usually be determined. However, the risk of premature birth is higher in women who are poor, have little education, and have poor nutrition or health or untreated illnesses or infections during pregnancy. The risk is lower in women who had early prenatal care. For unknown reasons, black women are significantly more likely than women of other racial groups to have a premature delivery. Other women at increased risk for premature delivery are those carrying more than one foetus and those who have serious or life-threatening disorders, including severe high blood pressure or kidney disease, preeclampsia or eclampsia, or infection of the uterus (chorioamnionitis).

Symptoms

Premature newborns usually weigh less than 5½ pounds. Physical features help doctors determine the newborn's gestational age (length of time spent in the uterus after the egg is fertilized). Underdeveloped Lungs: The lungs of the premature newborn may not have had enough time to fully develop before birth. Such newborns are likely to have respiratory distress syndrome. Respiratory distress syndrome occurs if the lungs are not mature enough to produce surfactant, a mixture of lipids (fats) and proteins that allows the air sacs of the lungs to remain open.

Underdeveloped Brain: The part of the brain that controls regular breathing may be so immature that the newborn has inconsistent breathing, with short pauses in breathing or periods during which breathing stops for 20 seconds or longer (apnea). The parts of the brain that control the mouth and throat are immature so the newborn cannot suck and swallow normally and will have difficulty coordinating feeding with breathing.

Brain Haemorrhage: Newborns born very prematurely are at increased risk of bleeding (haemorrhage) in the brain. Bleeding typically begins in an area called the germinal matrix and may extend into spaces within the brain called the ventricles. This form of haemorrhage is most likely to occur in those born very prematurely (before 32 weeks of pregnancy) and if there were problems during labour or delivery or breathing problems (such as respiratory distress syndrome) after birth. Depending on the size of the haemorrhage, newborns may have no symptoms or may experience lethargy, seizures, or even persistent unconsciousness (coma). Newborns with small or moderate-sized haemorrhages usually develop normally. Those with very large haemorrhages are at higher risk of dying or of having learning disorders or other brain-related problems later in life.

Abnormal Blood Sugar: Because premature newborns have difficulty maintaining normal blood sugar (glucose) levels, they are often treated with intravenous glucose solutions or given small frequent feedings.

Without regular intake of sugar, a newborn may develop low blood sugar levels (hypoglycemia). Most newborns with hypoglycemia do not develop symptoms. Others may become listless with poor muscle tone, feed poorly, or become jittery. Rarely, seizures may develop. These newborns are also prone to developing high blood sugar levels (hyperglycemia) if they receive too much sugar intravenously. Most newborns with hyperglycemia do not develop symptoms.

Underdeveloped Immune System: Newborns who are born very prematurely have low levels of antibodies, which cross the placenta from mother to the foetus during the latter part of pregnancy and offer protection from infection. Therefore, the risk of developing infections, especially infection in the blood (sepsis), is higher in premature newborns. The use of special devices for treatment, such as catheters and ventilators, further increases the newborn's risk of developing serious infections.

Underdeveloped Kidneys: Before delivery, waste products produced in the foetus are removed by the placenta and then excreted by the mother's kidneys. After delivery, the newborn's kidneys must take over these functions. Kidney function is poor in newborns who are born very prematurely but improves as the kidneys mature. A newborn with underdeveloped kidneys is likely to have difficulty regulating the amount of salt and water in the body.

Underdeveloped Digestive Tract and Liver: Initially, premature newborns may have difficulty with feedings. Not only do they have immature sucking and swallowing reflexes, but also their small stomach empties slowly. Very premature newborns may develop a serious injury to the inner surface of the intestines (necrotizing enterocolitis).

In premature newborns, the excretion of bilirubin may be impaired. Thus, premature newborns, even more than term newborns, tend to become jaundiced in the first few days after birth because of the build-up of bilirubin in their blood. Usually, the jaundice is mild and resolves as the newborn takes larger amounts of feedings and has more frequent bowel movements. Rarely, very high levels of bilirubin accumulate and put the newborn at risk for developing kernicterus, a form of brain damage caused by deposits of bilirubin in the brain.

Difficulty Regulating Body Temperature: Because premature newborns have a large skin surface area relative to their weight, they tend to lose heat rapidly, especially if they are in a cool room or if there is a draft. A lowering of body temperature results in a markedly increased rate of the body's metabolism, as the newborn attempts to maintain normal body temperature.

Prevention

The best way for premature birth to be prevented is for the expectant mother to take good care of her own health. She should eat a nutritious diet and avoid cigarettes, alcohol, and drugs. Ideally, she should receive early and regular prenatal care so that any complications of pregnancy can be recognized and treated. If it seems probable that early labour is about to start, an obstetrician may administer drugs (such as magnesium sulfate or ritodrine) to the mother to slow or stop contractions. Corticosteroids such as betamethasone or dexamethasone may also be given to the mother to accelerate maturation of the foetus's lungs. Corticosteroids also significantly reduce the risk of brain haemorrhage if the newborn is born prematurely.

Treatment and Prognosis

Treatment involves managing the complications, such as respiratory distress syndrome and high bilirubin levels. Very premature newborns are fed intravenously until they can tolerate tube feedings and finally feedings by mouth. A premature newborn may need to be hospitalized for days, weeks, or months. Over recent decades, the survival of premature newborns has improved dramatically. For most premature newborns, the long-term prognosis is very good, and they develop normally. However, those born extremely early (often before 28 weeks of pregnancy) are at an increased risk of death and of serious problems, including mental retardation, cerebral palsy, epilepsy, or blindness. Fortunately, only a minority of extremely premature newborns who survive have these problems. A larger percentage have normal intelligence, but many have learning disorders that eventually require special help.

RESPIRATORY DISTRESS SYNDROME

Respiratory distress syndrome is a breathing disorder of premature newborns in which the air sacs (alveoli) in a newborn's lungs do not remain open because the production of surfactant is absent or insufficient. For a newborn to be able to breathe easily, the air sacs in the lungs must be able to remain open and filled with air. Normally, the lungs produce a mixture of lipids (fats) and proteins called surfactant. Surfactant acts as a wetting agent and lines the surface of the air sacs, where it lowers the surface tension and allows the air sacs to remain open throughout the respiratory cycle. Usually, production of surfactant begins after about 34 weeks of pregnancy. The more premature the newborn, the greater the likelihood that respiratory distress syndrome will develop after birth.

Respiratory distress syndrome occurs almost exclusively in premature newborns and is more common in those whose mother has diabetes.

Symptoms and Diagnosis

In an affected newborn, the lungs are stiff and the air sacs tend to collapse completely, emptying the lungs of air. In some very premature newborns, the lungs may be so stiff that the newborn is unable to begin breathing at birth. More commonly, the newborn tries to breathe, but because the lungs are so stiff, severe respiratory distress occurs. Respiratory distress is manifested by visibly labored breathing, including retractions of the chest below the rib cage, flaring of the nostrils during breathing in, and "grunting" during breathing out. Because a good portion of the lung is airless, the newborn has low blood oxygen levels, which cause a bluish discolouration to the skin (cyanosis). Over a period of hours, the respiratory distress tends to become more severe, as the small amount of surfactant in the lungs is used up and increasing numbers of air sacs collapse and also as the muscles used for breathing tire and become weak. Eventually, without treatment, the newborn may suffer damage to the brain and other organs from a lack of oxygen or may die.

Diagnosis of respiratory distress syndrome is based on the symptoms and on abnormal chest x-ray results in a premature newborn.

Prevention and Treatment

The risk of respiratory distress syndrome is greatly reduced if delivery can be safely delayed until the foetal lungs have produced sufficient surfactant. The obstetrician can perform amniocentesis, in which some amniotic fluid is withdrawn into a syringe and analyzed for the adequacy of surfactant production. If production is not adequate but premature delivery cannot be avoided, the obstetrician may give the mother injections of a corticosteroid drug (betamethasone or dexamethasone). The corticosteroid crosses the placenta into the foetus and accelerates the production of surfactant. Within 48 hours of starting the injections, the foetal lungs mature to the point that respiratory distress syndrome will not develop after delivery or, if it does, is likely to be milder.

After delivery, a newborn with mild respiratory distress syndrome may require only supplemental oxygen, which is given through an oxygen hood or through a tube placed in the nose. A newborn with severe respiratory distress syndrome may require oxygen delivered by continuous positive airway pressure (CPAP-breathing spontaneously against positive pressure oxygen or air administered through tubes placed in both nostrils).

In a very sick infant, a tube may need to be passed into the windpipe (intubation), and the infant's breathing supported with mechanical ventilation.

Use of a surfactant preparation can be lifesaving and reduces complications, such as rupture of the lungs (pneumothorax). The surfactant preparation acts in the same way that natural surfactant does. Surfactant may be given immediately after birth in the delivery room to attempt to prevent respiratory distress syndrome or in the early hours after birth to a premature newborn who already has symptoms of this disorder. A newborn who is intubated can receive surfactant through the tube in the windpipe. Surfactant treatments may be repeated several times over the first days until respiratory distress syndrome resolves.

RETINOPATHY OF PREMATURITY

Retinopathy of prematurity is a disease in which the small blood vessels in the back of the eye (retina) grow abnormally. In newborns born very prematurely, growth of the blood vessels supplying the retina may stop for a period of time. When growth resumes, it occurs in a disorganized fashion. During disorganized rapid growth, the small blood vessels may bleed and eventually lead to scarring. In the most severe cases, this process may ultimately result in detachment of the retina from the back of the eye and loss of vision. High blood oxygen levels may also increase the risk of retinopathy of prematurity.

The newborn who is developing retinopathy of prematurity does not have symptoms, and diagnosis depends on careful examination of the back of the eyes by an eye specialist (ophthalmologist). Routinely, therefore, an ophthalmologist examines the eyes of premature newborns who weigh less than 1, 500 grams at birth starting 4 or more weeks after delivery. Eye examinations are repeated every 1 to 2 weeks as needed, until growth of the blood vessels in the retina is complete. Infants who develop severe retinopathy must have eye examinations, at least yearly, for the rest of their lives. If detected early, retinal detachment can occasionally be treated to avoid complete loss of vision in the affected eye.

Prevention, Treatment, and Prognosis

In a premature newborn who needs oxygen, the oxygen use is monitored carefully to prevent excessive oxygen levels in the blood that would put the newborn at increased risk of retinopathy of prematurity. Alternatively, the oxygen levels can be indirectly monitored using a pulse oximetre, which measures the level of oxygen in the blood going through a finger or toe.

Retinopathy is usually mild and resolves spontaneously, but the eyes need to be monitored by an ophthalmologist until blood vessel growth is mature. For very severe retinopathy of prematurity, laser treatment is applied to the outermost portions of the retina. This treatment stops the abnormal growth of blood vessels and decreases the risk of retinal detachment and loss of vision.

SEPSIS

Sepsis is bacterial infection in the blood. Newborns, especially premature ones, are at much higher risk of sepsis than are children and adults because of their immature immune system. Premature newborns also lack certain antibodies against specific bacteria; these antibodies usually cross the placenta from the mother late in pregnancy. Another important risk factor for sepsis is the use of intravenous lines and ventilators.

The most common type of bacteria causing sepsis in the newborn around the time of birth is Group B streptococcus. Sepsis that occurs later while the newborn is being cared for in the neonatal intensive care unit (NICU) is most likely to be caused by a type of staphylococcus (coagulase negative).

SMALL FOR GESTATIONAL AGE (SGA)

A newborn, whether delivered preterm, term, or postterm, whose weight is less than that of 90% of babies of the same gestational age at birth (below the 10th percentile) is considered small for gestational age. There are several causes for this condition. In many cases, the newborn may be small simply because of genetic factors, such as having small parents (less commonly, a specific genetic syndrome associated with small stature may be involved). In other cases, the placenta may have functioned poorly, so that the foetus did not receive adequate nutrients and growth was impaired. This may happen if the mother has high blood pressure, preeclampsia, kidney disease, or long-standing diabetes. A viral infection, such as cytomegalovirus acquired before birth, may be responsible. Foetal growth may also have been impaired if the mother smoked or used alcohol or illicit drugs during the pregnancy. Unless they have a genetic syndrome or viral infection, most small-for-gestational-age newborns have no symptoms. If the foetal growth was impaired because of poor placental function and inadequate nutrition, the newborn's growth may accelerate when provided with good nutrition after delivery. Some small-for-gestational-age newborns remain small as children and adults.

THYROID DISORDERS

These disorders occur if the thyroid gland produces too little thyroid hormone (hypothyroidism) or too much thyroid hormone (hyperthyroidism). Hypothyroidism: If untreated, hypothyroidism in the newborn results in poor growth and mental delay, eventually resulting in mental retardation.

The most common cause of hypothyroidism in the newborn is complete absence or underdevelopment of the thyroid gland. Initially, the newborn has no symptoms. Later, the newborn may have lethargy, poor appetite, constipation, a hoarse cry, umbilical hernia (a bulging of the abdominal contents where the umbilicus penetrates the abdominal wall), and slow growth. Eventually, the infant may develop coarse facial features and an enlarged tongue.

Early treatment can prevent mental retardation. For this reason, a blood test is performed in the hospital after birth on all newborns to measure thyroid hormone levels. Treatment is with thyroid hormone.

Hyperthyroidism: Rarely, a newborn may have hyperthyroidism, or neonatal Graves' disease. This generally occurs if the mother has Graves' disease during pregnancy or has been treated for it before pregnancy. In Graves' disease, the woman's body produces antibodies that stimulate the thyroid gland to produce increased blood levels of thyroid hormone. These antibodies cross the placenta and similarly affect the foetus. The result in an affected newborn is too high a metabolic rate, with rapid heart rate and breathing, irritability, and excessive appetite with poor weight gain.

The newborn, like the mother, may have bulging eyes (exophthalmos). If the newborn has an enlarged thyroid gland (goiter), the gland may press against the windpipe and interfere with breathing. A very rapid heart rate can lead to heart failure. Graves' disease is potentially fatal if not recognized and treated. Doctors suspect hyperthyroidism by the typical symptoms and confirm the diagnosis by measuring elevated levels of thyroid hormone and the thyroid-stimulating antibodies from the mother in the newborn's blood.

Newborns with hyperthyroidism are treated with drugs, such as propylthiouracil, that slow the production of thyroid hormone by the thyroid gland. Treatment is needed for only a few months because the antibodies that cross the placenta from the mother only last in the infant's bloodstream for this long.

TRANSIENT TACHYPNEA

Transient tachypnea of the newborn (transient rapid breathing, neonatal wet-lung syndrome) is temporary difficulty with breathing and low blood oxygen levels due to excessive fluid in the lungs after birth.

This disorder usually occurs in newborns born a few weeks before term or at term. It is more common after a caesarean section delivery. It is especially likely to occur if the mother has not been in labour before delivery (for example, a mother who has a scheduled caesarean section). Before birth, the air sacs of the lungs are filled with fluid. Immediately after birth, the fluid must be cleared from the lungs so that the air sacs can fill with air and the newborn can establish normal breathing. Some of the fluid is squeezed out of the lungs by pressure on the chest during a vaginal delivery. More of the fluid is rapidly reabsorbed directly by the cells lining the air sacs and from which it is immediately transported into the bloodstream. If this fluid transfer does not occur rapidly, then the air sacs continue to be partially filled with fluid and the newborn has difficulty breathing.

A newborn with transient tachypnea has respiratory distress with rapid breathing, drawing in of the chest wall during breathing in and "grunting" during breathing out, and may develop a bluish discolouration of the skin (cyanosis) if the blood oxygen levels become low. A chest x-ray shows abnormal results. Most newborns with transient tachypnea recover completely within 2 to 3 days. Treatment with oxygen is usually needed, although some newborns may need continuous positive airway pressure (CPAP-breathing spontaneously against positive pressure oxygen or air administered through tubes placed in the newborn's nostrils) or assistance with a ventilator.

LEVELS OF NEONATAL CARE (LEVEL I, II & III)

LEVEL I (PRIMARY CARE)

The inpatient services in a Level I (primary care) perinatal unit should embrace the LDR/LDRP model of care. Facilities should have all the resources required to meet the needs of low-risk pregnancies where there is no predictable neonatal intervention required.

Maternal

- Ability to manage pregnancies where the mother has had no prior perinatal mortality or low birth-weight infants, no significant medical disease, no significant pregnancy complications now or in the past, foetal growth seems adequate
- Maternal-foetal assessment; to include identification of at risk pregnancies (with early consultation).
- Ultrasound - capability for detailed anatomical scan in second trimester and biophysical profile.
- Availability of obstetric procedures/laboratory tests and diagnostic imaging.
- Provision of care for healthy mothers and their newborns with a gestational age at or over 36 weeks gestation and/or > 2.5 Kg.
- Appropriate consultation with medical staff responsible for newborn care when anticipated obstetric or neonatal problems exist.

Treatments: Labour and Birth Area

- Foetal monitoring available on a continuous basis.
- IV available 24 hrs/day.
- ability to perform a caesarean section within approximately 30 minutes.
- manage pregnancy with one previous lower segment caesarean section.

Newborn

- Care for the healthy newborn at or over 36 weeks gestation and/or >2.5Kg.
- Observation and management of transient conditions (e.g. hypothermia, hypoglycemia responding to enteral feeds, respiratory distress with reducing or no oxygen requirement, hyperbilirubinemia).
- Provision of newborn resuscitation according to the Neonatal Resuscitation: National Guidelines. This should include:

1. A formal NRP program for all personnel who care for (or may care for) infants as part of their work responsibilities. These personnel may include ER medical

and nursing staff, respiratory therapists in addition to perinatal medical/nursing/midwifery staff.

2. Designation of an in-house neonatal resuscitation team at all times with clearly defined responsibilities. Of the two people available for resuscitation of the newborn as their sole responsibility in the delivery room, one must be able to intubate and administer fluids and medications.

- Stabilization, initiation and maintenance of assisted ventilation until transfer.
- Ability to accept transfers of infants including home births with conditions that are expected to resolve within a short period of time (e.g. breastfeeding establishment, phototherapy).

Treatments: Newborn

Availability of skilled individuals to perform the following treatments:

- Continuous monitoring of: cardiorespiratory, 02 saturation, non-invasive BP measurement
- O2 therapy
- Endotracheal intubation
- Catheterization of umbilical vein
- Venipuncture
- Initiation of intravenous therapy
- Lumbar puncture
- Initiation of assisted manual or mechanical ventilation until transfer

LEVEL II (SECONDARY CARE)

The inpatient services provided at Level II (secondary care) should have all the functional capabilities contained in hospitals that provide Level I care. In addition, Level II facilities should be equipped to meet and handle maternal-foetal patients of moderate-risk.

Maternal

Consultation should be considered with an obstetrician and/or neonatologist/paediatrician in order to provide optimum care for the mother and/or newborn. These patients may be managed by continuing collaborative care and delivery in an obstetrical unit with a Level II neonatal unit, or they may be returned to the care of the referring caregiver with a suggested plan of management for the remainder of the pregnancy.

Ability to manage pregnancies that present with the following risk factors:

- Diabetes, Class A (gestational) or Class B
- Hypertension requiring drug therapy or with proteinuria
- Renal disease without hypertension and without renal function impairment premature rupture of membranes or premature labour (> 32wks)
- APH, single event and ceased
- Twin pregnancy-two sacs
- Cervical incompetence
- Breech (36 weeks +)
- Polyhydramnios
- Primigravada (age 35+) or less than 16 years
- Post-date pregnancy (10 days past dates)
- History of genetic disease in family (genetic amniocentesis or counseling required)
- History of prior still birth or neonatal death or premature delivery
- Haemoglobin <90g/L or haemoglobinopathy trait
- Maternal obesity >100kg at first visit
- Significant tobacco, alcohol, drug intake
- grand multipara (>5)
- Large for dates >90 percentile
- Previous uterine surgery including Caesarean section
- Other significant medical illness
- Placenta previa >32 wks
- Foetal anomalies not requiring immediate intervention

Maternal Intensive Care

ICU 24-hour capability:

- Monitoring: oxygen saturation monitoring ECG invasive monitoring including S-G and arterial lines.
- Provision of ventilation.
- Ability to manage significant hypertension, hypotension and DIC.

Neonatal

- Care for the healthy newborn.
- Availability of health care personnel trained in neonatal resuscitation available for every delivery, including the skill of intubation.
- Care of newborns born to mothers of Grade B risk.
- Resuscitation and stabilization of all neonates born in hospital initial and ongoing care for stable infants >1250 gm or >30 weeks gestational age.
- Care for moderately ill newborns who have problems that are expected to resolve rapidly.
- Including those transferred from level I or home birth.
- Initiation and maintenance of short-term ventilation (24 hrs); mandatory consultation with a neonatologist for infants < 1500g and notification of the Level III outborn facility for all ventilated infants.

Treatments: Newborn

Availability of skilled individuals to perform the following procedures/ treatments:

- Continuous monitoring of: cardiorespiratory status, O_2 saturation, transcutaneous O_2/CO_2, non-invasive BP measurement.
- Endotracheal intubation.
- Catheterization of umbilical artery and vein.
- Venipuncture.
- Lumbar puncture.
- Initiation and maintenance of short term assisted ventilation.
- Administration of surfactant.
- Insertion of chest tube.
- Initiation and maintenance of intravenous therapy.
- Arterial puncture.
- Gavage feeding.
- Initiation, maintenance, and monitoring of total parenteral nutrition (TPN).

- Administration and monitoring of low flow oxygen.
- Therapeutic drug monitoring

LEVEL III - (TERTIARY CARE)

Inpatient services in a Level III (tertiary care) perinatal unit need to provide a full range of services from normal to high-risk maternal/ neonatal care.

Inpatient services in a Level III outborn neonatal unit (tertiary care) need to provide the full range of services for high-risk neonatal care.

Maternal

High-risk pregnancies are those complicated to the extant that the foetus or the mother would benefit from tertiary care. Where doubt exists, appropriate consultation with a tertiary care facility should occur. Generally, these patients should be receiving care at a Level III (tertiary care) centre for antenatal care and delivery.

Ability to manage pregnancies that present with any of the following Grade C risk factors:

- Renal disease with hypertension +/- reduced function.
- Early uncontrolled premature labour (<32 weeks gestational age).
- Premature rupture of membrane (+/- sepsis) (<32 weeks gestational age and > 23 weeks antepartum bleeding, continuing or repeated (<32 weeks gestational age) heart disease with symptoms.
- Haemoglobinopathy.
- Rhesus isoimmunization (with antibodies).
- Foetal anomalies requiring immediate neonatal intervention.

Based on the judgment of the care provider, treatment may be provided at a Level II perinatal centre with appropriate consultation:

- Diabetes Class C, D, F, R, or significantly complicated (e.g. renal function impairment).
- Severe hypertension with significant proteinuria.
- Severe foetal growth arrest (<10th percentile) and or oligohydramnious.

Newborn

Inborn Units

- Resuscitation, stabilization and ongoing care of all neonates born in hospital.
- Identification and timely transfer of infants with congenital malformations or other disorders who may require special diagnostic procedures, paediatric subspecialty consultation, or surgical care or consultation not available in facility.
- Acceptance of transfers of infants from level I or II units when appropriate within regionalized system.

Outborn Units

- Provision of all required care for infants exceeding the capabilities of level I and II units.
- Provision of intensive care for neonates requiring re-admission after discharge from original hospital or after home birth.
- Acceptance of appropriate transfers from Level III inborn units (as defined in inborn units).
- Coordination and management of timely and appropriate transfers of infants requiring Level III care.

MAINTENANCE OF REPORTS AND RECORDS

Neonatal nursing is a specialty in the health care profession where nurses provide direct patient care to high-risk newborn babies. They access the patients' health problems and needs, and use mathematics to calculate medication and nutrition based on the patient's very low weight. Knowledge of the sciences is required to understand the function of the human body. Neonatal nurses operate high tech equipment in the neonatal intensive care unit such as ventilators and incubators. Nurses must also keep precise medical records on each infant patient to help the physician provide proper medical care.

Following is the technique for record keeping of neonates:

PAST HISTORY

Peri-conceptual History

- Was there any parental illness around time of conception that may be relevant?

- Was child conceived naturally or by assisted reproduction?
- If relevant, establish whether child is adopted (or in foster care) with due sensitivity to the child's awareness of the facts

History of Pregnancy

Any factors relevant to foetal wellbeing should be recorded. For example:

- Antenatal infections (for example rubella)
- Rhesus incompatibility and haemolytic disease
- Exposure to prescribed, recreational drugs or over the counter medication
- Any maternal illness or problems in pregnancy

Peri-natal History

Factors pertinent to the child's health should be identified. For example:

- Gestation
- Duration of labour
- Mode of delivery
- Birth weight
- What if any resuscitation required
- Birth injury
- Congenital malformations identified

Neonatal Period

Relevant examples include:

- Jaundice
- Fits
- Febrile illnesses
- Bleeding disorders
- Feeding problems

Other Relevant Past History

This will include:

- Any subsequent illnesses, surgery, accidents or trauma
- Results and any concerns from screening tests at child health clinics or school

- Immunisation record
- Travel details

Developmental History

- Parental recall of major milestones will usually give important information (such as sitting up, crawling, walking, talking, toilet training, reading).
- It may be useful to ask how the child's progress and milestones compare with siblings and peers.
- Observations from other carers (school, nursery and extended family) may be helpful.

Current Medication

- Prescribed medication
- OTC medication
- Recreational drug or solvent use- in teenagers such information is much more likely to be forthcoming if the patient is seen alone and reassured confidentiality will be maintained
- Complementary formulations

It is worth remembering that the parent's memory of medication may not be accurate. Corroboration may need to be sought.3 Pharmacists, GP computerised practice records and health visitors may be useful sources of additional information.

Drug Intolerances, Adverse Drug Reactions and Allergies

It is important to enquire further about any allergy. Minor adverse reactions can often be labelled inappropriately as allergies.

FAMILY HISTORY

- Relevant history. For example:
  - — Previous miscarriages or stillbirths
  - — Diabetes mellitus
  - — Hypertension
  - — Renal disease
  - — Seizures
  - — Jaundice
  - — Congenital malformations
  - — Infections such as tuberculosis

- Whether siblings and parents are all alive and well?
- Consider conditions which may have a genetic component (such as ischaemic heart disease and cerebrovascular disease). Occasionally it is appropriate to address risk factors (such as familial hypercholesterolaemia) during childhood.
- Consanguinity occurs more commonly in some cultures and may be relevant to inherited disease (particularly autosomal recessive conditions).
- It can be useful to present findings by using a two-generation family tree.

REFERENCES

Ehrenreich, Barbara and English, Derdre. Witches, Midwives and Nurses: A History of Women Healers The Feminist Press, 1973.

Enkin, Murray, Keirse, Marc J.N.C., Renfrew, Mary and Neilson, James. 2nd Edition.

Gaskin, Ina May. Spiritual Midwifery The Farm 1978.

Goer, Henci. Bergen and Gervey, . Obstetric Myths Versus Research Realities 1995.

Gordon, Linda. Woman's Body, Woman's Right: A Social History of Birth Control in America. New York: Grossman, 1977.

Graham, Harvey. Eternal Eve, the History of Gynaecology and Obstetrics Doubleday & Company, 1951.

Hartley, Carla. Helping Hands: The Apprentice Workbook.

Janssen, Holt, Patricia A, and Myers, Susan J License "Midwife-Attended, Out-of-Hospital Births in Washington State: Are They Safe? " Birth 1994: 21(3):141-148.

Kitzinger, Sheila. Homebirth. 1991. A commonsense guide to the alternatives to giving birth in the hospital.

7

High-risk Pregnancy

There is no formal or universally accepted definition of a "high-risk" pregnancy. Generally, however, a high-risk pregnancy involves at least one of the following: The woman or baby is more likely to become ill or die than usual, or complications before or after delivery are more likely to occur than usual.

Certain conditions or characteristics, called risk factors, make a pregnancy high risk. Doctors identify these factors and use a scoring system to determine the degree of risk for a particular woman. Identifying high-risk pregnancies ensures that women who most need medical care receive it. However a pregnancy can be considered a high-risk pregnancy for a variety of reasons. Factors can be divided into maternal and foetal. Maternal factors include age (younger than age 15, older than age 35); weight (pre-pregnancy weight under 100 lb or obesity); height (under five feet); history of complications during previous pregnancies (including stillbirth, foetal loss, preterm labour and/or delivery, small-for-gestational age baby, large baby, pre-eclampsia or eclampsia); more than five previous pregnancies; bleeding during the third trimester; abnormalities of the reproductive tract; uterine fibroids; hypertension; Rh incompatability; gestational diabetes; infections of the vagina and/or cervix; kidney infection; fever; acute surgical emergency (appendicitis, gallbladder disease, bowel obstruction); post-term pregnancy; pre-existing chronic illness (such as asthma, autoimmune disease, cancer, sickle cell anaemia, tuberculosis, herpes, AIDS, heart disease, kidney disease, Crohn's disease, ulcerative colitis, diabetes).

Most women will see one healthcare provider during pregnancy, either an obstetrician, a midwife, or a nurse practitioner. Women who have a medical problem may need to see a medical specialist as well. Women diagnosed with a high-risk pregnancy may also need the expert advice and care of a perinatologist. A perinatologist is a medical doctor (obstetrician) who specializes in the care of women who are at high risk for having problems during pregnancy. Perinatologists care for women who have pre-existing medical problems as well as women who develop complications during pregnancy.

DIAGNOSIS

A woman with a high-risk pregnancy will need closer monitoring than the average pregnant woman. Such monitoring may include more frequent visits with the primary caregiver, tests to monitor the medical problem, blood tests to check the levels of medication, amniocentesis, serial ultrasound examination, and foetal monitoring. These tests are designed to track the original condition, survey for complications, verify that the foetus is growing adequately, and make decisions regarding whether labour may need to be induced to allow for early delivery of the foetus.

TREATMENT

Treatment varies widely with the type of disease, the effect that pregnancy has on the disease, and the effect that the disease has on pregnancy. Additional tests may help determine the need for changes in medication or additional treatment.

PROGNOSIS

The prognosis depends in large part on the specific medical condition. Some medical conditions make it difficult to get pregnant and lead to a higher risk of problems in the baby. An example of this type of condition is thyroid disease. In thyroid disease, the thyroid gland (located in the neck) may produce too much or too little thyroid hormone. Abnormal levels of thyroid hormone can cause problems in pregnancy and affect the health of the baby. Fortunately, thyroid disease can be treated with medication. As long as the level of thyroid hormone is controlled throughout pregnancy, there should be no problems for mother or baby.

There are many medical conditions that usually do not interfere with pregnancy, but are themselves affected by pregnancy. This group includes asthma, epilepsy, and ulcerative colitis. For example, some women with ulcerative colitis experience a worsening of their symptoms during pregnancy, while others will have no change or may get better during pregnancy. The same is true of asthma; some women notice that their asthma symptoms are better during pregnancy, some find their asthma worse, and some women notice no change in symptoms during pregnancy.

No one understands why this is so, but due to this unpredictability, all women with chronic illnesses should be monitored carefully throughout pregnancy.

There is also a group of medical conditions that can have a major impact on pregnancy. Women with lupus (disease caused by alterations in the immune system that result in inflammation of connective tissue and organs) or kidney disease face real risks during pregnancy. Pregnancy can cause their symptoms to worsen significantly and can lead to serious illness. Because these diseases can affect the mother's ability to supply oxygen and nutrients to the baby through the placenta, they can cause problems for the baby as well. These babies may not be able to grow and gain weight properly (intrauterine growth retardation). There is also an increased risk of stillbirth.

Diabetes is a medical condition that is both affected by pregnancy and affects pregnancy. Diabetes can lead to miscarriages, birth defects, and stillbirths. When a woman monitors her blood sugar carefully and treats high levels with insulin, the risk of these negative outcomes drops a great deal. Unfortunately, pregnancy makes diabetes much harder to control. In general, blood sugar and the need for insulin to control it rise throughout pregnancy.

Most medical conditions do not lead to complications in pregnancy. With frequent visits to healthcare providers, and careful attention to medication, women with medical problems usually enjoy healthy, successful pregnancies. There are a few medical conditions that can cause health risks to both mother and baby during pregnancy. Women with these medical problems should consider these risks before deciding to become pregnant. Many of these women will benefit from the care of a perinatologist during pregnancy. Only rarely (in the case of severe heart disease, for example) are the risks to the mother so high that she should not consider pregnancy at all.

PREVENTION

A pre-pregnancy visit with a healthcare provider is especially important for a woman who has a medical problem. The doctor will discuss how women with this condition usually fare during pregnancy. For some diseases (such as lupus), pregnancy can mean increased risk of health problems for mother and baby.

Sometimes, the medication a woman needs to control a medical condition can cause problems for the baby. There may be another medication available that is safer for use in pregnancy. In some cases there is no other medication, and a woman must weigh the risks to the baby when deciding whether or not to become pregnant.

A woman who has not had a pre-pregnancy visit should contact a healthcare provider as soon as she learns she is pregnant. Often, the provider will schedule the first prenatal visit within a day or two, instead of waiting until eight to 10 weeks of pregnancy. This is because certain medical conditions can increase the risk of miscarriage. The provider will want to be sure that any medication is adjusted properly to increase the chance of having a successful pregnancy.

SCREENING AND ASSESSMENT

Monitoring the baby's well-being in the uterus in pregnancy is often undertaken using a cardiotocograph (CTG) machine. A CTG assesses the pattern of the baby's heartbeats alongside the size of the mother's contractions. However, this is not a very accurate test on its own. So monitoring the baby's movements has also been suggested as a useful addition to predict babies in difficulty. This is because a reduction in foetal movement sometimes precedes a baby's death. It is thought that if the oxygen supply to the baby through the afterbirth (placenta) is insufficient, the baby responds by moving less often. As foetal movement patterns may vary considerably, multiple foetal activities might be a better predictor of poor outcome. Consequently, the biophysical profile (BPP) and modified biophysical profile (MBPP) have been introduced. The BPP uses ultrasound to assess (1) foetal movement, (2) tone, (3) breathing and (4) the amniotic fluid volume that surrounds the baby. In addition, the baby's heartbeat is monitored over a 20-minute period using a CTG machine. This produces a paper tracing of the baby's heart rate, the mother's contractions and when the baby moves. Sometimes a modified BPP is used first (MBPP), involving the CTG trace and the amniotic fluid volume only. If this indicates a possible abnormality, then the full BPP is used. This review of trials compared the BPP (or MBPP) with conventional monitoring (CTG only) on pregnancy outcome in high-risk pregnancies.

Nursing assessment begins with a thorough history and physical examination. In addition, the woman is offered screening for HIV antibodies.

Review the woman's history for risk factors, such as unsafe sex practices, multiple sex partners, and injectable drug use. Also have the woman complete a risk assessment survey. In addition, question the woman about flu-like symptoms such as a low grade fever, fatigue, sore throat, night sweats, diarrhea, cough, skin lesions, or muscle pain. Perform a complete physical examination.

Obtain the woman's weight and determine if she has lost weight recently. Assess for signs and symptoms of sexually transmitted infections (STIs), such as vulvovaginal candidiasis, bacterial vaginosis, HSV, chancroid, CMV, or Chlamydia because of increased risk for STIs. Testing is essential because treatments are available that can reduce the likelihood of perinatal transmission and maintain the health of the woman.

ULTRASONIC, CARDIO TOMOGRAPHY, NST, CST, NON-INVASIVE & INVASIVE

Ultrasonography in pregnancy should be performed only when there is a valid medical indication. Indications for a first-trimester ultrasound (performed before 13 weeks and 6 days of gestation) include:

- To confirm the presence of an intrauterine pregnancy
- To evaluate a suspected ectopic pregnancy
- To evaluate vaginal bleeding
- To evaluate pelvic pain
- To estimate gestational age
- To diagnosis or evaluate multiple gestations
- To confirm cardiac activity
- As adjunct to chorionic villus sampling, embryo transfer, or localization and removal of an intrauterine device
- To assess for certain foetal anomalies, such as anencephaly, in patients at high risk
- To evaluate maternal pelvic or adnexal masses or uterine abnormalities
- To screen for foetal aneuploidy
- To evaluate suspected hydatidiform mole.

Standard Examination

A standard ultrasound includes an evaluation of foetal presentation, amniotic fluid volume, cardiac activity, placental position, foetal biometry, and foetal number, plus an anatomic survey. A standard examination of foetal anatomy includes the following essential elements:

- Head, face and neck (cerebellum, choroid plexus, cisterna magna, lateral cerebral ventricles, midline falx, cavum septi pellucidi, upper lip)
- Chest (heart)
- Abdomen (stomach, kidneys, bladder, umbilical cord insertion site into the foetal abdomen, umbilical cord vessel number)
- Spine (cervical, thoracic, lumbar, and sacral spine)
- Extremities (presence or absence of legs and arms)
- Sex (medically indicated in low-risk pregnancies only for the evaluation of multiple gestations).

Limited Examination

A limited examination does not replace a standard examination and is performed when a specific question requires investigation (e.g., to confirm foetal heart activity in a patient experiencing vaginal bleeding or to establish foetal presentation during labour). A limited examination may be performed during the first trimester to evaluate interval growth, estimate amniotic fluid volume, evaluate the cervix, and assess the presence of cardiac activity.

Specialized Examination

A detailed or targeted anatomic examination is performed when an anomaly is suspected on the basis of history, laboratory abnormalities, or the results of either the limited or standard examination. Other specialized examinations might include foetal Doppler ultrasonography, biophysical profile, amniotic fluid assessment, foetal echocardiography, or additional biometric measurements. Specialized examinations are performed by an operator with experience and expertise in such ultrasonography who determines that components of the examination on a case-by-case basis.

Indications for a second and third trimester ultrasound include the following:

- Estimation of gestational age
- Evaluation of foetal growth
- Evaluation of vaginal bleeding
- Evaluation of cervical insufficiency
- Evaluation of abdominal and pelvic pain
- Determination of foetal presentation
- Evaluation of suspected multiple gestation

- Adjunct to amniocentesis or other procedure
- Significant discrepancy between uterine size and clinical dates
- Evaluation of pelvic mass
- Examination of suspected hydatidiform mole
- Adjunct to cervical cerclage placement
- Evaluation of suspected ectopic pregnancy
- Evaluation of suspected foetal death
- Evaluation of suspected uterine abnormality
- Evaluation for foetal well-being
- Evaluation for premature rupture of membranes of premature labour
- Evaluation for abnormal biochemical markers
- Follow-up evaluation of a foetal anomaly
- Follow-up evaluation of placental location for suspected placenta previa
- Evaluation in those with a history of previous congenital anomaly
- Evaluation of foetal condition in late registrants for prenatal care
- To assess for findings that may increase the risk of aneuploidy
- To screen for foetal anomalies.

HIGH RISK APPROACH

Pregnant women require routine prenatal care to help ensure their health and the health of the foetus. Also, evaluation is often required for symptoms and signs of illness. Common symptoms that are often pregnancy-related include vaginal bleeding, pelvic pain, vomiting, and lower-extremity edema.

Follow-up visits should occur at about 4-wk intervals until 28 wk, at 2-wk intervals from 28 to 36 wk, and weekly thereafter until delivery. Prenatal care includes screening for disorders, taking measures to reduce foetal and maternal risks, and counseling.

During the initial visit, a full medical history is obtained. It includes previous and current disorders and drug use (therapeutic, social, and illicit), presence of risk factors for complications of pregnancy, and obstetric history, with the outcome of all previous pregnancies, including maternal and foetal complications (e.g., gestational diabetes, preeclampsia, congenital malformations, stillbirth). Family history should include all chronic disorders in family members to identify possible hereditary disorders. During subsequent visits, queries focus on interim developments, particularly vaginal bleeding or fluid discharge, headache, changes in vision, edema of face or fingers, and changes in frequency or intensity of foetal movement.

Gravidity is the number of confirmed pregnancies; a pregnant woman is a gravida. Parity is the number of deliveries after 20 wk. Multifoetal pregnancy is counted as one in terms of gravidity and parity. Abortus is the number of pregnancy losses (abortions) before 20 wk regardless of cause (e.g., spontaneous, therapeutic, or elective abortion; ectopic pregnancy). Sum of parity and abortus equals gravidity. Parity is often recorded as 4 numbers: number of term deliveries (after 37 wk), number of premature deliveries (> 20 and < 37 wk), number of abortions, and number of living children. Thus, a woman who is pregnant and has had one term delivery, one set of twins born at 32 wk, and 2 abortions is gravida 5.

A full general examination, including height and weight, is done first. In the initial obstetric examination, speculum and bimanual pelvic examination is done, noting the presence of lesions or discharge as well as colour and consistency of the cervix; also, foetal heart rate and, in patients presenting later in pregnancy, lie of the foetus are assessed. Pelvic capacity can be estimated clinically by evaluating various measurements with the middle finger during bimanual examination. If the distance from the underside of the pubic symphysis to the sacral promontory is > 11.5 cm, the pelvic inlet is almost certainly adequate. Normally, distance between the ischial spines is ≥ 9 cm, length of the sacrospinous ligaments is 4 to ≥ 5 cm, and the subpubic arch is ≥ 90°.

During subsequent visits, BP and weight assessment is important. Obstetric examination focuses on uterine size, fundal height (in cm above the symphysis pubis), foetal heart rate and activity, and maternal diet, weight gain, and overall well-being. Speculum and bimanual examination is usually not needed unless vaginal discharge or bleeding, leakage of fluid, or pain is present.

If a woman has Rh-negative blood, she may be at risk of developing Rh0(D) antibodies, and the foetus may be at risk of developing erythroblastosis foetalis. Rh0(D) antibody levels should be measured in pregnant women at 18 to 20 wk and again at about 26 to 28 wk. Additional measures may be necessary to prevent development of maternal Rh antibodies.

Generally, women are routinely screened for gestational diabetes between 24 and 28 wk. If women have risk factors for gestational diabetes, they are screened in the 1st trimester. Risk factors include gestational diabetes or a macrosomic neonate (weight > 4500 g at birth) in a previous pregnancy, unexplained foetal losses, a family history of diabetes, a history of persistent glucosuria, and body mass index (BMI) > 30 kg/m2. Screening uses a 50-g, 1-h glucose tolerance test.

Drugs and vitamins that are not medically indicated should be. Vaccines for measles, mumps, rubella, and varicella should not be used during. The hepatitis B vaccine can be safely used if indicated, and the influenza vaccine is given to women who are in the 2nd or 3rd trimester during influenza season. Women should not use alcohol and tobacco and should avoid exposure to secondhand smoke. They should also avoid exposure to chemicals or paint fumes, direct handling of cat litter (due to risk of toxoplasmosis), prolonged temperature elevation (e.g., in a hot tub or sauna), and exposure to people with active viral infections (e.g., rubella, parvovirus infection [fifth disease], varicella). Women with substance abuse problems should be monitored by a specialist in high-risk pregnancy.

Women should be advised to seek evaluation for unusual headaches, visual disturbances, pelvic pain or cramping, vaginal bleeding, rupture of membranes, extreme swelling of the hands or face, diminished urine volume, any prolonged illness or infection, or persistent symptoms of labour. Multiparous women with a history of rapid labour should notify the physician at the 1st symptom of labour.

LEVELS OF CARE; PRIMARY, SECONDARY AND TERTIARY LEVELS

There are three different levels of newborn care available at different hospitals. These are referred to as low-risk care, specialty care, and subspecialty care. The level of care is based on the specific needs of the newborn baby. After a baby is born, mother and newborn baby may require different levels of care but every effort will be made to keep them together at the same hospital. However, some seriously ill newborn babies must be transported to a hospital that provides a higher level of care.

LOW-RISK CARE (LEVEL I)

Hospitals provide care for low-risk women and their babies throughout and after childbirth. After childbirth, these hospitals provide postpartum care for both the mother and her newborn baby. They must be able to resuscitate and stabilize newborn babies if necessary, and evaluate and care for them until they are discharged from hospital. They stabilize and transfer newborn babies and mothers who need specialty or subspecialty care to an appropriate facility. They also provide nursing care to newborn babies who have been returned to low-risk care from a specialty or subspecialty hospital.

Neonatal Transport

Some premature and newborn babies with serious health problems are born in hospitals providing low-risk care, that cannot give the required level of care. They are transferred to a specialty or subspecialty hospital with the appropriate facilities by a transport team. The transport team generally includes at least two of the following people:

- Transport physician
- Transport nurse
- Transport respiratory therapist

All these people have expertise in the emergency transport of newborn babies. The transport team stabilizes the newborn baby for transport, and delivers neonatal intensive care to the newborn baby during the transfer from the birth hospital to the specialty or subspecialty hospital.

SPECIALTY CARE (LEVEL II)

Hospitals that provide specialty care services have the same responsibilities as low-risk care hospitals, and they also offer a number of extra services. They take care of high-risk mothers and newborn babies, some of whom are transferred in from other hospitals. Specialty care hospitals care for premature babies born at more than 32 weeks gestation and/or weighing 1500 g (3 lbs 5 oz) or more.

They also care for other newborn babies with health problems that are expected to improve quickly. Some specialty care hospitals have neonatal intensive care units (NICUs) with paediatricians and doctors called neonatologists who specialize in the care of newborn babies.

Reasons to transfer a newborn baby from low-risk care to specialty care include premature labour after 32 weeks, foetal growth restriction with low levels of amniotic fluid in the womb, anticipated minor congenital abnormalities, a form of severe high blood pressure in the mother called pre-eclampsia, a problem with the placenta called placenta previa, or an inflammation of the foetal membranes called chorioamnionitis.

Specialty hospitals are also able to stabilize very ill newborn babies s and transfer them to subspecialty hospitals if necessary.

SUBSPECIALTY CARE (LEVEL III)

Hospitals that provide subspecialty care services care for newborn babies of all risk categories. These include those who are transferred from low-risk care or specialty care hospitals. Newborn babies who should be treated in subspecialty care hospitals include:

- Babies who require complex care upon delivery
- Babies with serious birth defects
- Premature babies born at less than 32 weeks of pregnancy
- Babies with a birthweight of less than 1500 g (3 lbs 5 oz)

After childbirth, sometimes the mother needs to continue receiving care at a hospital that provides subspecialty services while the baby is well enough to be treated at another hospital. Conversely, sometimes the mother gives birth and stays in the hospital where her baby was born while her baby is transported to a hospital that provides subspecialty services.

This forced separation presents challenges for the mother, her newborn baby, and the father. The parents may feel that they cannot bond very well with their baby, but they should keep in mind that bonding takes place over a period of weeks or months, well after the time that their baby is back home. There may be challenges in terms of travelling between hospitals, the cost of obtaining accommodations close to the baby's hospital, and arranging for child care for older brothers or sisters.

DISORDERS OF PREGNANCY

Usually, labour and delivery occur without any problems. Serious problems are relatively rare, and most can be anticipated and treated effectively. However, problems sometimes develop suddenly and unexpectedly. Regular visits to a doctor or certified midwife during pregnancy make anticipation of problems possible and improve the chances of having a healthy baby and safe delivery.

HYPER-EMESIS GRAVIDARUM

As many as 90% of all pregnant women will experience some nausea and vomiting during the first three months of pregnancy. This is often called morning sickness (or pregnancy sickness), but will usually occur more often than just the morning.

Some women (1-10% of pregnant women) can develop the condition called hyperemesis gravidarum (HG). This is when the nausea and/or vomiting becomes so severe that the woman loses a large amount of weight. This can result in not enough water in the body (dehydration) and the body may not get enough nutrients to function properly. If HG becomes severe and/or is left untreated, it can be dangerous for both the mother and the baby.

Causes

The cause of HG is not completely understood, but there are several factors being researched that seem to contribute to it. These vary for each woman and may for each pregnancy:

- Rapidly changing hormone levels during early pregnancy
- The physical and emotional stress of pregnancy on the body
- Food in the stomach empties more slowly
- Stomach contents may move backwards into the esophagus (the tube that goes from the mouth to the stomach)
- Lack of certain vitamins and nutrients
- Infections (increased levels of bacteria) in the stomach
- Increased levels of other hormones like thyroid
- Changes in the immune function of the body
- Increased sense of smell and sensitivity to food texture/taste

Treatments

- If severe dehydration occurs, intravenous fluids (by vein) may need to be given in the hospital, clinic or at home.
- Many doctors prefer not to give any medicines during pregnancy, if possible. However, when a woman has HG, the risk of using certain medicines is much less than the risk of malnutrition and significant weight loss from HG. Many of the following medicines have been used for years and are known not to harm the baby.

BLEEDING IN EARLY PREGNANCY

Vaginal bleeding during pregnancy can be scary. It's not always a sign of trouble, however. In fact, most women who experience vaginal bleeding during pregnancy - particularly during the first trimester - go on to deliver healthy babies.

Bleeding During the First Trimester

Many women experience light vaginal bleeding during the first 12 weeks of pregnancy. Possible causes of vaginal bleeding during early pregnancy include:

- Implantation. A few women may notice a small amount of vaginal bleeding very early in pregnancy, about 10 to 14 days after fertilization. This "implantation bleeding" happens when the fertilized egg attaches to the lining of uterus. It's usually earlier, spottier and lighter in colour than a normal menstrual period, and it doesn't last long. Some women mistake this light bleeding for a period and don't realize they're pregnant.
- Cervical changes. When pregnant, more blood flows to the cervix. The pregnant women may experience harmless vaginal bleeding after contact to the cervix, such as after sex or a pelvic exam.
- Miscarriage. Up to 15 percent of known pregnancies end in miscarriage. Vaginal bleeding is the primary sign of miscarriage. But bleeding doesn't necessarily mean having a miscarriage. Remember, most women who experience vaginal bleeding during pregnancy go on to deliver healthy babies.
- Ectopic pregnancy. Sometimes an embryo implants somewhere outside the uterus, usually in a fallopian tube. This is known as an ectopic pregnancy. An embryo implanted outside the uterus can't survive. And without treatment, life-threatening blood loss is possible. In addition to vaginal bleeding, an ectopic pregnancy may cause abdominal or pelvic pain.
- Molar pregnancy. Rarely, an abnormal mass - instead of a baby - forms inside the uterus after fertilization. Vaginal bleeding is the most common sign of a molar pregnancy.
- Infection. Some cervical infections cause bleeding in early pregnancy.

Bleeding During the Second or Third Trimester

As the cervix begins to thin out and relax in preparation for labour, the thick plug of mucus that seals the opening of the cervix is dislodged.

When this happens, you may notice a thick or stringy discharge that may be tinged with blood. This "bloody show" is a normal sign of impending labour that may occur up to a week or two before delivery.

A bloody show near the end of pregnancy isn't cause for concern. But other causes of bleeding during the second or third trimester are more worrisome, including:

- Miscarriage. Vaginal bleeding is the primary sign of miscarriage. Although miscarriage is most common during the first trimester, a risk still exists in the second trimester.
- Preterm labour. Light bleeding in the second or third trimester may be a sign of preterm labour, especially when accompanied by regular contractions, dull backache or pelvic pressure.
- Problems with the cervix. A cervical infection, inflamed cervix or growths on the cervix may cause vaginal bleeding in the second or third trimester. Occasionally, light bleeding may be a sign that the cervix is opening prematurely (cervical incompetence). This can lead to preterm birth.
- Placenta previa. Painless, bright red vaginal bleeding in the second or third trimester may indicate placenta previa - a serious problem in which the placenta partly or completely covers the opening to the birth canal. The bleeding may stop at some point, but it nearly always recurs days or weeks later.
- Placental abruption. Rarely, the placenta begins to separate from the inner wall of the uterus before birth. This may cause bleeding that's scant, heavy or somewhere in between. The bleeding is usually accompanied by abdominal pain.
- Uterine rupture. Rarely, the uterus tears open along the scar line from a prior C-section. This may cause vaginal bleeding, intense abdominal pain and abdominal tenderness. If uterus ruptures - either before or during labour - an emergency C-section is needed to prevent life-threatening complications.

Depending on the cause of the bleeding and various other factors, treatment may include bed rest or medication.

ECTOPIC

The word "ectopic" means "out of place." In an ectopic pregnancy, the fertilized egg implants outside of the uterus and begins to grow. Sadly, an ectopic pregnancy cannot result in the birth of a baby. Without prompt treatment, it can cause serious bleeding and threaten the life of the pregnant woman. Ectopic pregnancy is treated either with drug therapy or surgery. About 50 to 80 percent of women who have had an ectopic pregnancy go on to have a normal pregnancy.

PREGNANCY, VESICULAR MOLE

In a molar pregnancy, the early placenta grows abnormally into a mass of cysts (called a hydatidiform mole). The embryo does not form at all or is malformed and cannot survive. About 1 in 1, 500 pregnancies is molar. An ultrasound exam can diagnose a molar pregnancy. The woman then has surgery to remove the molar tissue from the uterus. In some cases, molar tissue can turn into choriocarcinoma, a rare form of cancer. Fortunately, this cancer has a very high cure rate. Most women with molar pregnancies go on to have healthy pregnancies later. The risk of reoccurrence is only about 1 to 2 percent.

ANTE-PARTUM HAEMORRHAGE

In a molar pregnancy, the early placenta grows abnormally into a mass of cysts (called a hydatidiform mole). The embryo does not form at all or is malformed and cannot survive. About 1 in 1, 500 pregnancies is molar. An ultrasound exam can diagnose a molar pregnancy. The woman then has surgery to remove the molar tissue from the uterus. In some cases, molar tissue can turn into choriocarcinoma, a rare form of cancer. Fortunately, this cancer has a very high cure rate. Most women with molar pregnancies go on to have healthy pregnancies later. The risk of reoccurrence is only about 1 to 2 percent.

UTERINE ABNORMALITY AND DISPLACEMENT

The cardinal ligaments provide the major support for the uterus and vagina. These ligaments may be unduly stretched if the foetus is large or if forceps delivery is attempted before full cervical dilation. If the cardinal ligaments do not return to normal after delivery, the uterus will sag backward and downward into the vagina. The uterus usually forms an acute angle with the axis of the vagina, which in itself tends to prevent proplase. Proplase of the uterus occurs when the cardinal ligaments and other supporting structures (e.g., uterosacral ligaments) relax and the relationship of the axis of the uterus to that of the vagina is altered.

Congenital defects account for descensus (prolapse) of the uterus in infants and nulliparas, but childbirth injury is responsible for its gradual development in multiparas. Cystocele and rectocele, which almost always accompany uterine prolapse, enlarge and pull down on the uterus and cervix, adding to the stress on the weakened cardinal ligaments. The more severe prolapse are seen in postmenopausal women when tissue atrophy eliminates whatever residual support existed. Degrees of prolapse are classified as follows:

- First-degree prolapse. Cervix is situated between the level of the ischial spines and the vaginal introitus.
- Second-degree prolapse. Cervix protrudes through introutius, but corpus remains within the vagina.
- Third-degree prolapse. Complete prolapse; cervix and body of uterus protrude through vagina, and vagina is inverted. The extent of the defect is best evaluation by asking the woman to strain while lying down, by exerting traction on the cervix with a tenaculum, or by examining her while she is an upright position.
- Procidentia. Uterus, vaginal vault, rectum, and bladder, and perhaps the posterior cul-de-sac as well, protrude.

Symptoms of uterine prolapse reflects sensations produced by the weight of the descending structures and their protrusion through the vaginal introitus. Third-degree prolapse may eventuate in cervical ulceration and bleeding. Transvaginal correction of the defect is preferable, but in selected individual (e.g., those who are aged) a pessary may be inserted to stabilized the uterus. The goals of operative procedures are:

- To correct the cystocele and rectocele,
- Return the uterus to a forward position,
- Shorten the elongated cervix, and
- Shorten the cardinal ligaments.

Several procedures accomplish these goals:

- Manchester-Fothergill: amputation of the cervix, shortening of the cardinal ligaments, and plastic repair of the vagina.
- Vaginal hysterectomy.
- Colpocleisis (Le Fort's procedure): obliteration of the vagina by approximation of the anterior and posterior walls.

RETROVERSION AND LATERAL DISPLACEMENT

Displacement indicates a movement from front to back or from side to side, rather than a descent, as in prolapse. The two types of displacement are:

- A change in the long axis of the uterus, for example, anteflexion, malposition, and retroflexion, and
- A change in the direction of the long axis of the uterus in relation to the vaginal canal, for example, lateral retroversion, and retrocession.

Most positional differences are simple anatomic variations. They are asymptomatic and have no clinical significance. Retroversion is the most common simple displacement caused by factors that are congenital or acquired after childbirth. Cul-de-sac disease may be responsible and is of clinical significance. Lateral displacement may signal adnexal disease such as large ovarian tumor on the opposite side.

The supporting ligaments that hold the uterus in anteversion are the round and uterosacral ligaments. The uterosacral ligaments pull the cervix backward and upward; the round ligaments hold the fundus in the anterior position. These ligaments gradually regain their length and return the uterus to anteversion in two thirds of women within approximately 2 months after delivery; in one third of women the uterus remains retroverted. Uncomplicated retroversion as a sequel to childbirth is rarely symptomatic; low backache is not a symptom. Occasionally it may be difficult to conceive because the cervix points toward the anterior vaginal wall and away from the posterior fornix containing seminal fluid. Retrodisplacement is also clinically significant because it must occur first before the uterus can prolapse.

Infrequently, chronic pelvic congestion may accompany a chronically retroverted uterus and is credited as the cause of deep pelvic and low back pain, difficulty with evacuation of the rectum, menstrual abnormalities associated with an exaggeration of premenstrual tension, and dyspareunia. The uterus may become boggy and congested, and the tubes and ovaries (often containing multiple follicular cysts) often prolapse posteriorly into the cul-de-sac. Surgical correction is necessary only if the woman has symptoms that may be related to uterine position. A properly placed pessary replaces the uterus in the anterior position. If symptoms are relieved, it can assumed that uterine displacement had contributed to the symptoms. Even through pessaries are retained for short periods of time, the woman needs to follow principle of good hygiene to avoid vaginal infection.

- Some women can be taught to remove the pessary at night, cleanse it, and replace it when they get up in the morning. This practice helps to reduce the likelihood of pressure necrosis from irritation against the vaginal wall.

- If the pessary is always to be left in place, regular douching may be recommended to remove the increased secretions its presence may cause and to help prevent infection.
- The woman is encouraged to visit her health care provider frequently while the pessary is in place.

Pessary in place to hold posterior vaginal fornix, with it, attached cervix well backward and upward in pelvis.

GENITAL FISTULAS

A fistula is an abnormal or unnatural communication between one hollow viscus and another or from one hollow viscus to the outside. Genital fistulas are located between the bladder and the genital tract (vesicovaginal, vesicocervical, vesicouterine), and between the ureter and the vagina (ureterovaginal), and between the rectum or sigmoid colon and other structures (entrovesical, entrouterine, entrovaginal).

Etiologic Factors

- Congenital anomaly,
- Gynecologic surgery,
- Obstetric trauma,
- Cancer,
- Radiation therapy,
- Gynecologic trauma,
- Infection

Discussion of obstetric-related urinary tract and rectovaginal fistulas as follows:

URINARY TRACT FISTULAS

The most common urinary tract fistula (vesicovaginal) forms in the anterior vaginal wall. Historically, necrosis of the vesicovaginal septum from pressure during delayed labour was responsible for the fistula formation; this is seldom the case today because such labours would dictate caesarean delivery.

Today, operative injury near the uterovesical junction during radical hysterectomy for cancer is the primary cause of a fistula between the uterus and the bladder.

The woman with this abnormal opening is partially or completely incontinent, and urine passes through the vagina. A transvaginal surgical repair is possible in most cases.

RECTOVAGINAL FISTULAS

The most common causes of this abnormal communication between the rectum and vagina are infection in the episiotomy, a suture placed through the rectal wall during repair, or an unrecognized rectal injury during parturition or vaginal repair.

Fistulas may form subsequent to extension of cervical cancer or radiation therapy. Trauma-induced fistulas are usually located near the introitus; those induced by cancer tend to be located higher in the reproductive structures. Surgical repair is possible but could be complicated by infection, which delays healing or causes the repair to breakdown. Preoperative preparation is necessarily prolonged to allow for 2 days of liquid diets, enemas, and antibiotic therapy. A temporary colostomy may be indicated before surgical correction of a complicated rectovaginal fistula.

GENERAL NURSING CARE

Nursing care of women with pelvic relaxation problems and fistulas requires sympathetic understanding and encouragement because the women's emotional reactions are often intense. Women with vesicovaginal or rectovaginal fistulas may become withdrawn because of embarrassment about odors and soiling of their clothing beyond their control. The nurse needs to use a very sensitive approach in suggesting hygienic practices that reduce bad odors.

If the woman has a rectovaginal fistula, there is a constant oozing of fecal material into the vagina, which may be temporarily lessened by giving a high enema; preoperatively, the woman is encouraged to do this before going out of the house. A soft rubber catheter is used if enemas are given in the preoperative period and should be directed carefully on the side of the rectum opposite the fistula. Although a constipating diet will give temporary relief by discourage fecal material from entering the vagina through the fistula, Constipation will eventually cause pressure and may possibly aggravate the condition; it may even cause the fistula to enlarge. Therefore the woman is advised against restricting diet and fluids in an effort to control bowel action. After surgery, enemas are contraindicated until healing is complete.

PERIOPERATIVE CARE

It is fruitless to perform surgery until inflammation and induration have subside. This preoperative period may extend to 3 to 4 months. Surgical repair is made through a suprapubic incision into the bladder.

The fistulous tract is then dissected out and closed. In the first postoperative week the woman can expect drainage from the bladder through both a suprapubic and a urethral catheter, usually connected to a suction apparatus set at gentle pressure is mandatory.

- Urinary and vaginal drainage are noted.
- Vaginal douches may be ordered; douching is accomplished gently and with gentle fluid pressure.
- Bed rest or restriction to the hospital room may be needed for several days because the drainage tubes need to be suctioned.
- The nurse is challenged to institute measure to prevent physical complications of immobility (especially pneumonia, D.V.T, constipation) and emotional discomfort from sensory deprivation.
- Repair of fistulas is not always successful, and repeat surgeries may be needed.
- The nurse needs to employ a variety of techniques and understanding patience when a woman's anxiety and irritation are expressed.
- The woman needs encouragement from nursing and medical staff, and she needs assurance that they understand her problem.
- Perineal cleansing is done at least twice daily and after each voiding and defecation.
- Local application of an ice pack helps to reduce swelling and promotes comfort. Ice packs are always covered before application to the skin A disposable glove filled with ice serves as an adequate ice pack and is easily made and inexpensive to use.
- An indwelling catheter attached to continuous drainage may be in place for 24 to 48 hours.
- Urinary output and character of urine are monitored.
- After removal of the catheter, the woman is encouraged to void in the usual way.
- Within 7 to 10 days following surgery, daily vaginal douching with normal saline may be prescribed.
- Whether douches are ordered immediately after surgery or at a late date, sterile equipment and sterile solution is used.

- Discharge planning includes instruction for continued douching at least once per day, following by a tub bath.
- Laxative are to be keep stools soft and prevent constipation to minimize stress on the surgical site.
- The woman is encouraged to follow up her medical care by keeping scheduled appointments.

DISEASES COMPLICATION PREGNANCY

Numerous diseases may complicate pregnancy. The most important of those that affect placental development and function are herein reviewed. With some of these complications of pregnancy, the placental findings may simply be confirmatory of the disease. With others, placental pathology may be the first indication of an abnormality. Despite many reports of diseases that complicate pregnancy, associated placentas are often not examined, or they are not reported in the descriptions. That is unfortunate because those placentas could aid in diagnosis and knowledge of the pathogenesis of these conditions. Moreover, a better understanding of the placenta could allow us better insight into the mechanisms of the effects that certain conditions have on the foetus.

MEDICAL AND SURGICAL CONDITIONS

Virtually any maternal medical or surgical condition can complicate the course of a pregnancy and/or be affected by the pregnancy. In addition, conditions arising in pregnancy can have adverse effects on the mother and/or the foetus. For example, babies born prematurely account for>50% of perinatal morbidity and mortality; an estimated 5% of women will describe bleeding of some extent during pregnancy, and in some patients the bleeding will endanger the mother. Elective major surgery should be avoided during pregnancy. Normal uncomplicated pregnancy does not alter operative risk except as it may interfere with the diagnosis of abdominal disorders and increase the technical problems of intra-abdominal surgery. Abortion is not a serious hazard after operation unless peritoneal sepsis or other significant complications occur. During the first trimester, congenital anomalies may theoretically be induced in the developing foetus by hypoxia.

INFECTIONS

Infections are a part of normal life. We all suffer from the odd coughs and colds, and many women have experienced troublesome thrush (yeast infections) or cystitis. Pregnancy is a time when some infections are more common than usual, and a time when other infections can present a particular risk either to the woman or her unborn baby. This article will review the more common and problematic infections that might affect pregnancy.

Coughs, Colds & Flu

Women are just as likely to get these during pregnancy as outwith this time. They are little threat to the pregnancy itself and all that is needed is symptom relief: lots of fluids, rest and TLC. Inhaled decongestants are safe, but cough linctus should be avoided. It is quite safe to take paracetamol up to normal maximum doses (1g, four times per day). If a cough becomes productive with green phlegm, this may mean a bacterial infection needing antibiotics.

Vaginal Infections

Thrush: Pregnancy makes a woman more likely to get a thrush infection, most commonly caused by the yeast Candida albicans. This yeast is commonly found in the vagina in up to 16% of non-pregnant women and 32% during pregnancy. It does not always cause symptoms and only requires treatment if it causes troublesome itching, soreness or the typical thick, white discharge. It is more common in second and subsequent pregnancies, in the third trimester, during summer months, following a course of antibiotics and in diabetic women. Treatment with Clotrimazole (Canesten) vaginal suppositories is usually effective. The tablet treatment Fluconazole (Diflucan) is not advised during pregnancy.

Men can be affected by thrush, it causing a redness and soreness of the glans of the penis, with a pin-point spotty appearance. Thrush affecting men is a lot less common than for women and it is even less frequent for a man to act as a 'reservior' of infection where the woman keeps getting it back from him. It is not necessary for partner to get treatment unless they have symptoms.

Group B Streptococcus (GBS): Group B streptococcus is a bacterium that around 15-20% of pregnant women carry in the vagina, usually causing no problems at all. In a small number of cases, the bug is passed to the baby during delivery and it can lead to a blood-borne infection or even meningitis. Treatment is usually only advised in one of a number of 'high risk' scenarios. These include: early labour (before 37 weeks), prolonged or early rupture of the membranes, if there is a temperature during labour or if a previous baby has been affected with the condition. The treatment involves antibiotics through a drip during labour - tablet treatment cannot reliably eradicate the infection.

Sexually Transmitted Infections

Both chlamydia and gonorrhoea infections can pass to the baby during delivery causing eye infections. Gonorrhoea is quite rare, occurring in less than 1 per 1000 women. Chlamydia is more common, affecting around 5% of pregnancies. It can also lead to chest infections in the baby or infections of the lining of the womb for the mother after delivery. Both of these infections are treatable during pregnancy but a second swab should be taken afterwards to confirm that they are cleared. It is most important to screen and treat sexual partners, otherwise they will pass the infection back again.

Genitourinary medicine clinics (previously known as STD or VD clinics) have come a long way since the 1970's. They are really sexual health clinics and many young women use them for smear tests, contraceptive advice or any unusual vaginal itch or discharge - not necessarily sexually transmitted. They have facilities not available to GP's, obstetricians or gynaecologists and are the best place to go for any vaginal discharge that proves troublesome to clear. Testing for HIV infection is routine in some hospitals, but is not usual outside of high-risk areas. If lady feel that she may have been at risk, any GUM or hospital clinic will be able to arrange one, often the same day if necessary. HIV infection passes to the baby in about 15% of cases, but this can be reduced to 8% with drug treatment and perhaps even lower with an elective caesarean section, so there is definitely a benefit to knowing for sure.

Urinary Tract (Water) Infections

Urinary tract infections (UTI's) are more common during pregnancy than at other times, mostly because of a slowing down of the urine flow on its way from the kidney to the bladder. Around 1 in 25 women get a UTI during pregnancy, the common symptoms being a discomfort or burning sensation on passing urine, an aching pain over the bladder or needing to pass water very frequently. This last symptom is unfortunately very common in pregnancy anyway and is not very reliable in making the diagnosis. If the infection passes up to the kidneys and into the blood stream (pyelonephritis or septicaemia) it causes loin pain, vomiting, a fever and can even start premature labour.

By treating early UTI's, kidney infections and their complications can be prevented. The infection is diagnosed by looking at the urine under a microscope and seeing if a bug can be grown from the sample. This can also confirm which antibiotic is the best to use. A mild infection is treated with a course of antibiotic tablets for at least a week, but a more severe one would need admission to hospital, intravenous antibiotics and rest. After one UTI, further infections are more common and monthly checks on the urine are suggested to see if one is developing even before symptoms appear.

Genital Herpes

Herpes infections affect about 10% population, though only in one third of cases is an actual diagnosis as such made. It usually presents initially with a flu-like illness, followed by an outbreak of vulval sores, which are very painful and swollen glands in the groin. By a week to 10 days later these have usually healed over. Sometimes the initial attack is mistaken for a thrush infection, just causing an itch or soreness, seemingly responding to cream or pessaries. Occasionally it is completely without symptoms at all. The first (primary) attack is usually the most painful. The herpes virus stays in the nerve in the spine and can reactivate causing a secondary attack. This occurs on average at 3-4 months after the first one, and recurrences return on average 2-3 times per year, but this is extremely variable.

The risk of herpes to pregnancy is greatest if the primary attack occurs after 28 weeks. The mother's initial antibody response can take up to 12 weeks to fully develop. Secondary attacks are much less of a risk. The risk of herpes is passing the infection to the baby at the time of delivery. Primary attacks also can lead to early labour or poor growth. Because of these risks, a caesarean section is usually advised at term if a primary attack occurs during pregnancy after 28 weeks, or if there is an active secondary attack at the time of labour.

Toxoplasmosis

Toxoplasmosis is caused by a parasite called toxoplasma gondii. This is found in different forms in raw meat, within cats that eat raw meat and their faeces. Toxoplasmosis infection is common in both men and women outside of pregnancy, however it is infection during pregnancy that is of most concern as it can lead to infection in the unborn infant: congenital toxoplasmosis. Around 30% of women will have already had a toxoplasma infection before pregnancy. It typically causes a flu-like illness with swollen glands in the neck. Most people are unaware that it was in fact toxoplasmosis.

In only about 30-40% of women who catch toxoplasmosis during pregnancy, does the infection pass to the unborn baby. The actual risk appears to be related to the gestation at which it is acquired. It is greatest in the third trimester at 70%, whereas in early pregnancy only 15% of infants will become infected.

Toxoplasmosis infection may lead to miscarriage, stillbirth, or survival with growth problems, blindness, water on the brain (hydrocephalus), brain damage, epilepsy, or deafness. If a woman is found to have acquired toxoplasmosis during pregnancy, she will be offered an ultrasound scan to look for signs of foetal infection. After 20 weeks gestation, she may be offered a definitive test - cordocentesis. This involves a scan and blood sample being taken from the umbilical cord.

Although toxoplasmosis is quite serious when it occurs, it is relatively rare. Women with cats do not need to get rid of them when they become pregnant; it is just necessary to take a few precautions. Be sure to only eat meat that has been cooked right through. Wash hands, cooking utensils and food surfaces after preparing raw meat and wash all the soil from fruit and vegetables before eating. Keep raw meat and cooked foods on separate plates. If possible get someone else to clean out the dirty cat litter or use gloves and wash hands afterwards. Always use gloves when gardening and wash hands afterwards.

Chicken Pox

It's not uncommon for women who are pregnant to come into contact with someone who has chicken pox. This can cause great worry, but it is uncommon for there to be a problem. Firstly, if lady have definitely had chicken pox before, there is no risk to the baby. In any case, even if lady doesn't recall having had chicken pox, it is likely you have antibodies (80% do) from a silent infection. Sometimes the laboratory can use the stored blood taken at booking to speed this up.

Risks to the baby are important at the following two times, only if mum gets chicken pox:

- Before 20 weeks - risk of chicken-pox syndrome. This is actually quite rare. Up until 14 weeks the risk is about 0.4%, whereas between 14-20 weeks it is 2%. If a woman has VZ-Ig treatment after being exposed, the risk is even lower.
- Mum's rash developing within a week before delivery to a month afterwards. It takes about a week for mum to pass the protective antibodies to the baby, so if born before that time, the baby is at risk of overwhelming infection after birth.

Between 20 weeks and term there is no risk to the baby. VZ-Ig is a form of antibody treatment that can reduce the risk of chicken-pox syndrome and should be given by 10 days after the initial attack.

GYNAECOLOGICAL DISEASES COMPLICATING PREGNANCY

Disorders that affect the female reproductive system are called gynecologic disorders. Breast disorders are often also considered gynecologic disorders.

Preventive healthcare includes having regular gynecologic examinations, even when no symptoms are present, and screening tests. Screening tests are done before people have any symptoms to check for disorders that can be prevented or treated effectively if recognized early. Women should have a gynecologic evaluation every year starting at about age 13 to 15. For all women who are sexually active, the evaluation should include a pelvic examination. For younger women who are not sexually active, this evaluation may not include a pelvic examination. Beginning about 3 years after first vaginal intercourse or at age 21, the pelvic examination should include cervical cytology testing (such as a Papanicolaou or Pap test) to detect precancerous changes of the cervix.

For gynecologic care, a woman should choose a health care practitioner with whom she can comfortably discuss sensitive topics, such as sex, birth control, pregnancy, and problems related to menopause. The practitioner may be a gynaecologist, an internist, a nurse-midwife, or a general, family, or nurse practitioner.

Gynecologic evaluation of young and teenage girls can sometimes be done by their pediatrician. However, if the pediatrician cannot set aside time for the girl to speak privately about personal concerns or is reluctant to provide gynecologic care, another health care practitioner should be found for this care.

The gynecologic visit is the time to ask the practitioner questions about reproductive and sexual function and anatomy, including safe sex practices, such as the use of condoms to minimize the risks of sexually transmitted infections.

PREGNANCY INDUCED HYPERTENSION & DIABETES, TOXEMIA OF PREGNANCY, HYDRAMNIOS

Pregnancy-induced Hypertension (PIH)

Pregnancy-induced hypertension (PIH) is a form of high blood pressure in pregnancy. It occurs in about 5 percent to 8 percent of all pregnancies. Another type of high blood pressure is chronic hypertension - high blood pressure that is present before pregnancy begins. Pregnancy-induced hypertension is also called toxemia or preeclampsia. It occurs most often in young women with a first pregnancy. It is more common in twin pregnancies, in women with chronic hypertension, preexisting diabetes, and in women who had PIH in a previous pregnancy.

Usually, there are three primary characteristics of this condition, including the following:

- High blood pressure (a blood pressure reading higher than 140/90 mm Hg, or a significant increase in one or both pressures).
- Protein in the urine.
- Edema (swelling).

Eclampsia is a severe form of pregnancy-induced hypertension. Women with eclampsia have seizures resulting from the condition. Eclampsia occurs in about one in 1, 600 pregnancies and develops near the end of pregnancy, in most cases. HELLP syndrome is a complication of severe preeclampsia or eclampsia. HELLP syndrome is a group of physical changes including the breakdown of red blood cells, changes in the liver, and low platelets (cells found in the blood that are needed to help the blood to clot in order to control bleeding).

Causes

The cause of PIH is unknown. Some conditions may increase the risk of developing PIH, including the following:

- Pre-existing hypertension (high blood pressure)
- Kidney disease
- diabetes
- PIH with a previous pregnancy
- Mother's age younger than 20 or older than 40
- Multiple fetuses (twins, triplets)

With high blood pressure, there is an increase in the resistance of blood vessels. This may hinder blood flow in many different organ systems in the expectant mother including the liver, kidneys, brain, uterus, and placenta. There are other problems that may develop as a result of PIH. Placental abruption (premature detachment of the placenta from the uterus) may occur in some pregnancies. PIH can also lead to foetal problems including intrauterine growth restriction (poor foetal growth) and stillbirth.

If untreated, severe PIH may cause dangerous seizures and even death in the mother and foetus. Because of these risks, it may be necessary for the baby to be delivered early, before 37 weeks gestation.

Symptoms

The following are the most common symptoms of high blood pressure in pregnancy. However, each woman may experience symptoms differently. Symptoms may include:

- Increased blood pressure
- Protein in the urine
- Edema (swelling)
- Sudden weight gain
- Visual changes such as blurred or double vision
- Nausea, vomiting
- Right-sided upper abdominal pain or pain around the stomach
- Urinating small amounts
- Changes in liver or kidney function tests

Diagnosis

Diagnosis is often based on the increase in blood pressure levels, but other symptoms may help establish PIH as the diagnosis. Tests for pregnancy-induced hypertension may include the following:

- Blood pressure measurement
- Urine testing
- Assessment of edema
- Frequent weight measurements
- Eye examination to check for retinal changes
- Liver and kidney function tests
- Blood clotting tests

Treatment

Specific treatment for pregnancy-induced hypertension will be determined by the physician based on:

- Pregnancy, overall health, and medical history
- Extent of the disease
- Tolerance for specific medications, procedures, or therapies

- Expectations for the course of the disease
- Opinion or preference

The goal of treatment is to prevent the condition from becoming worse and to prevent it from causing other complications. Treatment for pregnancy-induced hypertension (PIH) may include:

- Bed-rest (either at home or in the hospital may be recommended).
- Hospitalization (as specialized personnel and equipment may be necessary).
- Magnesium sulfate (or other antihypertensive medications for PIH).
- Foetal monitoring (to check the health of the foetus when the mother has PIH) may include:
  - — Foetal movement counting - keeping track of foetal kicks and movements. A change in the number or frequency may mean the foetus is under stress.
  - — Nonstress testing - a test that measures the foetal heart rate in response to the foetus' movements.
  - — Biophysical profile - a test that combines nonstress test with ultrasound to observe the foetus.
  - — Doppler flow studies - type of ultrasound that uses sound waves to measure the flow of blood through a blood vessel.
- Continued laboratory testing of urine and blood (for changes that may signal worsening of PIH).
- Medications, called corticosteroids, that may help mature the lungs of the foetus (lung immaturity is a major problem of premature babies).
- Delivery of the baby (if treatments do not control PIH or if the foetus or mother is in danger). Caesarean delivery may be recommended, in some cases.

Early identification of women at risk for pregnancy-induced hypertension may help prevent some complications of the disease. Education about the warning symptoms is also important because early recognition may help women receive treatment and prevent worsening of the disease.

Toxemia of Pregnancy

Pregnancy toxemia is caused by the sudden extra demand for energy by the fast-growing kids or lambs in the last few weeks of pregnancy. Seventy percent of foetal growth occurs during the last few weeks. The disease is not normally observed in ewes carrying singles. It is usually seen when the ewe is carrying two or more lambs. Does and ewes that are too fat often will experience pregnancy toxemia. At the time when the kids or lambs are growing very rapidly, increasing amounts of space and energy are needed, in addition to the protein and energy needed for maintenance of the doe or ewe. The increase in feedstuffs high in energy must be supplied on a daily basis. Does or ewes consuming large amounts of hay need a greater internal space in the rumen, which causes decreasing space for growth of the kids or lambs in the uterus. In meeting the nutritional needs of the kids or lambs, the doe or ewe will metabolize or break down fat resources from her body to maintain pregnancy. This rapid breakdown of body stores of energy produces ketones (a toxic by-product) and lady soon observe the symptoms of the disease. Maintaining does or ewes in a medium body condition rather than overly fat condition early in pregnancy will help keep down the disease.

Transmission

Pregnancy toxemia is not a transmittable disease from one doe or ewe to another, however, flocks or herds experiencing the disease may appear to be infectious because the plane of nutrition and management throughout pregnancy is similar. This shortage of energy in the diet may cause these symptoms in several does or ewes, especially those carrying twins or triplets.

Treatment and Prevention

The treatment of pregnancy toxemia is usually unsuccessful. Providing energy in the form of molasses or syrup generally does not suffice. Treatment with propylene glycol at 60 to 90 ml (2 to 3 oz) twice daily may help. Caesarean section to deliver the kids or lambs early will sometimes save the doe or ewe and the kids or lambs if they are near term. Corticosteroids may be used to abort the doe or ewe to prevent the loss of the dam. Kids or lambs will die shortly following the diagnosis of pregnancy toxemia due to lack of nutritional transfer from the doe or ewe to them. The sooner the kids or lambs are born, the less likely the doe or ewe will die.

Grain is a high source of available energy. Feeding 1-2 lbs. of grain daily along with high quality legume hay during the last four to six weeks of pregnancy will help prevent pregnancy toxemia. If the does or ewes are large, it may be necessary to increase the grain from 50% to 100%. Feeding grain first and having ample space at the feeders for each doe or ewe to get her share of the grain followed by hay feeding may help. Protein requirements should also be balanced, but protein level in the feed is not related to pregnancy toxemia. Exercising the doe or ewe is quite helpful especially in the cold winter months when feeding is in drylot. Hay can be placed in feeders quite a distance from the barn to force the does or ewes to walk to the feed to increase their exercise.

Hydramnios

Hydramnios is a condition in which there is too much amniotic fluid around the foetus. It occurs in about 3 to 4 percent of all pregnancies. It is also called polyhydramnios. Severe hydramnios may signal a problem with the foetus, such as a central nervous system or gastrointestinal defect. In rare cases, it can lead to early labour or even foetal death. Mild hydramnios is more common, and doesn't signal a problem. In fact, extra fluid that appears during the second trimester is likely to return to a normal range without treatment.

Causes

There are several causes of hydramnios. Generally, either too much fluid is being produced or there is a problem with the fluid being taken up, or both. Factors that are associated with hydramnios include the following:

Maternal factors:

- Diabetes- If lady have diabetes and having trouble managing it properly, you can end up with high fluid levels. She will probably be given a glucose test to see if diabetes is the cause. Such cases are usually mild and relatively easy to resolve by getting the diabetes under control.

Foetal factors:

- Gastrointestinal abnormalities that block the passage of fluid.
- Abnormal swallowing due to problems with the central nervous system, such as neural tube defects or chromosomal abnormalities.
- Twin-to-twin transfusion syndrome- Polyhydramnios is especially likely in the case of twin-to-twin transfusion syndrome, where the donor twin may suffer from too little amniotic fluid, while the recipient twin is creating too much.

- Heart failure.
- Congenital infection (acquired in pregnancy).

Symptoms

The following are the most common symptoms of hydramnios. However, each woman may experience symptoms differently. Symptoms may include:

- Rapid growth of uterus
- Unusual discomfort in the abdomen - due to the extra pressure
- Wild fluctuations in weight;
- Increased back pain;
- Extreme swelling in feet and ankles
- Uterine contractions

The symptoms of hydramnios may resemble other medical conditions. Always consult physician for a diagnosis. In women with oligohydramnios, it is particularly important to not smoke, get a very good diet, rest a bit more and observe and report any signs or symptoms of preterm labour.

Diagnosis

In addition to a complete medical history and a physical examination, hydramnios is usually diagnosed with ultrasound by measuring pockets of fluid to estimate the total volume. A score of 25 centimetres (cm) or above is considered high. A normal score for the third trimester is 5 to 25 cm. In some cases, ultrasound is also helpful in finding a cause of hydramnios, such as multiple pregnancy or a birth defect.

Treatment

Specific treatment for hydramnios will be determined by physician based on:

- Pregnancy, overall health, and medical history
- Extent of the condition
- Tolerance for specific medications, procedures, or therapies
- Expectations for the course of the condition
- Opinion or preference

Treatment for hydramnios may include:

- Close monitoring the amount of amniotic fluid and frequent follow-up visits with the physician

- Medication. In certain cases, doctor may prescribe a prostaglandin inhibitor like Indomethacin, which has been shown to reduce the baby's urine output.
- Amnioreduction - amniocentesis to remove some of the amniotic fluid; this procedure may need to be repeated.
- Delivery: Once labour begins, the large gush of fluid leaving the uterus means having an increased risk of placental abruption or umbilical cord prolapse. Both of these problems can cut off the baby's oxygen supply and may require an emergency caesarean section.

The goal of treatment is to relieve the mother's discomfort and continue the pregnancy.

RH INCOMPATIBILITY

Rh incompatibility is an important factor which often leads to various pregnancy complications and so, if lady come to know about her pregnancy, then, she should go through some blood tests in order to confirm the Rh factor. The blood tests will determine blood type and Rh factor. People with different blood types have different protein ratio on the surfaces of their red blood cells. There are four blood types- A, B, AB and O. Each of these four blood types is again classified on the basis of the presence of another protein on the surface of the red blood cell and this classification indicates the Rh factor. Those who have this additional protein, they are Rh positive.

Rh incompatibility refers to that problematic situation when a child is born to a couple of having opposite Rh factors. If a Rh negative woman and a Rh positive man conceive a baby, then, the baby usually suffers from various health problems. Most of the children born to Rh negative mother and Rh positive father are Rh positive. It is important to note that Rh incompatibility is not a danger in case of mother's first pregnancy. In this case, the blood of the foetus does not normally enter the mother's circulatory system during pregnancy.

But, there is a chance of intermingling of the mother's blood with the baby's at the time of delivery. And, if it happens, then, the mother's body would recognize the Rh protein as foreign substance and would start producing antibodies against the Rh proteins introduced in the mother's blood.

Rh incompatibility can also occur when an Rh negative pregnant woman gets exposed to the Rh protein in course of blood transfusions at the time of miscarriage and Ectopic pregnancy. But, today Rh incompatibility can be handled with proper medicine. The woman with the potentiality of developing Rh incompatibility is given two Rh immune-globuline shots during her first pregnancy.

The first one is given on 28th week of pregnancy and the second one is given within 72 hours of delivery. These shots act as vaccine and prevent the growth of antibodies in the mother's body and thereby reduce the chance of complications in the newborn and also in case of future pregnancies.

MENTAL DISORDERS

Many pregnant women experience psychiatric disorders in their childbearing years. Emerging research shows mental illness not only affects the mother's well-being but may also have significant effects on foetal outcomes. This review details what is known about the prevalence of mental illness during pregnancy as well as how such disorders may influence pregnancy outcomes. Maternal depression during pregnancy is an independent risk factor for low foetal birth weight and premature delivery, but other illnesses, such as anxiety disorders, eating disorders and psychotic illness, may also predict adverse birth outcomes. Possible behavioral, genetic and neuroendocrine mechanisms for these relationships are presented. Principles of treatment for psychiatric disorders during pregnancy are also discussed, with an emphasis on the role of the obstetrical provider.

Since the majority of these illnesses start before or during the child-bearing years, many pregnant women have significant psychiatric comorbidity. Most research has focused on the impact of stress, anxiety and depression on the developing foetus, but newer studies indicate that a wide variety of mental disorders can pose a risk for adverse pregnancy outcomes. In order to make appropriate decisions regarding whether, and how, to treat psychiatric symptoms during pregnancy, providers must understand what is known about the impact of untreated illness on the pregnancy and weigh these risks against potential risks from psychiatric medications used for treatment.

Preterm delivery (PTD) and low birth weight (LBW) continue to be significant risk factors for foetal and infant death and complications. If mental health affects timing of delivery or foetal growth there might be new approaches to improving perinatal outcomes. Despite widespread recognition that postpartum depression and postpartum psychosis present substantial risks for infant and child outcomes, the impact of antenatal mental illness on the foetus is less well understood. This review summarizes how psychiatric illness during pregnancy affects foetal outcomes and how obstetrical practitioners might use this information to provide optimal patient care.

The review also highlights the current research and gaps in understanding relationships between mental health and pregnancy outcomes and proposes key areas where additional research is needed.

ADOLESCENT PREGNANCY, ELDERLY PRIMI AND GRAND MULTIPARE

Child marriages are still prevalent today in India the results of which are girls becoming mothers in their teens. In addition to that, the recent spate of incidents of rape on minors and the rising levels of promiscuity among teenagers are also a cause of great concern as they lead to teenage pregnancies.

Also known as adolescent pregnancy, teenage pregnancy is one that occurs from puberty to the age of 19. Puberty is the stage of adolescence when a girl can sexually reproduce, however a young woman can become pregnant even before her first menstrual cycle. This is because ovulation, the release of an egg from the ovary, may occur before the first period. In the absence of adequate contraception the egg can become fertilized. And this is quite common in teenagers, as most of them do not use any birth control measures like condoms when they have sexual intercourse. Our own study conducted on 400 college students of Mumbai showed that most of the sexually active girls start worrying about contraceptives only after 6 months of sexual activity.

For a woman including a teenager to conceive it is not necessary that actual penetration takes place. This is because sperm can travel upwards from its presence in the area of the external genital area and result in pregnancy. It is therefore very important for teenagers to have proper knowledge and understanding of their body and its functions before they become sexually active. Responsible sexual behaviour prevents pregnancy.

Whether the pregnancy is due to marriage or sex between unmarried teenagers there are nevertheless some issues concerning the higher rates of nutritional and obstetric problems associated with adolescent pregnancy. Also, the ignorance and immaturity can result in higher morbidity and mortality among mothers and babies.

SYMPTOMS OF PREGNANCY

The symptoms of a teenage pregnancy are not different from a normal pregnancy. They include:

- Missed period
- Fatigue
- Nausea/vomiting
- Breast enlargement and breast tenderness
- Irregular vaginal spotting or bleeding
- Stomach cramping
- Increased drowsiness and moodiness

In spite of experiencing these symptoms many teenagers do not tell anyone and as such often go unnoticed by friends and family. Unfortunately, the teenager with irregular periods may not even realize that she is pregnant until well into the fifth month of pregnancy - when she starts feeling the baby's movements.

DIAGNOSIS

Any teenage girl who experiences irregular or absent periods or any of the symptoms is advised to undergo a pregnancy test. This should be done by the doctor even if she does not admit to have had sexual intercourse. An early diagnosis of pregnancy helps the teenager to adjust emotionally and physically. Also, early prenatal care is essential.

Usually, pregnancy is associated with weight gain but if nausea and vomiting are significant there could be weight loss. Further, pelvic examination by a gynaecologist may reveal bluish or purple colouration of vaginal walls, bluish or purple colouration and softening of the cervix, and softening and enlargement of the uterus. Finally, an ultrasound may be done to confirm the presence and current status of the pregnancy.

CAUSE FACTORS

The ultimate "cause" of teenage pregnancy is unprotected intercourse. A sexually active teenager who does not use contraception has a 90% chance of becoming pregnant within one year. Potential behaviour patterns for a teenage girl becoming pregnant include:

- Early dating behaviour
- High-risk behaviours (smoking, alcohol and substance abuse)
- Lack of a support group or few friends

- Unhealthy environment at home
- Stress and depression
- Delinquency/criminal behaviour
- Living in a community where early childbearing is common and viewed as the norm rather than as a cause for concern
- Exposure to domestic or sexual violence
- And most important, financial constraints

MULTIPLE PREGNANCY

Multiple pregnancy is a pregnancy with two or more fetuses. Names for these include the following:

- Twins - 2 fetuses
- Triplets - 3 fetuses
- Quadruplets - 4 fetuses
- Quintuplets - 5 fetuses
- Sextuplets - 6 fetuses
- Septuplets - 7 fetuses

While multiples account for only a small percentage of all births (about 3 percent), the multiple birth rate is rising.

CAUSES

There are many factors related to having a multiple pregnancy. Naturally occurring factors include the following:

- Heredity: A family history of multiple pregnancy increases the chances of having twins.
- Older age: Women over 30 have a greater chance of multiple conception. Many women today are delaying childbearing until later in life, and may have twins as a result.
- High parity: Having one or more previous pregnancies, especially a multiple pregnancy, increases the chances of having multiples.
- Race: African-American women are more likely to have twins than any other race. Asian and Native Americans have the lowest twinning rates. Caucasian women, especially those over age 35, have the highest rate of higher-order multiple births (triplets or more).

Other factors that have greatly increased the multiple birth rate in recent years include reproductive technologies, including the following:

- Ovulation-stimulating medications such as clomiphene citrate and follicle stimulating hormone (FSH) help produce many eggs, which, if fertilized, can result in multiple babies.
- Assisted reproductive technologies such as in vitro fertilization (IVF) and other techniques help couples conceive. These technologies often use ovulation-stimulating medications to produce multiple eggs which are then fertilized and returned to the uterus to develop.

Multiple pregnancy usually occurs when more than one egg is fertilized and implants in the uterus. This is called fraternal twinning and can produce boys, girls, or a combination of both. Fraternal multiples are simply siblings conceived at the same time. However, just as siblings often look alike, fraternal multiples may look very similar. Fraternal multiples each have a separate placenta and amniotic sac.

Sometimes, one egg is fertilized and then divides into two or more embryos. This is called identical twinning and produces all boys, or all girls. Identical multiples are genetically identical, and usually look so much alike that even parents have a hard time telling them apart. However, these children have different personalities and are distinct individuals. Identical multiples may have individual placentas and amniotic sacs, but most share a placenta with separate sacs. Rarely, identical twins share one placenta and a single amniotic sac. Being pregnant with more than one baby is exciting and is often a happy event for many couples. However, multiple pregnancy has increased risks for complications.

SYMPTOMS

The following are the most common symptoms of multiple pregnancy. However, each woman may experience symptoms differently. Symptoms of multiple pregnancy may include:

- Uterus is larger than expected for the dates in pregnancy
- Increased morning sickness
- Increased appetite
- Excessive weight gain, especially in early pregnancy
- Foetal movements felt in different parts of abdomen at same time

DIAGNOSIS

Many women suspect they are pregnant with more than one baby, especially if they have been pregnant before. Diagnosis of multiple fetuses may be made early in pregnancy, especially if reproductive technologies have been used. In addition to a complete medical history and physical examination, diagnosis may be made by:

- Pregnancy blood testing: Levels of human chorionic gonadotrophin (hCG) may be quite high with multiple pregnancy.
- Alpha-fctoprotein: Levels of a protein released by the foetal liver and found in the mother's blood may be high when more than one foetus is making the protein.
- Ultrasound - a diagnostic imaging technique which uses high-frequency sound waves and a computer to create images of blood vessels, tissues, and organs. Ultrasounds are used to view internal organs as they function, and to assess blood flow through various vessels - with a vaginal transducer, especially in early pregnancy, or with an abdominal transducer in later pregnancy.

MANAGEMENT

Specific management for multiple pregnancy will be determined by physician based on:

- Pregnancy, overall health, and medical history
- Number of fetuses
- Tolerance for specific medications, procedures, or therapies
- Expectations for the course of the pregnancy
- Opinion or preference

DELIVERY

Delivery of multiples depends on many factors including the foetal positions, gestational age, and health of mother and fetuses. Generally, in twins, if both fetuses are in the vertex (head-down) position and there are no other complications, a vaginal delivery is possible. If the first foetus is vertex, but the second is not, the first foetus may be delivered vaginally, then the second is either turned to the vertex position or delivered breech (buttocks are presented first). These procedures can increase the risk for problems such as prolapsed cord (when the cord slips down through the cervical opening). Emergency caesarean birth of the second foetus may be needed. Usually, if the first foetus is not vertex, both babies are delivered by caesarean. Most triplets and other higher-order multiples are born by caesarean.

Vaginal delivery may take place in an operating room because of the greater risks for complications during birth and the need for caesarean delivery. Caesarean delivery is usually needed for fetuses that are in abnormal positions, for certain medical conditions of the mother, and for foetal distress.

CARE

Because many multiples are small and born early, they may be initially cared for in a special care nursery called the neonatal intensive care unit (NICU). Once babies are able to feed, grow, and stay warm, they can usually be discharged. Other babies, that are healthy at birth, may need only a brief check in a special care nursery.

Breastfeeding multiples is certainly possible and many mothers of twins and even triplets are successful in breastfeeding all of their babies. Lactation specialists can help mothers of multiples learn techniques for breastfeeding their babies separately and together, and to increase their milk supply. Mothers whose babies are unable to breastfeed because they are sick or premature can pump their breast milk and store the milk for later feedings.

Families with more than one baby need help from family and friends. The first two months are usually the most difficult as everyone learns to cope with frequent feedings, lack of sleep, and little personal time. Having help for household chores and daily tasks can allow the mother the time she needs to get to know her babies, for feedings, and for rest and recovery from delivery.

ABNORMALITIES OF PLACENTA & CORD

There are two major placental abnormalities. Placenta previa is a condition that occurs during pregnancy when the placenta is abnormally placed, and partially or totally covers the cervix. Placental abruption occurs when the placenta separates from the wall of the uterus prior to the birth of the baby. This can result in severe, uncontrollable bleeding (haemorrhage). The uterus is the muscular organ that contains the developing baby during pregnancy. The lowest segment of the uterus is a narrowed portion called the cervix. This cervix has an opening (the os) that leads into the vagina, or birth canal. The placenta is the organ that attaches to the wall of the uterus during pregnancy. The placenta allows nutrients and oxygen from the mother's blood circulation to pass into the developing baby (the foetus) via the umbilicalcord.

During labour, the muscles of the uterus contract repeatedly. This allows the cervix to begin to grow thinner (called effacement) and more open (dilatation). Eventually, the cervix will become completely effaced and dilated, and the baby can leave the uterus and enter the birth canal. Under normal circumstances, the baby will emerge through the mother's vagina during birth. In placenta previa, the placenta develops in an abnormal location. Normally, the placenta should develop relatively high up in the uterus, on the front or back wall. In about 1 in 200 births, the placenta will be located low in the uterus, partially or totally covering the os. This causes particular problems in late pregnancy, when the lower part of the uterus begins to take on a new formation in preparation for delivery. As the cervix begins to efface and dilate, the attachments of the placenta to the uterus are damaged, resulting in bleeding.

During a normal labour and delivery, the baby is born first. Several minutes to 30 minutes later, the placenta separates from the wall of the uterus and is delivered. This sequence is necessary because the baby relies on the placenta to provide oxygen until he or she begins to breathe independently. Placental abruption occurs when the placenta separates from the uterus before the birth of the baby. Placental abruption occurs in about 1 out of every 200 deliveries. African American and Latin-American women have a greater risk of this complication than do Caucasian women. It was once believed that the risk of placental abruption increased in women who gave birth to many children, but this association is still being researched.

While the actual cause of placenta previa is unknown, certain factors increase the risk of a woman developing the condition. These factors include:

- Having abnormalities of the uterus
- Being older in age
- Having had other babies
- Having a prior delivery by caesarean section
- Smoking cigarettes.

When a pregnancy involves more than one baby (twins, triplets, etc.), the placenta will be considerably larger than for a single pregnancy.

This also increases the chance of placenta previa. Placenta previa may cause a number of problems. It is thought to be responsible for about 5% of all miscarriages. It frequently causes very light bleeding(spotting) early in pregnancy. Sometime after 28 weeks of pregnancy (most pregnancies last about 40 weeks), placenta previa can cause episodes of significant bleeding. Usually, the bleeding occurs suddenly and is bright red. The woman rarely experiences any accompanying pain, although about 10% of the time the placenta may begin separating from the uterine wall (called abruptio placentae), resulting in pain. The bleeding usually stops on its own. About 25%of such patients will go into labour sometime in the next several days. Sometimes, placenta previa does not cause bleeding until labour has already begun. Placenta previa puts both the mother and the foetus at high risk. The mother is at risk of severe and uncontrollable bleeding (haemorrhage), with dangerous blood loss. If the mother's bleeding is quite severe, this puts the foetus at risk of becoming oxygen deprived. The foetus' only source of oxygen is the mother's blood. The mother's blood loss, coupled with certain changes that take place in response to that blood loss, decreases the amount of blood going to the placenta, and ultimately to the foetus. Furthermore, placenta previa increases the risk of preterm labour, and the possibility that the baby will be delivered prematurely.

The cause of placental abruption is unknown. However, a number of risk factors have been identified. These factors include:

- Older age of the mother
- History of placental abruption during a previous pregnancy
- High blood pressure
- Certain disease states (diabetes, collagen vascular diseases)
- The presence of a type of utérine tumor called aleiomyoma
- Twins, triplets, or other multiple pregnancies
- Cigarette smoking
- Heavy alcohol use
- Cocaine use
- Malformations of the uterus
- Malformations of the placenta
- Injury to the abdomen (as might occur in a car accident).

Treatment of placenta previa depends on how far along in the pregnancy the bleeding occurs. When the pregnancy is less than 36 weeks along, the foetus is not sufficiently developed to allow delivery without a high risk of complications. Therefore, a woman with placenta previa is treated with bed rest, blood transfusions as necessary, and medications to prevent labour. After 36 weeks, the baby can be delivered via caesarean section. This is almost always the preferred method of delivery in order to avoid further bleeding from the low-lying placenta. The first line of treatment for placental abruption involves replacing the mother's lost blood with blood transfusions and fluids given through a needle in a vein. Oxygen will be administered, usually by a mask or through tubes leading to the nose. When the placental separation is severe, treatment may require prompt delivery of the baby. However, delivery may be delayed when the placental separation is not as severe, and when the foetus is too immature to insure a healthy baby if delivered. The baby is delivered vaginally when possible. However, a caesarean section may be performed to deliver the baby more quickly if the abruption is quite severe or if the baby is in distress.

INTRA-UTERINE GROWTH RETARDATION

Intrauterine growth restriction (IUGR) is a term used to describe a condition in which the foetus is smaller than expected for the number of weeks of pregnancy. Another term for IUGR is foetal growth restriction. Newborn babies with IUGR are often described as small for gestational age (SGA). A foetus with IUGR often has an estimated foetal weight less than the 10th percentile. This means that the foetus weighs less than 90 percent of all other fetuses of the same gestational age. A foetus with IUGR also may be born at term (after 37 weeks of pregnancy) or prematurely (before 37 weeks).

Newborn babies with IUGR often appear thin, pale, and have loose, dry skin. The umbilical cord is often thin and dull-looking rather than shiny and fat. Babies with IUGR sometimes have a wide-eyed look. Some babies do not have this malnourished appearance but are small all-over.

CAUSES

Intrauterine growth restriction results when a problem or abnormality prevents cells and tissues from growing or causes cells to decrease in size. This may occur when the foetus does not receive the necessary nutrients and oxygen needed for growth and development of organs and tissues, or because of infection. Although some babies are small because of genetics (their parents are small), most IUGR is due to other causes. Some factors that may contribute to IUGR include the following:

- Maternal factors:
  - — High blood pressure
  - — Chronic kidney disease
  - — Advanced diabetes
  - — Heart or respiratory disease
  - — Malnutrition, anaemia
  - — Infection
  - — Substance abuse (alcohol, drugs)
  - — Cigarette smoking
- Factors involving the uterus and placenta:
  - — Decreased blood flow in the uterus and placenta
  - — Placental abruption (placenta detaches from the uterus)
  - — Placenta previa (placenta attaches low in the uterus)
  - — Infection in the tissues around the foetus
- Factors related to the developing baby (foetus):
  - — Multiple gestation (twins, triplets, etc.)
  - — Infection
  - — Birth defects
  - — Chromosomal abnormality

IUGR can begin at any time in pregnancy. Early-onset IUGR is often due to chromosomal abnormalities, maternal disease, or severe problems with the placenta. Late-onset growth restriction (after 32 weeks) is usually related to other problems.

With IUGR, the growth of the baby's overall body and organs are limited, and tissue and organ cells may not grow as large or as numerous. When there is not enough blood flow through the placenta, the foetus may only receive low amounts of oxygen. This can cause the foetal heart rate to decrease placing the baby at great risk.

Babies with IUGR may have problems at birth including:

- Decreased oxygen levels
- Low Apgar scores (an assessment that helps identify babies with difficulty adapting after delivery)
- Meconium aspiration (inhalation of the first stools passed in utero), which can lead to difficulty breathing
- Hypoglycemia (low blood sugar)
- Difficulty maintaining normal body temperature
- Polycythemia (too many red blood cells)

Severe IUGR may result in stillbirth. It may also lead to long-term growth problems in babies and children.

DIAGNOSIS

During pregnancy, foetal size can be estimated in different ways. The height of the fundus (the top of a mother's uterus) can be measured from the pubic bone. This measurement in centimetres usually corresponds with the number of weeks of pregnancy after the 20th week. If the measurement is low for the number of weeks, the baby may be smaller than expected.

Other diagnostic procedures may include the following:

- Ultrasound: Ultrasound (a test using sound waves to create a picture of internal structures) is a more accurate method of estimating foetal size. Measurements can be taken of the foetus' head and abdomen and compared with a growth chart to estimate foetal weight. The foetal abdominal circumference is a helpful indicator of foetal nutrition.
- Doppler flow: Another way to interpret and diagnose IUGR during pregnancy is Doppler flow, which use sound waves to measure blood flow. The sound of moving blood produces wave-forms that reflect the speed and amount of the blood as it moves through a blood vessel. Blood vessels in the foetal brain and the umbilical cord blood flow can be checked with Doppler flow studies.
- Mother's weight gain: A mother's weight gain can also indicate a baby's size. Small maternal weight gains in pregnancy may correspond with a small baby.

MANAGEMENT

Management of IUGR depends on the severity of growth restriction, and how early the problem began in the pregnancy. Generally, the earlier and more severe the growth restriction, the greater the risks to the foetus. Careful monitoring of a foetus with IUGR and ongoing testing may be needed.

Some of the ways to watch for potential problems include the following:

- Foetal movement counting - keeping track of foetal kicks and movements. A change in the number or frequency may mean the foetus is under stress.

- Nonstress testing - a test that watches the foetal heart rate for increases with foetal movements, a sign of foetal well-being.
- Biophysical profile - a test that combines the nonstress test with an ultrasound to evaluate foetal well-being.
- Ultrasound - a diagnostic imaging technique which uses high-frequency sound waves and a computer to create images of blood vessels, tissues, and organs. Ultrasounds are used to view internal organs as they function, and to assess blood flow through various vessels. Ultrasounds are used to follow foetal growth.
- Doppler flow studies - a type of ultrasound which use sound waves to measure blood flow.

TREATMENT

Although it is not possible to reverse IUGR, some treatments may help slow or minimize the effects. Specific treatments for IUGR will be determined by physician based on:

- Pregnancy, overall health, and medical history
- The extent of the disease
- Tolerance for specific medications, procedures, or therapies
- Expectations for the course of the disease
- Opinion or preference

Treatments may include:

- Nutrition: Some studies have shown that increasing maternal nutrition may increase gestational weight gain and foetal growth.
- Bedrest: Bedrest in the hospital or at home may help improve circulation to the foetus.
- Delivery: If IUGR endangers the health of the foetus, then an early delivery may be necessary.

Intrauterine growth restriction may occur, even when the mother is in good health. However, some factors may increase the risks of IUGR, such as cigarette smoking and poor maternal nutrition. Avoiding harmful lifestyles, eating a healthy diet, and getting prenatal care may help decrease the risks for IUGR. Early detection may also help with IUGR treatment and outcome.

NURSING MANAGEMENT OF MOTHERS WITH HIGH-RISK PREGNANCY

A pregnancy that has maternal or foetal complications requiring special medical attention or bed rest is considered to be high-risk. Complications, as used here, mean that the risk of illness or death before or after delivery is greater than normal for the mother or baby. Risk factors in pregnancy are those findings discovered during prenatal assessment that are known to have a potentially negative effect on the outcome of the pregnancy, either for the woman or the foetus. This evaluation determines whether or not the mother has characteristics or conditions that make her or her baby more likely to become sick or die during the pregnancy.

CAUSES AND SYMPTOMS

All risk factors do not threaten pregnancy to the same extent. The risk of complications is increased by smoking, poor nutritional habits, drug and alcohol abuse, domestic violence, prepregnancy maternal health status, psychosocial factors, prior health care, the presence of chronic medical problems in the mother, past history of repeated preterm delivery, multiple gestation, and abnormalities of the foetus or placenta. A woman with a high-risk pregnancy may have an earlier labour and delivery depending upon the foetal or maternal complication present and, likewise, present with symptoms dependent on the condition. Since the placenta supplies the baby with its nutrients and oxygen, any condition that threatens the blood supply to it threatens foetal development.

The threat of a preterm delivery is the most common reason for a referral to a perinatal centre, which is linked to obstetric and newborn services that provide the highest level of care for a pregnant woman and her baby. A preterm delivery may occur because of a premature rupture of membranes (the bag of water surrounding the baby breaks) or preterm labour. There is a strong correlation of vaginal or uterine infection with the pregnant woman's water breaking, and there are lab tests that can be predictive of a woman's risk of experiencing preterm labour.

According to a 2001 report from the U.S. Centres for Disease Control and Prevention, there were 29.6 deaths per 100, 000 births among African-American women between 1991 and 1997. The rate for women of Hispanic origin was 10.3, and for white women it was 7.3. The rate for Asian women was unavailable. The second most common causes of death in women are problems related to pregnancy and delivery, including blood clots that travel to the lungs, anaesthesia complications, bleeding, infection, and high blood pressure complications. A baby dies before, during, or after birth in 16 out of 1, 000 deliveries in the United States. Almost 50% of these deaths are stillbirths, which are sometimes unexplained. The rest of the deaths occur in babies up to 28 days old, and the leading cause of these is birth defects, followed by prematurity. Risk factors can be present before pregnancy occurs and others develop during pregnancy.

DIAGNOSIS

A risk-scoring sheet is utilized by many health care agencies during the prenatal assessment to establish if a woman may be at risk for complications during her pregnancy. This score sheet is implemented at the first prenatal visit, becomes a part of the woman's record, and is updated throughout the pregnancy as necessary. A woman's age affects pregnancy risk, as girls 15 years old and under are more likely to develop high blood pressure, protein in the urine and fluid accumulation (preeclampsia), or seizures (eclampsia). They also are more likely to have underweight or undernourished babies. A woman 35 or older has a greater risk of developing high blood pressure or diabetes, as well as a much higher risk of having a chromosomal abnormality such as Down syndrome. A woman shorter than five feet or a woman weighing less than 100 pounds before pregnancy has a greater risk of having a small or preterm baby.

Lab data and ultrasound are also utilized to determine high-risk pregnancies by specific blood tests and imaging of the baby. A pregnancy may begin as low risk and change to high risk secondary to complications determined from the ongoing assessment of the pregnant woman. Since many of these complications can be managed with proper treatment, it is essential that a pregnant woman keep her obstetric appointments.

TREATMENT

Treatment will vary, depending upon the maternal or foetal complication present. Generally, a woman with severe high-risk factors in pregnancy should be referred to a perinatal centre to obtain the highest level of care for herself and her baby. Interventions to improve health status might include nutritional assessment; physical examination; teaching modalities for smoking cessation, drug and alcohol programs; prescribing medications related to the condition or changing pre-pregnancy medications (known to cause problems in the foetus); serial ultrasounds to learn foetal status; amniocentesis; foetal transfusions; foetal surgery; antepartum testing; bed rest; home health care; hospitalization; and early delivery. In a postterm pregnancy (greater than 42 weeks), the death of a baby is three times more likely than that of a normal term pregnancy (37-40 weeks). The treatment in this case would be to induce labour before problems start to occur with an aging placenta.

Advances in the management of complications in high-risk pregnancies have provided women with a means of controlling their risks, which substantially increases the potential for a successful outcome. Since it is impossible to guarantee a good outcome in a normal pregnancy, it is even more difficult to ensure that a high-risk pregnancy will result in a healthy infant and mother. A woman who strictly adheres to the medical regimen established for her, however, will greatly increase her chances of a positive result.

HEALTH CARE TEAM ROLES

The pregnant woman's interview at her first visit the health care provider is conducted by the nurse, who obtains the data necessary to begin the high-risk screening. The physician or midwife caring for a pregnant woman should review the prenatal assessment sheet, order lab data, and obtain ultrasounds to determine if any risk factors are present. If it is determined that a woman has a high-risk pregnancy, she should be referred to a perinatologist for advanced care. This is the specialist who establishes and implements the medical regimen needed for the particular maternal/foetal complication and the interdisciplinary team associated with the perinatal centre works in its management. The perinatal team usually comprises a nutritionist, social worker, nurse educators, geneticists, ultrasonographers, and additional nursing staff who are responsible for the monitoring and supervising of ongoing team care of the patient.

PREVENTION

The early weeks of pregnancy are the most crucial ones for the foetus. Many women do not know they are pregnant until several weeks after conception, so education about the need for preconceptional care is essential. Preconception counseling guides a woman in planning a healthy pregnancy. These are some of the factors to which attention must be paid:

- Family history
- Medical history
- Past pregnancies

- Current medications
- Lifestyle
- Environment
- Infections

MAINTENANCE OF RECORDS AND REPORT

In high risk pregnancy cases the nurses should keep records of the pregnant women in following manner:

General

Is this a planned or desired pregnancy?

Menstrual History

- Age at which menarche occurred
- Start and end dates of most recent normal menstrual period
- Was most recent period like others in duration and amount of flow? (if not, determine dates of previous period)
- Was there any bleeding after most recent normal menstrual period?
- Contraceptives: type, when last used

Presumptive Symptoms of Pregnancy

- Fatigue
- Urinary frequency
- Breast tenderness, tingling or enlargement
- Nausea and vomiting

Current Symptoms

- Nausea and vomiting
- Weight loss or gain
- Headache
- Edema
- Abdominal pain
- Bleeding (determine amount)
- Vaginal discharge or fluid leakage (colour, odor)
- Urinary symptoms

- Constipation (usually a later symptom)
- Backache (usually a later symptom)
- Calculate estimated date of delivery: last normal menstrual period vs. uterine size

Assess client for risks in current pregnancy: infections (e.g., hepatitis B carrier, vaginal group B streptococcus [GBS] status), Rh antibody status (if negative, it is important to know father's blood group)

History of Previous Pregnancies

- Dates and locations of previous deliveries
- Period of gestation (term or preterm)
- Antepartum complications (e.g., preeclampsia, gestational diabetes, abruptio placentae)
- Labour history and complications
- Intrapartum complications (e.g., foetal distress)
- Delivery history (e.g., spontaneous vaginal delivery, caesarean section)
- Condition of infant (e.g., Apgar scores, if known)
- Postpartum complications

Other Relevant Information

- Medical and surgical history
- Family history (e.g., genetic disorders, neural tube defects, multiple gestation, congenital anomaly, mental retardation, bleeding disorders)
- Complete review of all systems
- Smoking, alcohol use, use of street drugs
- Use of medications (type, dosage, period of use, prescription or over the counter [OTC])

PHYSICAL EXAMINATION

General

- Apparent state of health
- Appearance of comfort or distress
- Colour (e.g., flushed, pale)
- Nutritional status (obese or emaciated)
- Facial edema

Vital Signs

- Temperature
- Heart rate
- Respiratory rate
- Blood pressure
- Foetal heart rate

Breasts

- Signs of infection
- Masses, tenderness
- Nipples: shape (e.g., inverted), erosion, discharge

Abdomen

- Striae
- Scars
- Measurement of fundal height, shape of fundus
- Agreement between fundal height and expected date of delivery
- Foetal position, presentation and movements
- Uterine tenderness or hardness
- Contractions (e.g., Braxton-Hicks)

Pelvis

- Perineal varicosities
- Vaginal bleeding, discharge (colour, odor, consistency)
- Cervical assessment
- Pelvic adequacy (if a primigravida)
- Hemorrhoids
- Muscular support in the pelvic floor (e.g., cystocele, rectocele)

Other Aspects

- Edema (facial, hands, pretibial, pedal)
- Reflexes
- Pregnancy test

REFERENCES

Kitzinger, Sheila. The Midwife Challenge Pandora, 1991.

Kitzinger, Shiela. The Experience of Childbirth. 3rd Edition . Penguin Books. 1972.

Hubbard, Ruth, Mary Sue Henifin and Barbara Fried (eds.), Women Looking at Biology Looking at Women. Boston: G.K. Hall and Co., 1979.

Leep, Nicky, and Hunter, Billie. The Midwife's Tale . The untold story of birth in the 1920's , 1930's and 1940's in Britain.

Midwifery Today. Getting an Education: Paths to Becoming a Midwife 1995 (Midwifery Today, PO Box 2672-350, Eugene, OR, 97402. USA.

Mitford, Jessica. The American Way of Birth The Penguin Group, 1993.

Odent, Michel. Birth Reborn . Pantheon Books. New York, 1984 and 1990.

Posner, Judith. It's all in your head: feminist and medical models of menopause (strange bedfellows). Sex Roles. 5:170- 190.

Rothman, Barbara Katz. In Labor: Women and Power in the Birthplace 1991.

Steiger, Carolyn. Becoming a Midwife Hoogan House Publishing, 1987.

Ulrich, Laurel Thatcher. A Midwife's Tale . Vintage Books, New York, 1990.

Varney, Helen. Nurse Midwifery . 2nd Edition. Blackwell Scientific Publications. 1987.

8

Abnormal Labour

An abnormal labour may be referred to as dystocia, which simply means difficult labour or childbirth. In the active phase of the first stage or in the second stage of labour, an abnormal labour is identified when the rate of labour progress is slowed (protraction of labour) or stops altogether (arrest of labour). In order to determine if labour can be corrected to allow for vaginal delivery, the obstetrician must augment labour with oxytocin (Pitocin), a medication that stimulates the uterine contractions and is also used to induce labour. Definitions of abnormal labour are listed in Table below.

A few examples of abnormal labour patterns may help to understand how the diagnosis of abnormal labour is made:

- Protraction of Dilation. The cervix dilates from 4 to 6 centimetres over 3 or 4 hours. This rate of dilation is slow, even in a first-time pregnancy. The expected dilatation over this period of time would be from 4 centimetres dilated to 7 to 8 centimetres dilated.
- Arrest of Dilation. The cervix is found to be 6 centimetres dilated on two examinations, one or two hours apart. Thus, no cervical dilation has occurred during the period of observation.
- Arrest of Descent. The head of the foetus is found to be at the same station in the birth canal on two different examinations, one hour apart. Arrest of descent is a diagnosis made in the second stage, after the cervix is completely dilated.

UTERINE HYPOCONTRACTILITY

Labour may start out well, only later to stop or stall if the uterus fails to contract sufficiently. Sometimes this is caused by medications that lessen the intensity or frequency of the contractions. This type of abnormal labour is variously referred to as uterine inertia, uterine hypocontractility, or inadequate uterine power. Uterine hypocontractility is fairly common, especially in women having their first labour. In some centres that practice active management of labour, nearly 50% of all first pregnancies are treated with oxytocin to augment labour. However, uterine hypocontractility is less frequent in women who have previously been pregnant. These cases should be very carefully monitored before oxytocin is administered.

CEPHALO-PELVIC DISPROPORTION (CPD)

If the labour is still slow or stalled after oxytocin has been administered, the baby's head may simply be too large to fit through the birth canal. This condition is commonly called cephalo-pelvic disproportion (CPD). Vast experience has proven the only way to tell uterine hypocontractility from CPD is by trying to augment labour-uterine hypocontractility will be corrected and labour will progress normally, while labour will continue to stall in women with CPD. Women with CPD are delivered by caesarean section. With the proper use of oxytocin to augment labour, true CPD requiring caesarean section occurs in no more than 10 to 15% of women.

DYSTOCIA

Dystocia (antonym eutocia) is an abnormal or difficult childbirth or labour. Approximately a fifth of human labors have dystocia. Can also be related to livestock. Dystocia may arise due to incoordinate uterine activity, abnormal foetal lie or presentation, absolute or relative cephalopelvic disproportion, or (rarely) a massive foetal tumor such as a sacrococcygeal teratoma. Oxytocin is commonly used to treat incoordinate uterine activity. However, pregnancies complicated by dystocia often end with assisted deliveries including forceps, ventouse or, commonly, caesarean section. Recognized complications of dystocia include foetal death, respiratory depression, Hypoxic Ischaemic Encephalopathy (HIE), and brachial nerve damage. A prolonged interval between pregnancies, primigrad birth, and multiple birth have also been associated with increased risk for labour dystocia.

Shoulder dystocia is a dystocia in which the anterior shoulder of the infant cannot pass below the pubic symphysis, or requires significant manipulation to pass below the pubic symphysis.

Abnormalities of the Expulsive Forces

- Uterine forces insufficiently strong or inappropriately coordinated to efface & dilate the cervix (uterine dysfunction)

- Inadequate voluntary muscle effort during the second stage of labour
- Abnormalities of presentation, position, or development of the foetus
- Abnormalities of the maternal bony pelvis
- Abnormalities of the reproductive tract that form an obstacle to foetal descent
- Today, expression such as cephalopelvic disproportion and failure to progress are often used to describe these dysfunctional labour when caesarean delivery is necessary
- Cephalopelvic disproportion (CPD)
- Disparity between the dimensions of the foetal head and maternal pelvis to preclude vaginal delivery
- True CPD is rare and most CPD are due to malposition of the foetal head: asynclitism or extension of the bony diametres of the foetal head
- Inability to achieve vaginal delivery after reaching complete dilatation is a significant marker of true dystocia because it is likely to recur
- Failure to progress
- This term include lack of progressive cervical dilatation or lack of descent
- The CPD and failure to progress are not precise terms and we should use more
- Practical terms, such as protraction or arrest
- The woman must be in the active phase of labour to diagnose either of these disorders
- Active phase arrest in 5 % of term nulliparas, this incidence has not changed since the 1950s
- Inadequate uterine contractions (< 180 Montevideo units) were diagnosed in 80 % of women with active-phase arrest

MALPOSITIONS AND MALPRESENTATIONS

Foetal malpresentations are abnormalities of foetal position, presentation attitude, or lie. They collectively constitute the most common cause of foetal dystocia, occurring in approximately 5% of labours. Included in this category are persistent occiput posterior and occiput transverse positions, brow presentation, face presentation, transverse or oblique lies, and breech and compound presentation.

Vertex Malpositions

Occiput Posterior: The occiput posterior position may be normal in early labour, with about 10-20% of fetuses in occiput posterior position at onset of labour. In 87% of cases, the head rotates to the occiput anterior positions when it reaches the pelvic floor. If the head does not rotate, persistent occiput anterior position may result in dystocia. Interestingly, approximately two-thirds of cases of occiput posterior presentation at delivery occur through malrotation during the active phase of labour. The mechanism of this fetopelvic disproportion is partial deflexion of the foetal head. This partial deflexion increases the diametre that must engage in the pelvis. Occiput posterior presentation may result from a contracted anthropoid or android pelvis or insufficient uterine action. The use of epidural anaesthesia with higher rates of occiput posterior presentation.

PREMATURE LABOUR

Preterm labour is labour that begins before 37 completed weeks of pregnancy. Although the exact definitions may vary, preterm labour may include one, or more, of the following:

- Uterine contractions
- Rupture of the amniotic sac (membranes)
- Cervical dilatation (opening of the cervix)

Nearly 13 percent of all babies born are preterm.

Causes

Many factors can contribute to preterm labour. Although the exact cause of preterm labour is unknown in many cases, one major cause is premature rupture of membranes (breaking of the amniotic sac). Other related factors include the following:

- Maternal factors:
  - — Preeclampsia (also known as toxemia or high blood pressure of pregnancy)
  - — Chronic medical illness (such as heart or kidney disease)
  - — Infection (such as group B streptococcus, urinary tract infections, vaginal Infections, infections of the foetal/placental tissues)

— Drug abuse (such as cocaine)
— Abnormal structure of the uterus
— Cervical incompetence (inability of the cervix to stay closed during pregnancy)
— Previous preterm birth

- Factors involving the pregnancy:
  — Abnormal or decreased function of the placenta
  — Placenta previa (low lying position of the placenta)
  — Placental abruption (early detachment from the uterus)
  — Premature rupture of membranes (amniotic sac)
  — Hydramnios (too much amniotic fluid)
- Factors involving the foetus:
  — When foetal behaviour indicates the intrauterine environment is not healthy
  — Multiple gestation (twins, triplets, or more)
  — Erythroblastosis foetalis (Rh/blood group incompatibility)

Preterm birth is the greatest problem associated with preterm labour. Although most babies are born after 37 weeks, those born preterm are at increased risks for many complications.

According to the March of Dimes, about 13 percent of babies born in the US are born preterm, or before 37 completed weeks of pregnancy. Of the babies born preterm:

- 71 percent are born between 34 and 36 weeks of gestation (the time from conception to birth)
- About 13 percent are born between 32 and 33 weeks of gestation
- About 6 percent are born at less than 28 weeks of gestation

Premature babies are born before their bodies and organ systems have completely matured. These babies are often small, with low birthweight (less than 2, 500 grams or 5.5 pounds), and they may need help breathing, eating, fighting infection, and staying warm. Very premature babies, those born before 28 weeks, are especially vulnerable. Many of their organs may not be ready for life outside the mother's uterus and may be too immature to function well.

Symptoms

The following are the most common symptoms of preterm labour. However, each woman may experience symptoms differently. Symptoms may include:

- Uterine contractions, especially more than four in one hour
- Menstrual-type cramps
- Pelvic pressure
- Backache
- Intestinal upset
- Vaginal discharge of blood, mucus, or water

Diagnosis

If preterm labour is suspected, most women are evaluated in the labour and delivery area of the hospital. Usually, an electronic monitor is used to check the frequency, duration, and strength of contractions. This monitor has a transducer that is placed over abdomen with a belt. The contractions are transmitted and recorded by the monitor. The foetal heart rate may also be monitored at this time.

Other ways of assessing preterm labour may include the following:

- Cervical examination - an examination by a physician's gloved fingers of the cervix can help determine if the cervix has softened, shortened, thinned, or dilated (opened) - all signs of preterm labour.
- Ultrasound (with a vaginal transducer to measure the length of the cervix, or with an abdominal transducer to check the foetus and amniotic fluid levels)
- Testing for premature rupture of membranes (the amniotic sac)
- Testing for foetal fibronectin (FFN) - a protein that helps glue together the tissues of the placenta. FFN may be released when there is a disruption in these tissues or with infection. The protein is then found in cervical secretions where it can be sampled and tested.

TREATMENT FOR PRETERM LABOUR

Specific treatment for preterm labour will be determined by physician based on:

- Pregnancy, overall health, and medical history
- Extent of the condition
- Tolerance for specific medications, procedures, or therapies
- Expectations for the course of the condition
- Opinion or preference

Treatment for preterm labour may include:

- Bed-rest (either at home or in the hospital may be recommended)
- Hospitalization (as specialized personnel and equipment may be necessary)
- Tocolytic medications - medications to help slow or stop contractions. These may be given in an injection under the skin or intravenously (IV). Tocolytic medications often used include terbutaline and magnesium sulfate.
- Corticosteroid medications - medications that may help mature the lungs of the foetus. Lung immaturity is a major problem of premature babies.
- Cervical cerclage - a procedure used to suture the cervical opening. Cerclage is used for women with an incompetent cervix. This is a condition in which the cervix is physically weak and unable to stay closed during pregnancy.
- Antibiotics (to treat infection)
- Delivery - if treatments do not stop preterm labour or if the foetus or mother is in danger, delivery of the baby may occur. Caesarean delivery may be recommended in certain cases.

Prevention

Because of the tremendous advances in the care of sick and premature babies, more and more babies are surviving despite being born early and being very small. However, prevention of early birth is the best way of promoting good health for babies.

Prenatal care is a key factor in preventing preterm births and low birth-weight babies. At prenatal visits, the health of both mother and foetus can be checked. Because maternal nutrition and weight gain are linked with foetal weight gain and birth-weight, eating a healthy diet and gaining weight in pregnancy are essential. Prenatal care is also important in identifying problems and lifestyles that can increase the risks for preterm labour and birth. Some ways to help prevent prematurity and to provide the best care for premature babies may include the following:

- Identifying mothers at risk for preterm labour
- Prenatal education of the symptoms of preterm labour
- Avoiding heavy or repetitive work or standing for long periods of time which can increase the risk of preterm labour
- Early identification and treatment of preterm labour

Some women at high risk for preterm birth may be candidates for treatment with the hormone progesterone. This hormone and its derivative, 17-hydroxyprogesterone, are naturally produced by the placenta during pregnancy. Recent studies have shown promising results in reducing the risk of preterm birth in certain high-risk women who received these types of progesterone medications beginning in early pregnancy. More research is needed for this and other ways to help reduce the incidence of prematurity.

DISORDERS OF UTERINE ACTIONS

Labour is a dynamic process characterized by uterine contractions that increase in regularity, intensity, and duration, causing progressive dilatation and effacement of the cervix and descent of the foetus through the birth canal. The progress of labour is evaluated primarily through the birth canal. The progress of labour is evaluated primarily through estimates of cervical dilation and descent of the foetal presenting part.

Prolonged Labour

The latent phase of labour begins with the onset of regular contractions and extends to the beginning of the active phase of cervical dilation. The duration of the latent phase averages 6.4 hours in nulliparas and 4.8 hours in multiparas. The latent phase is abnormally prolonged if it lasts more than 20 hours in nulliparas or 14 hours in multiparas. Causes of prolonged latent phase include excessive sedation or sedation given before the end of the latent phase, the use of conduction or general anaesthesia before labour enters the active phase, labour beginning with an unfavorable cervix, uterine dysfunction characterized by weak, irregular, uncoordinated, and ineffective uterine contractions, and fetopelvic disproportion. Treatment options in prolonged latent phase primarily consist of therapeutic rest regimens or active sedation and hydration, 85% of patients spontaneously enter the active phase of labour, and further progression in dilation and effacement may be expected.

The prognosis for vaginal delivery after therapeutic measures is excellent. Patients with a prolonged latent phase of labour who respond to rest can be expected to deliver vaginally in nearly all cases. After abnormalities in the latent phase have been corrected, patients are not at nay greater risk of developing subsequent labour disorders than are patienst who have experienced a normal latent phase.

Precipitate Labour

Precipitate dilation occurs if cervical dilation occurs at a rate of 5 or more centimetres per hour in a primipara or at 10 cm or more per hour in a multipara. Precipitate descent occurs with descent of the foetal presenting part of 5 cm or more per hour in primparas and 10 cm or more per hour in multiparas.

Precipitate labour may result from either extremely strong uterine contractions or low birth canal resistance. Although the initiating mechanism for extraordinarily forceful uterine contractions is usually not known, abnormal contractions may be associated with administration of oxytocin. Strong uterine contractions (both in force and increased basal tone) may also accompany abruption placentae. Little known about causes of low birth canal resistance.

If oxytocin administration is the cause of abnormal contractions, it may simply be stopped. The problem typically resolves in less than 5 minutes. The patient should be placed in the lateral position to prevent any pressures on the inferior vena cava. If excessive uterine activity is associated with foetal heart rate abnormalities, and this pattern persists despite discontinuation of oxytocin, a β-mimetic such as 125-250 μg of terbutaline or ritodrine can be given slowly by intravenous injection if there are no contraindications. Magnesium sulfate has also been recommended to decrease uterine contractions. Physical attempts to retard delivery are absolutely contraindicated.

Maternal complications are rare if the cervix and birth canal are relaxed. However, when the birth canal is rigid and extraordinary contractions occur, uterine rupture may result. Lacerations of the birth canal are common. In addition, precipitate labour is one of the known antecedents of maternal amniotic fluid embolism. Thus enhanced maternal monitoring for this complication is imperative. Furthermore, the uterus that has been hypertonic with labour tends to be hypotonic postpartum, thereby predisposing to postpartum haemorrhage.

Perinatal mortality is increased secondary to hypoxia, possible intracranial haemorrhage, and risks associated with unattended delivery. Impeded placental exchange with resultant hypoxia is created by decreased uteroplacental blood flow as a result of the more frequent and more forceful contractions as well as by increased basal uterine tone.

Perinatal intracranial haemorrhage may result from trauma to the foetal head pushing against unyielding maternal tissue with contractions. Resuscitation equipment, baby warmers, and other supportive measures may not be readily available in cases of unattended delivery.

COMPLICATIONS OF THIRD STAGE: INJURIES TO BIRTH CANAL

In this stage of labour placental separation and expulsion take place; for the mother the main risks are haemorrhage during or after separation of the placenta, and retention of the placenta. Postpartum haemorrhage is one of the main causes of maternal mortality. The incidence of postpartum haemorrhage and retention of the placenta is increased if predisposing factors are present, such as multiple pregnancy or polyhydramnios, and complicated labour: augmentation of labour, obstructed labour, or vaginal operative delivery. Postpartum haemorrhage and placental retention also occur more frequently if these complications were present in the obstetric history of the woman. To a certain extent therefore it is possible to select during pregnancy and in the course of labour those women with an increased risk of complications in the third stage. But even in low-risk pregnancies and after an uneventful first and second stage of labour serious haemorrhage and/or placental retention may sometimes occur. The management of the third stage may influence the incidence of these complications, and the amount of blood lost.

OBSTETRICAL EMERGENCIES AND THEIR MANAGEMENT

It is now universally recognised that the most effective strategy for reduction in the risk of death due to complications of pregnancy and delivery is to provide emergency obstetric care services (EmOC) within the reach of all pregnant women. There are two reasons for the universal acceptance of this strategy. First, majority of female deaths due to complications of pregnancy and delivery are due to selected emergency situations that emerge after the onset of labour and immediately after the delivery. The second reason is that it is generally not possible to predict these emergencies well in advance so that appropriate care can be arranged well in time. There is however a gap of a few hours between the onset of and obstetric emergency and death. If adequate attention and care is provided to the woman in this period, she survives otherwise death is inevitable. This means that nearer the emergency obstetric services are to the woman in emergency, the greater is the probability that the woman receives necessary care ad treatment and greater is the probability that she survives.

In other words, the time elapsed in making available emergency obstetric care services to the woman in distress is crucial in preventing majority of the maternal deaths. In a situation where majority of deliveries occur at home and are conducted either by the members of the family or by untrained persons or by minimally trained traditional birth attendants, ensuring that the emergency obstetric care is available to the women in obstetric emergency in the shortest possible time is perhaps the most important challenge to the prevention of unwanted maternal deaths and reduction of maternal mortality.

The above considerations constitute the rationale for including availability and use of emergency obstetric care services as one of the integral components of the safe motherhood programme. Availability and use of emergency obstetric services has been identified as one of the important process indicators of the safe motherhood programme. Emergency obstetric care services have been divided into basic emergency obstetric care services and comprehensive emergency obstetric care services on the basis of 'signal functions'. A short well defined list of 'signal functions' is very useful in assessing the availability of emergency obstetric care services. There are eight 'signal functions' that have been suggested to assess the availability of emergency obstetric care services:

- Antibiotics (injectable)
- Oxytocics (injectable)
- Anticonvulsants (injectable)
- Manual removal of placenta
- Removal of retained products
- Assisted vaginal delivery
- Caesarean section
- Blood transfusion.

PRESENTATION AND PROLAPSE OF CORD

There are three varieties:

- Overt cord prolapse - if the presenting part of the foetus does not fit the pelvis snugly after membrane rupture, there is a risk that the umbilical cord can slip past and present at the cervix or descend into the vagina. This is known as overt cord prolapse. It represents an acute obstetric emergency as prolapse exposes the cord to intermittent compression compromising the foetal circulation. Depending on its duration and degree of compression, foetal hypoxia, brain damage and even death can occur. Exposure of the umbilical cord to air causes irritation and cooling, resulting in vasospasm of the cord vessels.

- Occult cord prolapse - where the umbilical cord lies alongside the presenting part.
- Funic presentation - where the cord can be felt to prolapse below the presenting part before membranes have ruptured. The cord may slip to one side of the head and disappear as the membranes rupture.

Risk Factors

- Multiparity
- Prematurity
- Low birth weight (<2.5 kg)
- Abnormal presentations (breech, oblique, transverse, unstable lie)
- Foetal congenital abnormality
- Cephalopelvic disproportion
- Pelvic tumours
- Low lying placenta or other abnormal placentation
- Polyhydramnios
- Macrosomia
- Multiple births (2nd twin at particular risk)
- High foetal station
- Long umbilical cord
- Obstetric interventions including amniotomy (before presenting part is engaged), use of scalp electrode or intrauterine pressure catheter and attempted external cephalic or internal podalic version

Signs

Cord prolapse may occur with no outward physical signs and a normal foetal heart trace.

- Abdominal examination: an ill-fitting or non-engaged presenting part should alert one to the possibility of cord prolapse.
- Vaginal examination (VE) - examine for the cord at every VE during labour and specifically after rupture of membranes if risk factors:

- — With an overt prolapse, the cord can be seen protruding from the introitus or loops of cord can be palpated within the vaginal canal. If the cord is pulsating, the foetus is alive.
- — Occult prolapses are rarely felt on pelvic examination and only indication may be foetal heart rate changes.
- — With a funic presentation, loops of cord are palpated through the membrane.

Whilst it is generally important to avoid digital examination of women in preterm labour, suspicion of cord prolapse is an important exception and speculum and/or digital exam should be swiftly undertaken in these circumstances.

Foetal Monitoring

- Whilst the foetus remains in good condition, variable foetal heart rate deceleration are seen during uterine contractions that promptly return to normal after contraction subsides.
- With prolonged and complete compression, bradycardia occurs.
- With deteriorating foetal status activity diminishes and eventually stops.

Have a high index of suspicion for cord prolapse, particularly if foetal monitoring changes occur soon after rupture of membranes, whether spontaneous or with amniotomy.

Investigations

Routine antenatal ultrasound is not adequately sensitive to detect cord presentation. Most suspected cord presentations do not develop into a cord prolapse at delivery.

Loops of cord in front of the presenting of the presenting part can be visualised using colour Doppler studies. This is not routinely done but can be used to serially examine women at high risk.

Management

Treat a prolapsed cord as an acute obstetric emergency.

- With an overt prolapse:
  - — If the foetus is viable, place mother in the knee-chest position (patient facing the bed, chest level to bed, knees tucked under chest, pelvis and buttocks elevated) or head-down tilt in the left lateral and apply upward pressure

against presenting part to lift the foetus away from the prolapsed cord. This can be done manually (gloved hand/ 2 fingers pushing upwards against the presenting part or once the presenting part is above the pelvic brim, using continuous suprapubic pressure in an upwards direction) or by filling the urinary bladder.

— Manual replacement of the prolapsed cord above the presenting part is not currently recommended. Avoid handling cord outside the vagina as this induces vasospasm.

— Proceed to emergency caesarean section as soon as possible.

— If available, give terbutaline 0.25 mg subcut to reduce contractions when there are persistent foetal heart rate trace abnormalities despite attempts to prevent cord compression manually and there may be delays in achieving delivery.

— Only proceed with vaginal delivery if delivery is imminent, the cervix is fully dilated and there are no contraindications.

This can be expedited with episiotomy/vacuum extraction or forceps.

- Ensure resuscitation is available for baby post-delivery.
- If the foetus has died, deliver in the manner that is safest for the woman.
- If an occult prolapse is suspected:
  — Place the mother in left lateral position.
  — If the foetal heart rate returns to normal, allow labour to continue with mother receiving O2 and foetal heart rate continuously monitored.
  — If foetal heart rate remains abnormal, expedite a rapid caesarean section.
- With funic presentation, a decision needs to be made between prompt elective caesarean section prior to membrane rupture or artificial rupture of membranes with full preparations for an emergency caesarean section in case the cord does become an overt prolapse on rupture.

In the community, cord prolapse is associated with a tenfold increase in perinatal mortality rate, compared to that occurring in hospital.

Prognosis

Perinatal mortality rate associated with cord prolapse of 91/1000. Prematurity and congenital abnormality are underlying factors in many cases. Even congenitally normal, full-term babies can die as a consequence of cord prolapse - home birth and delay in transfer to hospital have been identified as particular risks in these cases. The most common serious morbidities associated with cord prolapse relate to asphyxia: hypoxic brain injury and cerebral palsy. There are few long-term studies looking at long-term sequelae of cord prolapse.

Prevention

- Consider admission of all pregnant women with transverse, oblique or unstable lie from 37+6 weeks of gestation. Cord prolapses occurring in hospital have better outcomes than those occurring within the community. Advise these women that they will require rapid assessment if they start labour or have a spontaneous rupture of membranes and should seek help as soon as possible.
- Similarly, admit women with premature rupture of membranes and a non-cephalic presentation.
- Avoid artificial rupture of membranes (AROM) where possible. If an AROM is performed with a mobile presenting part, ensure arrangements have been put in place for an immediate emergency section should a cord prolapse occur.
- Whenever a VE or other obstetric procedure is performed following rupture of membranes with a high presenting part, avoid any upward pressure on the presenting part.
- Treat high-risk patients with constant foetal monitoring during delivery.

Amniotic Fluid Embolism

Normally, amniotic fluid does not enter the maternal circulation because it is contained safely within the uterus, sealed off by the amniotic sac. AFE occurs when the barrier between amniotic fluid and maternal circulation is broken and, possibly under a pressure gradient, fluid abnormally enters the maternal venous system via the endocervical veins, the placental site (if placenta is separated), or a uterine trauma site. Why this entry into maternal circulation occurs in some women and not in others is not clearly understood. The devastating consequence of circulating foetal debris (carried by amniotic fluid) occurs only rarely, even though during normal labour and delivery, caesarean deliveries, and minor traumatic procedures foetal tissue may pass into maternal circulation and cause no symptoms. That AFE develops in only a minute proportion of these women suggests that either it is an effect of the amount of exposure to foetal debris or the type of foetal debris (containing meconium or not) or that some maternal factors may play a significant role.

Predisposing factors once considered to be associated with AFE include placental abruption, uterine overdistention, foetal death, trauma, tumultuous or oxytocin-stimulated labour, multiparity, advanced maternal age, and rupture of membranes. However, in numerous documented cases of AFE, none of these conditions or demographic characteristics occurred or were applicable at the time of the event. Furthermore, a recent analysis of 46 verified cases of AFE did not substantiate most of these as associated factors; 12% of the cases occurred in women with intact membranes, 70% during labour, 11% after vaginal delivery, and 19% during caesarean delivery with or without labour.

Once the signs and symptoms are recognized and a presumptive diagnosis is made, supportive measures should be implemented promptly. In the event of cardiac arrest, the resuscitation team should follow standard Advanced Cardiac Life Support protocols for obstetric patients. Ideally, overall management of AFE should take place in an obstetric intensive care unit. Many hospitals lack obstetric intensive care units and so the patient must be cared for in a medical oı surgical intensive care unit. Critical care nurses without obstetric expertise often become anxious when caring for pregnant patients; however, the initial principles of dealing with obstetric emergencies are the same as for any emergency: airway, breathing, and circulation. The major difference for this particular emergency is the need to care for 2 patients.

The foetus should be monitored continuously for signs of compromise (preferably by an obstetric nurse with expertise in electronic foetal monitoring). Specific to pregnant women is the importance of positioning. In order to ensure optimal uterine perfusion throughout the management of AFE, the mother's hips should be displaced to the left to prevent the weight of the gravid uterus from compressing the inferior vena cava and compromising blood flow.

Rupture of Uterus

Uterine inversion during the acute postpartum period is a relatively rare complication. Severe post-partum haemorrhage and shock result from the uterine fundus collapsing. If unrecognized, this obstetric emergency could cause serious morbidity or death. The reported incidence of uterine inversion varies considerably in the literature. Most commonly, the frequency is reported to be approximately 1 in 2000 deliveries; however, a range of 1 in 4000 to 1 in several hundred thousand can be found. Maternal mortality has been reported to be as high as 15%. Treatment options for this obstetric complication are also quite varied. Several pharmacologic methods, as well as manual and surgical options, have been described for correcting an inversion. The most important aspect of treatment remains immediate recognition and prompt attention to its management.

SHOULDER DYSTOCIA

Shoulder dystocia needs to be distinguished from a mere difficulty with delivery of the shoulder. The latter occurs because of the prevailing delivery practice, with the mother in a semi-recumbent position on the delivery bed. There may be insufficient room for appropriate lateral i.e. downward flexion for delivering the anterior shoulder. In addition, the weight of the mother is in part taken on the sacrum which is therefore pushed upwards, thus decreasing the antero-posterior diametre of the pelvic outlet. Many of these cases require only a positional change, into left lateral, or kneeling, which frees the sacrum and allows lateral flexion.

Proper shoulder dystocia occurs when there is disproportion between the bisacromial diametre of the foetus and the anterioposterior diametre of the pelvic inlet. This results in the anterior shoulder becoming impacted behind the symphysis pubis.

Diabetic mothers have a threefold increased risk of shoulder dystocia because of a disproportionate increase in foetal abdominal circumference to head circumference. The presence of maternal diabetes together with macrosomia (defined here as > 4kg) is estimated to result in shoulder dystocia in a third of those delivering vaginally.

However, the event is difficult to predict, as half of all instances of shoulder dystocia occur in babies weighing less than 4kg. Furthermore, of the babies which do weigh over 4 kg, most are not detected as such clinically. Even an ultrasound scan often misses these babies because of its low sensitivity (60%) of detection of macrosomia in the third trimester.

Inducing the suspected large babies only increases the intervention rate and will not decrease the incidence of shoulder dystocia. A policy of caesarean sections for those babies predicted antenatally to weigh more than 4.2 kg increases the section rate but does not have a significant impact on the rate of shoulder dystocia. A prophylactic caesarean section policy on babies of 4-4.5kg would require more than a thousand sections to avert one brachial plexus injury.

Management

Early recognition/raised level of suspicion: Large baby, post dates, large maternal BMI, maternal diabetes, previous history of shoulder dystocia; prolonged 2nd stage, turtle neck sign.

Mc Roberts position: Femora are abducted, rotated outwards and flexed, so that thighs touch the mother's abdomen, with the aid of two assistants. The buttocks need to come over the edge of the bed, allowing the sacrum to rotate backwards. Apply suprapubic pressure: Another assistant puts hand laterally and pushes in direction that the baby is facing and posteriorly to try and disimpact the anterior shoulder. This is done at the same time as moderate traction of head. 91% of cases will be delivered by this stage.

Woods screw manoeuvre: Rotation of the posterior shoulder by 180 degrees to deliver the anterior shoulder from under the symphysis pubis. Rubin's manoeuvre is turning the baby in the opposite direction (reverse Woods manoeuvre). This has the advantage of abducting the shoulders, thereby decreasing the diametre.

Delivery of posterior arm: Insert hand into sacral hollow to identify the posterior shoulder, arm down to the wrist. Sweep this across the foetal chest, flexing the elbow, to deliver the arm posteriorly.

Zavanelli manoeuvre (cepahalic replacement): Manual return of the partially born, but undeliverable, foetus to the vagina for extraction by caesarian section. This is done by rotating the head back to the occiput anterior position, flexing the head with pressure on the occiput whilst using the other hand to replace the chin back into the vagina. Tocolytics can help the procedure (terbutaline 0.25mg sc)

Symphysiotomy: division of the fibrocartilagenous symphysis pubis. Using local anaesthetic, infiltrate the joint with the patient in the lithotomy position (thighs supported at no more than 90 degrees, so as not to put too great a strain on the sacroiliac joints). Use the index and middle fingers of the left hand on the posterior aspect of the symphysis. Push the indwelling catheter aside with the index finger and use the middle finger to monitor the action of the scalpel. The latter is used like a pencil, keeping it vertical and, using the entry point as a fulcrum, to bring the blade down towards the operator. Remove, turn 180 degrees and in original point to divide the upper half of the symphysis. If completed, the middle finger can fit into the space created by the separation.

OBSTETRICAL PROCEDURES AND OPERATIONS

There are many procedures and operations in obstetrics which are as follows:

INDUCTION OF LABOUR

Initiating labour in a pregnant woman without contractions seems to be a simple way to explain induction of labour. For many women, induction is becoming increasingly more common. In fact, induction has been on the increase during the past decade. In last decade, there has been a 77 percent increase in the number of inductions. Initiating labour can be very simple. It is becoming so commonplace that it can lull us into misusing the process of induction. Therefore, it is very important to have a medical reason to induce a patient.

Reasons to induce include:

- Overdue (at least one to two weeks)
- Toxemia (elevated blood pressure)
- Premature rupture of the amniotic sac
- Infection in the uterus (chorioamnionitis)
- Problems with the baby's growth
- Low amniotic fluid (oligiohydramnios)
- Excessively large baby (macrosomia)
- Prior poor obstetrical history (prior stillborn)
- Underlying medical condition in the mother (high blood pressure, kidney disease, heart disease, etc.)

This list represents the most common indications to deliver a baby. There are many other factors to consider when deciding to induce someone.

There is also a list of patients with certain conditions who should not be induced. These would include:

- Placenta previa (afterbirth in front of the baby's head)
- Prior classical c-section (incision is up and down on the uterus)
- Breech baby or other abnormal foetal positions (i.e., sideways)

- Foetal distress
- Active herpes infection

It is not logical to stress the importance of having a reason to induce a baby because the unexpected can happen and usually does. With regards to induction, it is not necessary that it doesn't always work according to plan. Not all attempts at delivery are successful. Sometimes, induction can increase the risk of caesarean section. Therefore, induction should be limited to real indications.

A woman who is uncomfortable near her due date may wish to be induced. She should be sympathized with her plight, but perhaps it would be better to reassure her that what she is feeling is normal rather than induce her.

After determining the need for induction, the physician must do a pelvic exam to evaluate cervical exam. Going back to the prepared childbirth classes for a moment, the cervix acts as the doorway to the uterus. It holds the baby inside for nine months. At some point in time, it begins the process of effacement (thinning out) and dilatation. The other important issue is how low the baby's head is in the birth canal. This is known as the station. The pelvic exam allows the practitioner to determine how ready is the women to labour. If he or she feels that the cervix is "ripe" then the women can be induced. For those with an unfavorable exam, other methods need to be utilized to help in preparation for labour. This specific group of women is going to need extra help. They should also realize that they are at higher risk of needing a caesarean section.

Cervical ripening agents are available to help thin out and dilate the cervix in advance of induction. These techniques help improve chances of a vaginal delivery. They also tend to make the induction easier. There are numerous ways to ripen the cervix. Presently, most physicians utilize a vaginal insert (Cervidil) or gel containing prostaglandin. Although prostaglandins have many functions, in obstetrics, they have a unique ability to soften and dilate the cervix without painful contractions. On occasion, they can also trigger labour or lead to over-stimulation of the uterus (known as hyperstimulation). This can cause foetal stress and potentially result in a caesarean section. These agents take at least six hours to work and are typically placed the night before labour is to begin. In many centres, including mine, we keep the patient in the hospital overnight and continually monitor them. Most of the time, the patient is able to sleep, but it isn't the best night of rest she could have. Other agents, including inflating a balloon in the uterus (a foley) and cervical dilators (laminaria) can trigger cervical ripening without the risk of hyperstimulation of the uterus. These agents tend to be less effective as cervical ripening agents, and they are more uncomfortable.

Risks of Induction

As it can be noticed throughout this discussion, there are some potential downsides to induction. Failed inductions do occur and lead to an increased number of caesarean sections. The cervical ripening agents can trigger foetal stress and c-sections as well. On rare occasions, the uterus can rupture.

Another issue regarding induction is the ability to monitor the contractions on a continual basis. Most obstetricians will require constant foetal monitoring while Pitocin is in use. In most settings, this will require the women to remain in bed. Some hospitals have monitoring systems that allow patients to walk during labour.

In short it can be said that induction of labour is a medical procedure. It should be done for those with a medical reason. In these cases, the benefits of the induction must outweigh the risks involved. If we have a complication associated with induction, we should be able to justify our decision based on the medical necessity of the procedure. For those who undergo a social induction, anything negative that transpires during the induction is hard to justify. Induction is a safe and effective procedure with a very important role in obstetrics. It should be used based upon sound medical judgment.

FORCEPS

The obstetric forceps is an instrument designed to assist the delivery of the baby's head. It is used either to expedite delivery or to overcome or correct certain abnormalities in the cephalopelvic relationship that interfere with advancement of the head in labour.

The primary functions of the forceps are traction (either for assistance in the terminal phase of labour or to deal with arrest of the head) and rotation (in cases in which there is no disproportion but the head presents with an unfavorable diametre). Forceps delivery may be indicated in the interests of mother or baby, and when properly performed it may be life-saving.

The obstetric forceps consists of two matched parts that articulate, or lock. Each part is composed of a blade, shank, lock, and handle. Each blade is so designed that it possesses 2 curves: the cephalic curve, which permits the instrument to be applied accurately to the sides of the baby's head, and the pelvic curve, which conforms to the curved axis of the maternal pelvis. The tip of each blade is called the toe.

The front of the forceps is the concave side of the pelvic curve. The blades are referred to as left and right according to the side of the mother's pelvis on which they lie after application. According to the rule of the forceps, the handle of the left blade is held in the left hand and the blade is applied to the left side of the mother's pelvis; the handle of the right blade is then held in the right hand and inserted so as to lie on the right side of the mother's pelvis. When the blades are inserted in this order, the right shank comes to lie atop the left so that the forceps articulate, or lock, as the handles are closed.

Physicians have been making modifications in one or more of the four basic parts since forceps were first invented. Although more than 600 kinds of forceps have been described only a few are currently in use. Obstetric forceps may be divided into two groups: classic forceps and special forceps. Classic forceps are those with the usual cephalic and pelvic curves and English lock; the Simpson and Elliot forceps are the prototypes. Special forceps are those designed to solve specific problems; those in modern use are the Piper, Kielland, and Barton forceps.

VACUUM VERSION

Vacuum extraction is an increasingly popular obstetric procedure in obstetrical practice. Use of the extractor complements that of forceps in many services, while in others it essentially replaces them. There are risks associated with any vaginal delivery. Both the forceps and the vacuum extractor are imperfect instruments. Even when used properly by well-meaning and skillful clinicians these instruments are capable of inflicting injury to both mother and baby. The cardinal rules pf instrumental delivery are simple: neither the vacuum extractor nor the forceps should ever be used without valid indication or by an operator uncertain of the clinical setting or of his or her skill or if true disproportion is suspected. Despite concerns, vacuum extraction is a safe obstetric procedures. Nonetheless, vacuum operations require careful attention to detail and considerable practice to minimize risk while achieving the benefits of atraumatic vaginal delivery.

MANUAL REMOVAL OF PLACENTA

The need for manual removal of the placenta can arise after any vaginal delivery, and midwives should be trained to carry it out at primary health care and at first referral level. The longer the placenta is retained, the greater the hazards, death in these cases being due to shock from haemorrhage and infection. It is best if manual removal of the placenta is carried out within the first hour after delivery. In some circumstances, the placenta may be retained for 48 hours or longer before the woman reports for treatment. In such cases severe anaemia and septicaemic shock may ensue and treatment is best provided at a tertiary level hospital.

CAESAREAN SECTION

The decline in maternal, and to a lesser extent foetal, mortality is mainly due to the tremendous impact that delivery by caesarean section has had on obstetrics. The procedure has, however, come to be abused. Many unnecessary operations are performed on a daily basis all over the world, to a degree not often seen in other surgical procedures. While the introduction of intrapartum monitoring has increased the proportion of caesarean sections compared to total deliveries all over the world the rise has not resulted in more favourable perinatal outcomes.

The indications for caesarean section are usually maternal, foetal or physician-related factors - or a mixture of the three. In our study, the most common indications were failure to progress, foetal distress and cephalopelvic disproportion. These findings agree with other recently published data. Multiple pregnancy and breech presentation are additional factors contributing to the rise in abdominal deliveries (a sad reflection, perhaps, on the "progress" of obstetrics) - although neither of them is an absolute indication.

Each case should be thoroughly evaluated to determine the possibility for normal vaginal delivery. Foetal macrosomia, a problem common to diabetic mothers, presents a dilemma as to the appropriate mode of delivery. Expert, well-considered opinion should be sought, rather than taking the often more convenient option of exposing the mother to an unnecessary operation.

The routine use of prophylactic antibiotics is associated with fewer postoperative complications - especially in emergency procedures and high-risk patients. If the patient has already had one caesarean section, most obstetricians are only too willing to perform an abdominal delivery at the first hint of a problem, an attitude that should be discouraged. Vaginal delivery following a previous caesarean section is not inappropriate, provided the reason for the previous section is not a recurrent one. Liberman et al., in a recently published study, noticed an increase in the number of males born by caesarean section compared with females.

Another recent study reports an increased risk of lowered fertility, uncompleted pregnancy (ectopic pregnancy, possible miscarriage), complications in the next pregnancy (including placental complications), and health problems in the next infant. Because of the previously mentioned tendency of obstetricians to almost automatically decide for caesarean section if the patient's previous delivery was also by caesarean section, it will be difficult to substantially decrease the current high rate of repeat caesarean births. Preventive efforts should therefore be directed to decreasing the incidence of primary caesarean deliveries.

DESTRUCTIVE OPERATIONS

Unduly prolonged obstructed labour with the foetus jammed in the pelvic cavity beyond any hope of spontaneous delivery is not seen in the developed countries today. But such a situation is prevalent in the developing countries across the continents. It plagues thousands of women every year and accounts for 8% of maternal deaths in developing countries. In India 70% of our population lives in rural areas with barely any modern obstetric facilities. Antenatal care is mostly not available or not availed of for various reasons. Home deliveries with untrained female attendant is almost a norm. In India 50% deliveries lack skilled or trained assistance. When labour gets obstructed due to contracted pelvic and foetal malformation or malpresentation the pauturient, as an inevitable last recourse, is taken to the nearest primary health centre (PHC) which is often quiet a distance away requiring time consuming arduous journey. The arriving parturient often merits the description of a woman in neglected obstructed labour with a dead foetus and distressed mother with dehydration, advanced infection and a uterus desperately trying to surmount the obstruction. The PHCs, more often than naught, lack necessary skilled obstetric and anesthetic services, and adequate surgical and ancilliary facilities like blood transfusion to deal with the ordeal of the suffering parturient who just needs a simple craniotomy or cleidotomy or a difficult decapitation or evisceration or a prompt caesarean section with all its morbidity. Caesarean delivery is often resorted to as an easier way out in preference to destructive operations, often for want of training and skill in conducting these rewarding procedures.

NURSING MANAGEMENT OF WOMEN UNDERGOING OBSTETRICAL OPERATIONS AND PROCEDURES

The safety of a woman undergoing surgery depends on good preparation and anticipation of potential complications. The woman must be fully informed as to what is going to be done to her, the reasons for the procedures and the possible complications. With good planning most procedures will be successful for both the patient and the medical team. Most women who undergo either obstetric or gynaecological surgery are young and healthy.

It is important that the woman knows what procedure is going to be done, why and the possible complications. Informed consent can only be obtained by someone who understands these issues. Information leaflets written in conjunction with patient groups and in languages other than English can be of great help in ensuring that women are well informed about both the procedure and common complications.

Good nursing management is vital because the woman can be very frightened of going to theatre and a calm nursing approach is needed at that time.

Regular observations of blood pressure, pulse, respirations and vaginal loss need to be carried out on return to the ward. Constant reassuring and an informative approach by the nursing staff is a major contributing factor to a good postoperative recovery. Health education regarding personal hygiene, both in hospital and at home will help patient to understand how to care for the newborn. Some women do feel very emotional following an operation and this should be recognized as normal by nurse and reassurance and support given. A happy, relaxed atmosphere on the ward can help to make women feel cared for and can make their stay a positive experience.

REFERENCES

Buchan, William., Advice to Mothers. Philadelphia: 1804.

Culpeper, Nicholas., Directory for Midwives., London: 1651-1777.

Blunt, John., Man-Midwifery Dissected., London: 1763.

Hunter, William., The Anatomy of the Human Gravid Uterus., Birmingham: 1774.

Nihell, Elizabeth., A Treatise on the Art of Midwifery: Setting Forth Various Abuses Therein, Especially as to the Practice with Instruments., London: 1760.

Raynalde, Thomas., The Byrth of Mankynd., London: 1545.

Sharp, Jane., The Midwives Book, Or the Whole Art of Midwifery Discovered., London: 1671.

Smellie, William., An Abridgement of the Practice of Midwifery: and a Set of Anatomical Tables with Explanations., Worcester: 1786.

9

Abnormalities during Postnatal Periods

The postnatal period begins from birth and ends when the baby is six weeks of age. The postnatal period is a very special time where women undergo the transition into motherhood. For during pregnancy it can be very difficult to comprehend just what being mother will be like. However once the baby is born women have no option but to face major changes in their lives. The changes women undergo do not just include the physical changes that occur from the birth, but social and psychological changes as well. Each woman's experience is different. However it is not unusual for a woman to take time emotionally and personally feel to like they have 'become a mother'. A woman's experience as new mother is shaped by her past experiences. These experiences include the nature of her baby, prior experience with babies and the amount of support available to her.

Commonly women feel that the experience of mothering a new baby is very challenging. Women often feel drained as their role is all consuming. Tiredness is a common problem. Some women find that they feel alone or isolated - this is particularly evident in women who have worked full time and have not built a support network. Women also report a sense of loss. Be that a loss of time, freedom or loss of control. However once women grow in their confidence of parenting their new baby - the challenges begin to ease. By acquiring knowledge and skills about caring for a newborn baby - women are able to work it out and enjoy this wonderful part of life.

ASSESSMENT AND MANAGEMENT OF WOMAN WITH POSTNATAL COMPLICATIONS

Women's health nurses provide a service to well women. Clinical functions are performed in the context of nursing practice which emphasizes enhancing women's knowledge and choices about their own health through providing information, discussion, counselling and referral. All women who have abnormal pathology on clinical examination are referred appropriately.

PUERPERIAL INFECTIONS

The term puerperal infection refers to a bacterial infection following childbirth. The infection may also be referred to as puerperal or postpartum fever. The genital tract, particularly the uterus, is the most commonly infected site. In some cases infection can spread to other points in the body. Widespread infection, or sepsis, is a rare, but potentially fatal complication.

Puerperal infection affects an estimated 1-8% of new mothers in the United States. Given modern medical treatment and antibiotics, it very rarely advances to the point of threatening a woman's life. An estimated 2-4% of new mothers who deliver vaginally suffer some form of puerperal infection, but for caesarean sections, the figure is five-10 times that high.

Deaths related to puerperal infection are very rare in the industrialized world. It is estimated three in 100, 000 births result in maternal death due to infection. However, the death rate in developing nations may be 100 times higher.

Postpartum fever may arise from several causes, not necessarily infection. If the fever is related to infection, it often results from endometritis, an inflammation of the uterus. Urinary tract, breast, and wound infections are also possible, as well as septic thrombophlebitis, a blood clot-associated inflammation of veins. A woman's susceptibility to developing an infection is related to such factors as caesarean section, extended labour, obesity, anaemia, and poor prenatal nutrition.

The primary symptom of puerperal infection is a fever at any point between birth and 10 days postpartum. A temperature of 100.4°F (38°C) on any two days during this period, or a fever of 101.6°F (38.6°C) in the first 24 hours postpartum, is cause for suspicion. An assortment of bacterial species may cause puerperal infection. Many of these bacteria are normally found in the mother's genital tract, but other bacteria may be introduced from the woman's intestine and skin or from a healthcare provider.

The associated symptoms depend on the site and nature of the infection. The most typical site of infection is the genital tract.

Endometritis, which affects the uterus, is the most prominent of these infections. Endometritis is much more common if a small part of the placenta has been retained in the uterus. Typically, several species of bacteria are involved and may act synergistically--that is, the bacteria's negative effects are multiplied rather than simply added together. Synergistic action by the bacteria can result in a stubborn infection such as an abscess. The major symptoms of a genital tract infection include fever, malaise, abdominal pain, uterine tenderness, and abnormal vaginal discharge. If these symptoms do not respond to antibiotic therapy, an abscess or blood clot may be suspected.

Other causes of postpartum fever include urinary tract infections, wound infections, septic thrombophlebitis, and mastitis. Mastitis, or breast infection, is indicated by fever, malaise, achy muscles, and reddened skin on the affected breast. It is usually caused by a clogged milk duct that becomes infected. Infections of the urinary tract are indicated by fever, frequent and painful urination, and back pain. An episiotomy and a caesarean section carry the risk of a wound infection. Such infections are suggested by a fever and pus-like discharge, inflammation, and swelling at wound sites.

Diagnosis

Fever is not an automatic indicator of puerperal infection. A new mother may have a fever owing to prior illness or an illness unconnected to childbirth. However, any fever within 10 days postpartum is aggressively investigated. Physical symptoms such as pain, malaise, loss of appetite, and others point to infection.

Many doctors initiate antibiotic therapy early in the fever period to stop an infection before it advances. A pelvic examination is done and samples are taken from the genital tract to identify the bacteria involved in the infection. The pelvic examination can reveal the extent of infection and possibly the cause. Blood samples may also be taken for blood counts and to test for the presence of infectious bacteria. A urinalysis may also be ordered, especially if the symptoms are indicative of a urinary tract infection.

If the fever and other symptoms resist antibiotic therapy, an ultrasound examination or computed tomography scan (CT scan) is done to locate potential abscesses or blood clots in the pelvic region. Magnetic resonance imaging (MRI) may be useful as well, in addition to a heparin challenge test if blood clots are suspected. If a lung infection is suspected, a chest x ray may also be ordered.

Treatment

Antibiotic therapy is the backbone of puerperal infection treatment. Initial antibiotic therapy may consist of clindamycin and gentamicin, which fight a broad array of bacteria types. If the fever and other symptoms do not respond to these antibiotics, a third, such as ampicillin, is added. Other antibiotics may be used depending on the identity of the infective bacteria and the possibility of an allergic reaction to certain antibiotics.

Antibiotics taken together are effective against a wide range of bacteria, but may not be capable of clearing up the infection alone, especially if an abscess or blood clot is present. Heparin is combined with the antibiotic therapy in order to break apart blood clots. Heparin is used for five-seven days, and may be followed by warfarin for the following month. If the infection is complicated, it may be necessary to surgically drain the infected site. Infected episiotomies can be opened and allowed to drain, but abscesses and blood clots may require surgery.

Prognosis

Antibiotic therapy and other treatment measures are virtually always successful in curing puerperal infections.

Prevention

Careful attention to antiseptic procedures during childbirth is the basic underpinning of preventing infection. With some procedures, such as caesarean section, a doctor may administer prophylactic antibiotics as a preemptive strike against infectious bacteria.

BREAST ENGORGEMENT & INFECTIONS

Engorgement is a swelling of the breasts caused by expanding veins and the pressure of new milk. Many, but not all women experience engorgement usually two to six days after delivery. Immediately after birth, the mother produces colostrum, a yellow, sticky fluid secreted by the breasts that provides nutrition and protection against infections. Colostrum contains more protein, less sugar and much less fat than mature breast milk.

Engorgement usually happens when the breasts switch from colostrum to mature milk (often referred to as when the milk "comes in"). However, engorgement can also happen later if lactating women miss several nursings and not enough milk is expressed from the breasts. The degree of engorgement usually lessens with each child. First-time mothers often suffer more from engorgement than women who are nursing their second or third child, because the time it takes for the mature milk to "come in" seems to shorten with each child.

When the breasts switch from colostrum to mature milk, some feeling of fullness, swelling, and discomfort are normal. However, when breasts become engorged, they are more prone to infections, and therefore, preventative measures should be taken to avoid and reduce engorgement. Preventative measures and remedies for engorgement: Many doctors and lactation consultants agree that the best way to prevent engorgement is to nurse often. Some suggest not going more than three hours without nursing and not skipping night feedings.

When breasts are severely engorged, the baby often cannot latch on property. Pumping or manually expressing some breast milk can help reduce engorgement, allowing the baby to suckle, which will help alleviate the swelling and prevent future episodes. Also, some women find a warm shower just before a feeding helps relieve some discomfort and facilitate let down. Massaging the breasts as the baby nurses can help get out as much milk as possible.

UTI (URINARY TRACT INFECTION IN PREGNANCY)

UTI is common during pregnancy, apparently because of urinary stasis, which results from hormonal ureteral dilation, hormonal ureteral hypoperistalsis, and pressure of the expanding uterus against the ureters. Asymptomatic bacteriuria occurs in about 15% of pregnancies and sometimes progresses to symptomatic cystitis or pyelonephritis. Frank UTI is not always preceded by asymptomatic bacteriuria. Asymptomatic bacteriuria, UTI, and pyelonephritis increase risk of preterm labour and premature rupture of the membranes.

Urinalysis and culture at initial evaluation are routinely done to check for asymptomatic UTI. Diagnosis and treatment of symptomatic UTI is not changed by pregnancy, except drugs that may harm the foetus are avoided. Antibacterial drug selection is based on individual and local susceptibility and resistance patterns, but cephalexin, nitrofurantoin, or trimethoprim-sulfamethoxazole are usually good initial empiric choices.

After treatment, proof-of-cure cultures are required. Women who have pyelonephritis or have had > 1 UTI may require suppressive therapy, usually with trimethoprim-sulfamethoxazole or nitrofurantoin, for the rest of the pregnancy. In women who have bacteriuria with or without UTI or pyelonephritis, urine should be cultured monthly.

THROMBOEMBOLIC DISORDERS IN PREGNANCY

In the present world and specially in some developed nations, thromboembolic disorders-deep venous thrombosis or pulmonary embolism-are a leading cause of maternal mortality. During pregnancy, risk is increased because venous capacitance and venous pressure in the legs are increased, resulting in stasis, and because pregnancy causes a degree of hypercoagulability.

However, most thromboemboli develop postpartum and result from vascular trauma during delivery. Caesarean section also increases risk. Symptoms of thrombophlebitis or their absence do not accurately predict the diagnosis, disease severity, or risk of embolization. Thromboembolic disorders can occur without symptoms, with only minimal symptoms, or with significant symptoms. Also, calf edema, cramping, and tenderness, which may occur normally during pregnancy, may simulate Homans' sign.

Diagnosis and Treatment

Diagnosis of DVT is usually by Doppler ultrasonography. In the postpartum period, if Doppler ultrasonography and plethysmography are normal but iliac, ovarian, or other pelvic venous thrombosis is suspected, CT with contrast is used.

Diagnosis of PE is increasingly being made by helical CT rather than ventilation-perfusion scanning, because it involves less radiation and is equally sensitive. If the diagnosis of PE is uncertain, pulmonary angiography is required.

If DVT or PE is detected during pregnancy, the anticoagulant of choice is a low mol wt heparin (LMWH). LMWH, because of its molecular size, does not cross the placenta. It does not cause maternal osteoporosis or thrombocytopenia, which can result from prolonged (? 6 mo) use of unfractionated heparin. Warfarin crosses the placenta and may cause foetal abnormalities or death. Indications for thrombolysis during pregnancy are the same as for patients who are not pregnant. If PE recurs despite effective anticoagulation, surgery, usually placement of an inferior vena cava filter just distal to the renal vessels, is indicated.

If patients developed DVT or PE during a previous pregnancy or have an underlying thrombophilic disorder, they are treated with prophylactic LMWH 5000 units sc bid beginning at the first diagnosis of pregnancy and continuing until 6 wk postpartum.

POSTPARTUM HAEMORRHAGE

Postpartum haemorrhage (PPH) is a potentially life-threatening complication of both vaginal and caesarean delivery. Traditionally, PPH was defined as blood loss greater than 500 mL in a vaginal delivery and greater than 1, 000 mL in a caesarean delivery. However, studies have revealed that an uncomplicated delivery often results in blood loss of more than 500 mL without any compromise of the mother's condition. These findings resulted in adoption of a broader definition for PPH. Any bleeding that results in signs and symptoms of hemodynamic instability, or bleeding that could result in hemodynamic instability if untreated, is considered PPH. Blood loss of greater than 1, 000 mL with an vaginal delivery or a decrease in postpartum hematocrit level greater than 10% of the prenatal value also can be considered PPH.

Temporally, PPH can be divided into (1) early PPH that occurs within 24 hours after delivery and (2) late PPH that occurs 24 hours to 6 weeks after delivery. The exact incidence of PPH is difficult to determine. A reasonable consensus is that 1-10% of pregnancies are complicated by PPH, with the actual number in the range of 2-4%.

- PPH can cause severe morbidity and mortality.
- According to CDC data, 17% of maternal mortality is due to haemorrhage. PPH is thought to be the cause in one third to one half of these cases.
- Possible complications include exposure to blood products, the need for surgical intervention, and the need for permanent sterilization to control bleeding.

In addition to asking the standard questions about the prenatal period, request information about previous episodes of PPH, prior caesarean section, parity, and history of multiple fetuses or polyhydramnios.

- Ascertain if the patient or family has a history of coagulation disorders or excessive bleeding with surgical procedures or menses.
- Obtain information about medications, with emphasis on medications for hypertension (calcium-channel blockers) or heart disease (e.g., digoxin, warfarin). This information is important if the coagulopathy develops and the patient requires transfusions.
- Determine if the placenta has already been delivered.

Causes

- The most frequent cause of PPH is uterine atony, a condition in which the uterine corpus does not constrict properly, allowing continued blood loss from the placental site. Risk factors for atony include the following:
  - Overdistended uterus (e.g., multiple gestation, foetal macrosomia, hydramnios)
  - Fatigued uterus (e.g., augmented or prolonged labour, amnionitis)
  - Obstructed uterus (e.g., retained placenta or foetal parts, placenta accreta)
- The second most frequent cause is trauma to the uterus, cervix, and/or vagina. Risk factors for trauma include the following:
  - Delivery of a large infant
  - Instrumentation or intrauterine manipulation (e.g., forceps, vacuum)
  - Vaginal birth after caesarean section (VBAC)
  - Episiotomy
- Disorders of coagulation and thrombocytopenia, preexisting or occurring during the second or third stage of labour, may be associated with excessive bleeding.
- Trauma during delivery may result in hematomas in the perineum or pelvis. These hematomas may be palpable and should be suspected if the patient has unstable vital signs and little or no external bleeding.
- Uterine inversion may be associated with haemorrhage of approximately 2 L. No definitive study findings have demonstrated the relationship between traction on the umbilical cord and uterine inversion, although many clinicians indicate that a correlation may exist.
- Uterine rupture may be associated with little vaginal bleeding, but it should be considered in the presence of severe abdominal pain and unstable hemodynamic findings.
- Other risk factors for PPH include the following:
  - Preeclampsia
  - Previous PPH
  - Asian or Hispanic ethnicity
  - Nulliparity or multiparity

ECLAMPSIA AND SUBIVOLUTION

By eclampsia only those cases of toxamia of pregnancy are understood that are attended by convulsions. These convulsions are independent of any disturbances in function of the kidneys. For this reason a patient with eclampsia should not be treated in the same way as on e with nephritis. The fits occur as a rule with approximately regular intervals and tend to stop spontaneously after an average of 12 hours. They are always about equal, epileptiformic, and cause spasms o f the vessels, in consequence of which disturbances of the circulation arise, which are the reason of the strong albuminuria and disturbances in the function of the kidneys and liver, haemorrhages in the retina in the placenta, brain etc.

The duration of the eclampsia is too short to enable us to combat success fully the r ea l intoxication. That is why we must try to stop the fits and to lengthen the intervals, firstly hynarcotics and secondly by venesections. Twenty-five percent of eclampsia cases occur

postpartum: moreover the course of the eclampsia ante-partum is exactly the same as durante partum and postpartum. Therefore forcerd labour and Cesarian section are of no use but only increase the danger to the patient.

PSYCHOLOGICAL COMPLICATIONS

As many as 80% of women experience some mood disturbances after pregnancy ("postpartum"). They feel upset, alone, afraid, or unloving toward their baby, and guilt for having these feelings. For most women, the symptoms are mild and go away on their own. But 10-20% of women develop a more disabling form of mood disorder called postpartum depression.

Baby Blues: The "baby blues" are a passing state of heightened emotions that occurs in about half of women who have recently given birth. This state peaks 3-5 days after delivery and lasts from several days to 2 weeks. A woman with the blues may cry more easily than usual and may have trouble sleeping or feel irritable, sad, and "on edge" emotionally. Because baby blues are so common and expected, they are not considered an illness. Postpartum blues do not interfere with a woman's ability to care for her baby. The tendency to develop postpartum blues is unrelated to a previous mental illness and is not caused by stress. However, stress and a history of depression may influence whether the blues go on to become major depression.

Postpartum depression: Postpartum depression is depression that occurs soon after having a baby. Some health professionals call it postpartum nonpsychotic depression. This condition occurs in about 10-20% of women, usually within a few months of delivery. Risk factors include previous major depression, psychosocial stress, inadequate social support, and previous premenstrual dysphoric disorder. Symptoms include depressed mood, tearfulness, inability to enjoy pleasurable activities, trouble sleeping, fatigue, appetite problems, suicidal thoughts, feelings of inadequacy as a parent, and impaired concentration. If lady experience postpartum depression, she may worry about the baby's health and well-being. She may have negative thoughts about the baby and fears about harming the infant (although women who have these thoughts rarely act on them). Postpartum depression interferes with a woman's ability to care for her baby. When a woman with severe postpartum depression becomes suicidal, she may consider killing her infant and young children, not from anger, but from a desire not to abandon them.

Postpartum (puerperal) psychosis is the most serious postpartum disorder. It requires immediate treatment. This condition is rare. A woman with this condition experiences psychotic symptoms within 3 weeks of giving birth. These include false beliefs (delusions), hallucinations (seeing or hearing things that are not there), or both. This condition is associated with mood disorders such as depression, bipolar disorder, or psychosis. Symptoms can include inability to sleep, agitation, and mood swings. A woman experiencing psychosis can appear well temporarily, fooling health professionals and caregivers into thinking that she has recovered, but she can continue to be severely depressed and ill even after brief periods of seeming well. Women who harbor thoughts of hurting their infants are more likely to act on them if they have postpartum psychosis. If untreated, postpartum psychotic depression has a high likelihood of coming back after the postpartum period and also after the birth of other children.

CAUSES

No specific cause has been found. Hormone imbalance is thought to play a role. Levels of the hormones estrogen, progesterone, and cortisol fall dramatically within 48 hours after delivery. Women who go on to develop postpartum depression may be more sensitive to these hormonal changes.

Other known risk factors are:

- Mental illness before pregnancy
- Mental illness, including postpartum depression, in the family

- Postpartum mental disorder after an earlier pregnancy
- Conflict in the marriage, loss of employment, or poor social support from friends and family
- Pregnancy loss such as miscarriage or stillbirth
- The risk of major depression after miscarriage is high for women who are childless. It occurs even in women who were unhappy about being pregnant.
- The risk for developing depression after miscarriage is highest within the first few months after the loss.

Childbirth is a time of great change for a woman. The adjustment to these changes can contribute to depression: Physical changes after delivery are:

- Many changes occur after delivery, including changes in muscle tone and difficulty losing weight.
- Many new mothers are very tired after giving birth and in the weeks afterwards.
- Soreness and pain in perineal area (area around the birth canal) makes many women uncomfortable. Physical recovery after cesarean delivery may take even longer than after vaginal delivery.
- Changes in hormones can affect mood.

Common emotional changes after delivery are:

- Feelings of loss of an old identity, feeling trapped at home
- Feeling overwhelmed with responsibilities of motherhood
- Feeling stress from changes in routine
- Feeling fatigue because of broken sleep patterns
- Feeling less attractive physically and sexually

A mother's age and the number of children she has had do not relate to her likelihood of getting postpartum depression.

SYMPTOMS

Symptoms usually appear any time from 24 hours to a few months after delivery. If mother have these, it is important to see a health care provider, who will look for other conditions that can cause similar symptoms.

- Sad mood, frequent crying
- Lack of pleasure or interest in activities that once gave pleasure
- Sleep disturbance
- Weight loss
- Loss of energy
- Agitation or anxiety
- Feelings of worthlessness or guilt
- Trouble concentrating or making decisions
- Thoughts of death or suicide
- Decreased interest in sex
- Feelings of rejection

Physical symptoms such as frequent headaches, chest pain, rapid heart beat, numbness, shakiness or dizziness, and mild shortness of breath suggest anxiety. Postpartum anxiety disorder is a separate disorder from postpartum depression, but the two often occur together.

TREATMENT

Postpartum depression is treated much like any other depression. Support, counseling ("talk therapy") and medicines can all help.

REFERENCES

Kerr-Wilson R H J, Parham G P and Orr J W (1983) The effect of a full bladder on labour Obstetrics and Gynaecology 62(3) 319-323

Clement S and Reed B (1999) To stitich or not to stitich? The Practising Midwife 2(4) 20-27

McCandlish R (2001) Routine perineal suturing:is it time to stop? MIDIRS Midwifery Digest 11:3 296-300

Odibo L (1997) Suturing of perineal trauma: how well are we doing - an audit British Journal of Midwifery 5(11) 690-692

Fleming V and Hagen S (1998) To suture or not to suture British Journal of Midwifery Letters 6(11) 737

10

High Risk Newborn

Every family looks forward to the birth of a healthy newborn. It is an exciting time with so much to look forward to. In some cases, though, unexpected difficulties and challenges occur along the way. Some newborns are considered high risk. This means that a newborn has a greater chance of complications because of conditions that occur during foetal development, pregnancy conditions of the mother, or problems that may occur during labour and birth. Some complications are unexpected and may occur without warning. Other times, there are certain risk factors that make problems more likely. Fortunately, advances in technology have helped improve the care of sick newborns. Under the care of specialized physicians and other healthcare providers, babies have much greater chances for surviving and getting better today than ever before.

ASSESSMENTS FOR NEWBORN BABIES

Each newborn baby is carefully checked at birth for signs of problems or complications. A complete physical assessment will be performed that includes every body system. Throughout the hospital stay, physicians, nurses, and other healthcare providers continually assess a baby for changes in health and for signs of problems or illness. Assessment may include:

APGAR SCORING

The Apgar score is one of the first checks of new baby's health. The Apgar score is assigned in the first few minutes after birth to help identify babies that have difficulty breathing or have a problem that needs further care. The baby is checked at one minute and five minutes after birth for heart and respiratory rates, muscle tone, reflexes, and colour.

Each area can have a score of zero, one, or two, with ten points as the maximum. A total score of ten means a baby is in the best possible condition. Nearly all babies score between eight and ten, with one or two points taken off for blue hands and feet because of immature circulation. If a baby has a difficult time during delivery, this can lower the oxygen levels in the blood, which can lower the Apgar score. Apgar scores of three or less often mean a baby needs immediate attention and care. However, only 1.4 percent of babies have APGAR scores less than seven at five minutes after birth.

Sign	Score = 0	Score = 1	Score = 2
Heart Rate	Absent	Below 100 per minute	Above 100 per minute
Respiratory Effort	Absent	Weak, irregular, or gasping	Good, crying
Muscle Tone	Flaccid	Some flexion of arms and legs	Well flexed, or active movements of extremities
Reflex/ Irritability	No response	Grimace or weak cry	Good cry
Colour	Blue all over, or pale	Body pink, hands and feet blue	Pink all over

BIRTHWEIGHT

A baby's birthweight is an important indicator of health. The average weight for term babies (born between 37 and 41 weeks gestation) is about 7 lbs. (3.2 kg). In general, small babies and very large babies are at greater risk for problems. Babies are weighed daily in the nursery to assess growth, fluid, and nutrition needs. Newborn babies may lose as much as 10 percent of their birthweight. This means that a baby weighing 7 pounds 3 ounces at birth might lose as much as 10 ounces in the first few days. Premature and sick babies may not begin to gain weight right away.

Most hospitals use the metric system for weighing babies.

MEASUREMENTS

Other measurements are also taken of each baby. These include the following:

- Head circumference (the distance around the baby's head): It is normally about one-half the baby's body length plus 10 cm

- Abdominal circumference: The distance around the abdomen
- Length: The measurement from crown of head to the heel

PHYSICAL EXAMINATION

A complete physical examination is an important part of newborn care. Each body system is carefully examined for signs of health and normal function. The physician also looks for any signs of illness or birth defects. Physical examination of a newborn often includes the assessment of the following:

- Vital signs:
  - — Temperature - able to maintain stable body temperature 98.6° F (37° C) in normal room environment
  - — Pulse - normally 120 to 160 beats per minute
  - — Breathing rate - normally 30 to 60 breaths per minute
  - — General appearance - physical activity, tone, posture, and level of consciousness
  - — Skin - colour, texture, nails, presence of rashes
  - — Head and neck:
- Appearance, shape, presence of molding (shaping of the head from passage through the birth canal)
- Fontanels (the open "soft spots" between the bones of the baby's skull)
- Clavicles (bones across the upper chest)
  - — Face - eyes, ears, nose, cheeks
  - — Mouth - palate, tongue, throat
  - — Lungs - breath sounds, breathing pattern
  - — Heart sounds and femoral (in the groin) pulses
  - — Abdomen - presence of masses or hernias
  - — Genitals and anus - for open passage of urine and stool
  - — Arms and legs - movement and development

GESTATIONAL ASSESSMENT

Assessing a baby's physical maturity is an important part of care. Maturity assessment is helpful in meeting a baby's needs if the dates of a pregnancy are uncertain. For example, a very small baby may actually be more mature than it appears by size, and may need different care than a premature baby.

An examination called The Dubowitz/Ballard Examination for Gestational Age is often used. A baby's gestational age often can be closely estimated using this examination. The Dubowitz/Ballard Examination evaluates a baby's appearance, skin texture, motor function, and reflexes. The physical maturity part of the examination is done in the first two hours of birth. The neuromuscular maturity examination is completed within 24 hours after delivery. Information often used to help estimate babies' physical and neuromuscular maturity are shown below.

PHYSICAL MATURITY

The physical assessment part of the Dubowitz/Ballard Examination looks at physical characteristics that look different at different stages of a baby's gestational maturity. Babies who are physically mature usually have higher scores than premature babies.

Points are given for each area of assessment, with a low of -1 or -2 for extreme immaturity to as much as 4 or 5 for postmaturity. Areas of assessment include the following:

- Skin textures (i.e., sticky, smooth, peeling).
- Lanugo (the soft downy hair on a baby's body) - is absent in immature babies, then appears with maturity, and then disappears again with postmaturity.
- Plantar creases - these creases on the soles of the feet range from absent to covering the entire foot, depending on the maturity.
- Breast - the thickness and size of breast tissue and areola (the darkened ring around each nipple) are assessed.
- Eyes and ears - eyes fused or open and amount of cartilage and stiffness of the ear tissue.
- Genitals, male - presence of testes and appearance of scrotum, from smooth to wrinkled.
- Genitals, female - appearance and size of the clitoris and the labia.

Neuromuscular Maturity

Six evaluations of the baby's neuromuscular system are performed. These include:

- Posture - how does the baby hold his/her arms and legs.
- Square window - how far the baby's hands can be flexed toward the wrist.

- Arm recoil - how far the baby's arms "spring back" to a flexed position.
- Popliteal angle - how far the baby's knees extend.
- Scarf sign - how far the elbows can be moved across the baby's chest.
- Heel to ear - how close the baby's feet can be moved to the ears.

A score is assigned to each assessment area. Typically, the more neurologically mature the baby, the higher the score.

When the physical assessment score and the neuromuscular score are added together, the gestational age can be estimated. Scores range from very low for immature babies (less than 26 to 28 weeks) to very high scores for mature and postmature babies.

All of these examinations are important ways to learn about baby's well-being at birth. By identifying any problems, baby's physician can plan the best possible care.

BIRTH DEFECTS

There are many different types of birth defects that place a newborn at higher risk and require clinical care by a physician or other healthcare professional. Listed below is main, for which we have provided a brief overview.

A "birth defect" is a health problem or physical change, which is present in a baby at the time he/she is born. Birth defects may be very mild, where the baby looks and acts like any other baby, or birth defects may be very severe. Some of the severe birth defects can be life threatening, where a baby may only live a few months, or may die at a young age (in their teens, for example).

Birth defects are also called "congenital anomalies" or "congenital abnormalities." The word "congenital" means "present at birth." The words "anomalies" and "abnormalities" mean that there is a problem present in a baby.

CAUSES

There are many reasons why birth defects happen. Most occur due to environmental and genetic factors, but often the cause is unknown.

Birth defects have been present in babies from all over the world, in families of all nationalities and backgrounds. Anytime a couple becomes pregnant, there is a chance that their baby will have a birth defect. Most babies are born healthy. In fact, 97 out of 100 babies are born healthy. Anytime a couple becomes pregnant, there is a 3 to 4 percent chance that their baby will have a birth defect. The 3 to 4 percent number is sometimes called the background rate for birth defects, or the population risk for birth defects. In a family where birth defects are already present in family members or the parents themselves, the chance for a couple to have a child with a birth defect may be higher than the background rate of 3 to 4 percent.

Genetic and Environmental Causes of Birth Defects

When a baby is born with a birth defect, the first question usually asked by the parents is "how did this happen?" Sometimes, this question cannot be answered. This can be very upsetting for parents because it is normal to seek an answer as to why baby has a health problem. For some birth defects, however, there is a known cause, which may have to do with either genetic or environmental factors, or a combination of the two. Here is some general information and terms related to the different causes of birth defects:

- Inheritance: Inheritance is a word used to describe a trait given to you or "passed on" to you from one of parents. Examples of inherited traits would be eye colour or blood type.
- Chromosome abnormalities: Chromosomes are stick-like structures in the center of each cell (called the nucleus) that contain genes.
- Single gene defects: Genes are what determine your traits. Sometimes, a child can inherit not only those genes responsible for their normal traits such as the colour of their eyes, but also disease causing genes that result in a birth defect.
- Multifactorial inheritance: Multifactorial inheritance means that "many factors" (multifactorial) are involved in causing a birth defect. The factors are usually both genetic and environmental.
- Teratogens: A teratogen is an agent, which can cause a birth defect. It is usually something in the environment that the mother may be exposed to during her pregnancy. It could be a prescribed medication, a street drug, alcohol use, or a disease that the mother has, which could increase the chance for the baby to be born with a birth defect.

Although some birth defects have a single abnormality, others have abnormalities in multiple body systems or organs. Birth defects may cause life-long disability and illness, and with some, survival is not possible.

Some birth defects, such as mental retardation, are non-treatable disabilities. However, many physical defects can be treated with surgery. Repair is possible with many defects including cleft lip or palate, and certain heart defects.

DIAGNOSIS

Many birth defects can be diagnosed before birth with special tests (prenatal diagnosis). Chromosomal abnormalities such as Down syndrome can be diagnosed before birth by analyzing cells in the amniotic fluid or from the placenta. Foetal ultrasound during pregnancy can also give information about the possibility of certain birth defects, but ultrasound is not 100 percent accurate, since some babies with birth defects may look the same on ultrasound as those without problems. A chromosome analysis, whether performed on a blood sample or cells from the amniotic fluid or placenta, is over 99.9 percent accurate.

Tests that help screen for birth defects include the following:

- Alpha-fetoprotein: This blood test measures the levels of alpha-fetoprotein (AFP), a protein released by the foetal liver and found in the mother's blood. AFP is sometimes called MSAFP (maternal serum AFP). AFP screening may be included as one part of a two, three, or four-part screening, often called a multiple marker screen. The other parts may include the following:
  - hCG - human chorionic gonadotropin (hCG) is a hormone secreted by the early placental cells. High hCG levels may indicate a foetus with Down syndrome (a chromosomal abnormality that includes mental retardation and distinct physical features).
  - Estriol - a hormone produced by the placenta and by the foetal liver and adrenal glands. Low levels may indicate a foetus with Down syndrome.
  - Inhibin - a hormone produced by the placenta.
- Chorionic villus sampling (CVS): A prenatal test that involves taking a sample of some of the placental tissue. This tissue contains the same genetic material as the foetus and can be tested for chromosomal abnormalities and some other genetic problems. Testing is available for other genetic defects and disorders depending on the family history and availability of laboratory testing at the time of the procedure. In comparison

to amniocentesis (another type of prenatal test), CVS does not provide information on neural tube defects such as spina bifida. For this reason, women who undergo CVS also need a follow-up blood test between 16 to 18 weeks of their pregnancy, to screen for neural tube defects.

- Amniocentesis: A procedure used to obtain a small sample of the amniotic fluid that surrounds the foetus to diagnose chromosomal disorders and open neural tube defects (ONTDs) such as spina bifida. Testing is available for other genetic defects and disorders depending on the family history and availability of laboratory testing at the time of the procedure. The American College of Obstetricians and Gynaecologists (ACOG) recommends amniocentesis around 15 weeks to 20 weeks of pregnancy for those women who are at increased risk for chromosome abnormalities, such as women who are over age 35 years of age at delivery, or those who have had an abnormal maternal serum screening test, indicating an increased risk for a chromosomal abnormality or neural tube defect. However, in some situations, amniocentesis may be performed as early as 14 weeks.
- Ultrasound: A diagnostic technique that uses high-frequency sound waves to create an image of the internal organs. Many birth defects can be detected with ultrasound.

Sometimes, birth defects are not diagnosed until physical examination of the baby after birth. To confirm the physical findings, a small blood sample can be taken and the chromosomes can be analyzed. This information is important in determining the risk for that birth defect in future pregnancies.

PREVENTION

Research is ongoing to find and treat the causes of many birth defects. Immunizations of the mother against certain infections, such as rubella, can prevent infection. Much has been learned about the dangerous effects of alcohol on the developing baby and women are now advised to not drink during pregnancy. In recent years, a strong link has been discovered between the lack of the B-vitamin folic acid and the development of neural tube defects such as spina bifida. Taking a vitamin containing sufficient folic acid before conception and in early pregnancy can often help prevent many serious defects.

BIRTH INJURY

Occasionally during the birth process, the baby may suffer a physical injury that is simply the result of being born. This is sometimes called birth trauma or birth injury.

CAUSES

A difficult birth or injury to the baby can occur because of the baby's size or the position of the baby during labour and delivery. Conditions that may be associated with a difficult birth include, but are not limited to, the following:

- Large babies: Birthweight over about 4, 000 grams (8 pounds, 13 ounces)
- Prematurity: Babies born before 37 weeks (premature babies have more fragile bodies and may be more easily injured)
- Cephalopelvic disproportion: The size and shape of the mother's pelvis is not adequate for the baby to be born vaginally
- Dystocia: Difficult labour or childbirth
- Prolonged labour
- Abnormal birthing presentation: Such as breech (buttocks first) delivery

COMMON BIRTH INJURIES

The following are common birth injuries:

- Caput succedaneum: Caput is a severe swelling of the soft tissues of the baby's scalp that develops as the baby travels through the birth canal. Some babies have some bruising of the area. The swelling usually disappears in a few days without problems. Babies delivered by vacuum extraction are more likely to have this condition.
- Cephalohematoma: Cephalohematoma is an area of bleeding underneath one of the cranial bones. It often appears several hours after birth as a raised lump on the baby's head. The body resorbs the blood. Depending on the size, most cephalohematomas take two weeks to three months to disappear completely. If the area of bleeding is large, some babies may develop jaundice as the red blood cells break down.
- Bruising/Forceps marks: Some babies may show signs of bruising on the face or head simply as a result of the trauma

of passing though the birth canal and contact with the mother's pelvic bones and tissues. Forceps used with delivery can leave temporary marks or bruises on the baby's face and head. Babies delivered by vacuum extraction may have some scalp bruising or a scalp laceration (cut).

- Subconjunctival haemorrhage: Subconjunctival haemorrhage is the breakage of small blood vessels in the eyes of a baby. One or both of the eyes may have a bright red band around the iris. This is very common and does not cause damage to the eyes. The redness is usually absorbed in a week to ten days.
- Facial paralysis: During labour or birth, pressure on a baby's face may cause the facial nerve to be injured. This may also occur with the use of forceps for delivery. The injury is often seen when the baby cries. There is no movement on the side of the face with the injury and the eye cannot be closed. If the nerve was only bruised, the paralysis usually improves in a few weeks. If the nerve was torn, surgery may be needed.
- Brachial palsy: Brachial palsy occurs when the brachial plexus (the group of nerves that supplies the arms and hands) is injured. It is most common when there is difficulty delivering the baby's shoulder, called shoulder dystocia. The baby loses the ability to flex and rotate the arm. If the injury caused bruising and swelling around the nerves, movement should return within a few months. Tearing of the nerve may result in permanent nerve damage. Special exercises are used to help maintain the range of motion of the arm while healing occurs.
- Fractures: Fracture of the clavicle or collarbone is the most common fracture during labour and delivery. The clavicle may break when there is difficulty delivering the baby's shoulder or during a breech delivery. The baby with a fractured clavicle rarely moves the arm on the side of the break. However, healing occurs quickly. As new bone forms, a firm lump on the clavicle often develops in the first 10 days. If the fracture is painful, limiting movement of the arm and shoulder with a soft bandage or splint may be helpful.

BLOOD TYPES IN PREGNANCY

Every person has a blood type, (O, A, B, or AB) and an Rh factor, either positive or negative. The blood type and the Rh factor simply mean that a person's blood has certain specific characteristics. The blood type is found as proteins on red blood cells and in body fluids. The Rh factor is a protein that is found on the covering of the red blood cells. If the Rh factor protein is present on the cells, the person is Rh positive. If there is no Rh factor protein, the person is Rh negative.

The following are the possible combinations of blood types with the Rh factors:

Blood Type	A	B	O	AB
Rh positive	A+	B+	O+	AB+
Rh negative	A-	B-	O-	AB-

Rh factors are genetically determined. A baby may have the blood type and Rh factor of either parent, or a combination of both parents. Rh factors follow a common pattern of genetic inheritance. The Rh positive gene is dominant (stronger) and even when paired with an Rh negative gene, the positive gene takes over.

- If a person has the genes + +, the Rh factor in the blood will be positive.
- If a person has the genes + -, the Rh factor will also be positive.
- If a person has the genes - -, the Rh factor will be negative.

A baby receives one gene from the father and one from the mother. More specifically, consider the following:

- If a father's Rh factor genes are + +, and the mother's are + +, the baby will have one + from the father and one + gene from the mother. The baby will be + + Rh positive.
- If a father's Rh factor genes are + +, and the mother's are - -, the baby will have one + from the father and one - gene from the mother. The baby will be + - Rh positive.
- If the father's genes are + - Rh positive, and the mother's are + - Rh positive, the baby can be:
- + + Rh positive
- + - Rh positive
- - - Rh negative
- If the father's genes are - -, and the mother's are + -, the baby can be

- + - Rh positive
- - - Rh negative
- If the father's genes are - -, and the mother's are - -, the baby will be:
- - - Rh negative

Problems with the Rh factor occur when the mother's Rh factor is negative and the baby's is positive. Sometimes, an incompatibility may occur when the mother is blood type O and the baby is either A or B.

BREASTFEEDING

Giving birth to a premature or other high-risk baby (or babies) does not mean mother cannot breastfeed. Actually, the opposite may be the case. There is even more reason to provide mother's own milk for, and eventually breastfeed, a premature or a sick newborn. Providing milk for baby lets her participate in baby's healthcare in a very crucial way. Because the benefits of mother's milk are so important to the high-risk newborn, mother is able to do something for baby that no one else can. Many neonatologists and NICU staff members now encourage mothers to provide their own milk for high-risk babies, even if those mothers do not intend to breastfeed later. As the mother of a high-risk newborn, you may have to overcome difficulties that a mother and full-term, healthy baby are unlikely to run into when learning to breastfeed. However, lady and her baby will learn to breastfeed. It simply may take a bit more patience and persistence. How soon lady and her baby can begin to breastfeed will depend on the maturity of baby's brain and body systems. Although a baby's gestational age influences the development of stable body systems and the development of the reflexes needed for oral feedings, a baby's physical condition may also affect when direct breastfeeding can begin.

Until baby is able to breastfeed, mother can express her milk (remove milk from her breasts) to establish and maintain breast milk production. Milk expression also allows high-risk baby to get the benefits of mother's milk as soon as his/her gastrointestinal tract is ready to handle gavage (tube) or oral (by mouth) feedings. Plan to continue to express her milk until she knows her baby is able to get all needed nourishment directly from her breasts.

BENEFITS OF MOTHER'S MILK

Nature designed human milk especially for human babies, and it is the ideal food for baby's first several months. Breast milk contains just the right balance of nutrients, and it contains them in the form that is most easily used by the human baby's immature body systems. Because it was developed for baby, milk also is gentlest on baby's systems.

Breast milk is rich in the nutrients that promote brain growth and nervous system development. Of course, it is also the perfect first food to help human baby achieve every aspect of ideal growth and development.

PRETERM MOTHER'S MILK

The milk of mothers who give birth prematurely is somewhat different than milk produced by women after a full-term baby's birth in the following ways:

- Nutrients: Several studies found more fat, protein, and the minerals sodium, chloride, and iron in "preterm milk" than in "term" milk. The variation in nutrient content seems to be of benefit for the preterm baby.

Generally, premature babies who receive their own mothers' milk develop better eye function. They, and other high-risk babies fed mothers' milk, usually perform better on different kinds of intelligence tests as they grow older. This is mostly due to certain types of fats (fatty acid chains) in human milk, which are not available in artificial formulas. Yet these fats have been shown to be especially important for the growth and development of a high-risk baby's eyes, brain, and nervous system.

During the last weeks of pregnancy, a baby builds a lot of body tissue. Because premature babies are born early, they must build this tissue after birth. Tissue building requires protein. Preterm milk has a bit more protein, and the protein is in a form that is more easily used by premature baby. Other extra proteins in preterm milk reflect higher levels of certain anti-infective properties, especially ones that protect babies against gastrointestinal and respiratory infections.

- Anti-infective properties: Only human milk is alive with many different kinds of disease-fighting factors that help prevent mild to severe infections in babies. Preterm milk has higher levels of these anti-infective properties. Antibodies in human milk directly protect against infection. Other anti-infective factors create an environment that is friendly to the "good" bacteria, referred to as "normal flora, " and unfriendly to "bad" bacteria, viruses, or parasites. Human milk also appears to have properties that help a baby's own immune system work best.

The anti-infective properties in mother's milk are especially beneficial for premature and other high-risk babies, since these babies are more likely to be exposed to, and pick up, infections more easily. Babies receiving their own mothers' milk are many times less likely to develop diarrhea and a severe intestinal illness called necrotizing enterocolitis (NEC) during their NICU stay. If any of these problems do occur, they are usually less severe for the baby receiving his own mother's milk. Babies that are fully, or almost-fully, breastfed and those receiving expressed breast milk also have significantly fewer GI, respiratory, ear, and urinary infections after hospital discharge.

- Easily digested: Since nature designed human milk for human babies, milk is the most easily digested food baby can receive. A nutritious, yet easily digested first food is important for any baby, but it is particularly beneficial for the immature digestive tract of a premature baby and the more sensitive systems of many other high-risk babies. Baby uses less energy, yet breaks milk down more completely into its basic ingredients, so the nutrients, anti-infective factors, and all the other "ingredients" in milk are more available to fuel baby's body functions and to promote growth and development.

MILK EXPRESSION

Ongoing, long-term milk production depends mostly on milk removal. The more often milk is removed, and the more completely it is removed, the more milk the breasts make. The opposite is also true. When milk is removed less often, or an insufficient amount is removed, the breasts get the signal to slow milk production and make less. Milk removal occurs when a baby effectively breastfeeds or through appropriate milk expression.

Effective breastfeeding requires effective sucking by the baby so that enough milk is transferred from the breast into the baby's mouth where it is swallowed. To suck effectively, a baby must latch deeply onto the breast and use the structures in his/her mouth to create intermittent (periodic) suction and compress the milk sinuses (enlarged area of milk ducts) lying beneath the areola (the area about 1 1/2 to 2 inches behind the nipple tip). Proper sucking signals the mother's body to release the hormone oxytocin. This results in greater transfer of milk with the milk-ejection reflex (MER), or milk "let down."

Milk Expression Methods

Milk transfer also can be accomplished through milk expression techniques. Generally, the milk-ejection reflex is triggered during milk expression sessions, especially if frequent and regular sessions occur. These include the following:

- Manual expression - a mother compresses the milk sinuses by hand to remove milk.
- Breast pumps - remove milk by creating suction; a few also have features that compress milk sinuses to some degree.

There is no "one size fits all" method for achieving effective breastfeeding with a high-risk baby, because each baby and each situation is different. Give high-risk baby extra time to learn to breastfeed, and let the baby set the pace for learning. Learning to breastfeed effectively is a process that may take days or weeks for premature and many other high-risk babies. However, mother and her baby can become a breastfeeding team if she is patient, persistent, and maintain a healthy perspective.

In general, a baby must be able to suck-swallow-breathe in a coordinated way to take food by mouth. Some of the signs that a baby is getting ready to do this include the following:

- Physical stability: A baby's condition should be stable so the baby can physically handle an "in arms" feeding.
- Non-nutritive sucking: A baby first displays rhythmic sucking on a pacifier, feeding tube, etc., in brief bursts of more than one suck per second.
- Gestational age: At about 32 weeks gestation, a baby will begin to display bursts of sucking, and around 34 weeks a rhythmic suck-swallow-breathe pattern develops.
- Wakeful state: A baby must remain awake - from drowsy to quiet alert to active - for brief periods, to feed by mouth.
- Oral reflexes: A baby must be able to tolerate touch to the mouth area and demonstrate the reflexes needed for oral feeding, such as rooting, sucking, cough, and gag reflexes.

Breastfeeding is usually less stressful for a high-risk infant, because the baby sets the pace - both for an individual feeding and for the process of learning to feed effectively. A baby's heart and respiratory rates, oxygen saturation level, and body temperature tend to remain more stable, and often improve, during breastfeeding. This stability of physical systems means breastfeeding takes less energy and it is less "work" for the high-risk baby. Of course, a baby must actually latch-on and actively suck to get milk during breastfeeding and this may take time for a baby to learn.

When bottle-feeding, milk drips in the baby's mouth and a baby must swallow it, ready or not.

Stages in Breastfeeding

The stages listed below, which describe a baby's progression to direct breastfeeding, are meant only as a guideline. Progress varies among high-risk babies. A baby might move quickly from one stage to another, or skip a stage altogether. On the other hand, a baby may sometimes seem to get "stuck" at one stage for a few days or weeks.

- Practice feedings: During the early stages of learning to breastfeed, high-risk baby may not take much, if any, milk during breastfeeding. The baby is only practicing the motions.
- Skin-to-skin contact (Kangaroo Care): A baby is likely to begin rooting or nuzzling at the breast, and may actually latch-on, when held skin-to-skin.
- "Empty breast" feeding: A mother may want to pump before skin-to-skin holding sessions once rooting and nuzzling are noted. Then, the baby can latch-on and practice without being overwhelmed by the milk "let-down" and lots of milk at once. Being overwhelmed can affect a baby's physical state, and mother's mental state.
- Progressive non-nutritive sucking sessions: A baby will advance at the breast from latching-on, to sucking in bursts, to occasionally coordinating suck-swallow-breathe. As baby shows more ability, mother will want to see what he/she can do with more milk in the breast. Pump until the let-down flow slows and then offer the breast. This prevents large amounts of milk that often come with let-down from overwhelming the baby, yet leaves plenty of milk in the breast for a feeding.

NUTRITIVE FEEDINGS

Nutritive feeding means baby is able to effectively remove milk from the breast and swallow enough for continued growth and development. This requires nutritive sucking. During nutritive sucking, a baby consistently coordinates suck-swallow-breathe. You should notice baby is sucking at a rate of one suck per second, with a pause for a breath after every few sucks. To take in enough milk, the baby must be able to continue with this pattern for at least 10 to 15 minutes. Quite likely, mother will hear baby swallowing milk, which sounds like a "k" sound in the back of his/her throat, for at least part of the feeding.

In addition to nutritive sucking, a breastfeeding baby must wake and cue to feed 8 to 12 times in 24 hours if nutritive feeding is to be accomplished. Usually, there is a progression of feeding cues and the baby's seems more and more tense until food is offered.

CARING FOR BABIES IN THE NICU

Although about 9 percent of all newborn babies require care in a NICU, giving birth to a sick or premature baby can be quite unexpected for any parent. Unfamiliar sights, sounds, and equipment in the NICU can be overwhelming.

WARMTH AND TEMPERATURE REGULATION

Babies are not as adaptable as adults to temperature change. A baby's body surface is about three times greater than an adult's, compared to the weight of his/her body. Babies can lose heat rapidly, as much as four times more quickly than adults. Premature and low birthweight babies usually have little body fat and may be too immature to regulate their own temperature, even in a warm environment. Even full-term and healthy newborns may not be able to maintain their body temperature if the environment is too cold.

When babies are cold-stressed, they use energy and oxygen to generate warmth. If skin temperatures drop just one degree from the ideal 97.7° F (36.5°C), a baby's oxygen use can increase by 10 percent. By keeping babies at optimal temperatures, neither too hot nor cold, they can conserve energy and build up reserves. This is especially important when babies are sick or premature.

MEANS TO KEEP BABIES WARM

There are several ways to keep babies warm, including the following:

- Immediate drying and warming after delivery: A baby's wet skin loses heat quickly by evaporation and can lose 2 to 3°F (Immediate drying and warming can be done with warm blankets and skin-to-skin contact with the mother, or another source of warmth such as a heat lamp or over-bed warmer.)
- Open bed with radiant warmer: An open bed with radiant warmer is open to the room air and has a radiant warmer above. A temperature probe on the baby connects to the warmer to regulate the amount of warming. When the baby is cool, the heat increases. Open beds are often used in the delivery

room for rapid warming. They are also used in the NICU for initial treatment and for sick babies who need constant attention and care. Babies on radiant warmer beds are usually dressed only in a diaper.

- Incubator/isolette: Incubators are walled plastic boxes with a heating system to circulate warmth. Babies are often dressed in a T-shirt and diaper.

Once a baby is stable and can maintain his/her own body temperature without added heat, open cribs or bassinets is used. Babies are usually dressed in a gown or T-shirt, a diaper, and a hat. A baby can lose large amounts of heat through his/her head. Often, a blanket is wrapped snugly around the baby, called swaddling.

NUTRITION AND FLUIDS

Feeding babies in the NICU is quite different from feeding healthy babies. When babies are sick or premature, they are often not well enough to breastfeed or take a bottle. Premature babies may not be able to suck effectively, or their gastrointestinal tracts may not be mature enough to digest feedings. Babies who are medically unstable are often unable to take regular feedings. Babies with umbilical catheters and those on mechanical ventilators may not be able to be fed because of the risk of aspiration (breathing food into the lungs).

Intravenous (IV) Fluids

Many babies in the NICU receive essential fluids and electrolytes through a tube in a vein called an IV. Some babies may need a special preparation called parenteral hyperalimentation, which contains nutrients they need until they are able to take milk feedings.

The contents of IV fluids and hyperalimentation are carefully calculated for each baby. Calories, protein, fats, and electrolytes including sodium, potassium, chloride, magnesium, and calcium are all important components. Babies need calories, protein, and fats for adequate growth and development. Fluids, electrolytes, and vitamins are necessary for functioning of body systems.

Blood tests help determine how much of each component a baby needs and the amount of each nutrient can be increased or decreased accordingly. Daily weights and keeping track of a baby's urine output also help monitor fluid needs.

Monitoring Baby's Electrolyte and Blood Levels

Some babies have too much or too little of certain electrolytes or other components in the blood. As a result, some of the common problems include the following:

- Hypernatremia: High amounts of sodium (salt) in the blood.
- Hyperkalemia: High amounts of potassium in the blood; can be diagnosed by blood test, or by changes in the baby's heart rate pattern.
- Hyperglycemia: High amounts of glucose (sugar) in the blood; diagnosed by blood tests, often done by heel stick; some babies may need insulin to control high glucose levels.
- Hypoglycemia: Low blood sugar; usually treated with IV fluids containing dextrose (another form of sugar).
- Hypocalcemia: Low calcium levels in the blood; usually treated with calcium in IV fluids.

Feeding Baby in the NICU

The following are some ways babies may be fed in the NICU:

- Gavage or tube feedings: Premature babies, especially those younger than 32 to 34 weeks gestation, often cannot be fed from the breast or bottle. Gavage or tube feedings may be needed until the baby learns to suck effectively. For gavage feedings, a small flexible tube is placed into a baby's nostril or mouth and passed down into the stomach. The tube is sometimes removed, but may be left in place if feedings are frequent.

At first, tiny amounts of breast milk or formula are given through the feeding tube. Because of their small stomach size, very tiny babies may be fed using a pump that slowly delivers the milk in small amounts. Larger babies are able to gradually take larger amounts at each feeding.

Before each tube feeding, a baby is checked for residual, the amount of milk in the stomach left over from the last feeding. If the amount of residual is too high, it may mean the baby is not digesting food well.

- Nipple feedings: Feeding from breast or bottle can begin as soon as babies are stable and are able to suck effectively. Baby may begin nipple feedings while still being tube fed. Even if a baby is able to nipple feed, it can be tiring. As baby increases the amount he/she can take by nipple, the amount in the tube feedings can be decreased.

TESTING AND LAB PROCEDURES

Babies in the newborn intensive care unit (NICU) need frequent examinations and monitoring as part of their care. Although many tests require drawing blood from baby, they are necessary to help monitor baby's condition and to identify potential problems.

Common tests or lab work in the NICU may include the following:

- Blood typing - to check the blood group (A, B, O) and the Rh factor (positive or negative).
- Testing for anaemia (too few red blood cells) or polycythemia (too many red blood cells).
- Testing for infection in the blood, urine, or spinal fluid.
- Blood gases to measure oxygen levels and carbon dioxide.
- Blood sugar.
- Electrolyte levels.
- X-rays (to check placement of tubes or view the condition of the !ungs, heart, or abdomen).

Intravenous Line and Tubes

Because most babies in the NICU are too small or sick to take milk feedings, medications and fluids are often given through their veins or arteries. Babies may also need frequent lab tests and measurements of blood oxygen levels. There are several ways a baby may receive fluids and medications and have blood drawn without additional needle sticks, including the following:

- Intravenous line (IV): Babies may have an IV placed in a hand, foot, or scalp, where veins are easily accessed. Tubing connects the IV to a bag containing fluids that are carefully delivered with a pump.
- Umbilical catheter: After the umbilical cord is cut at birth, newborn babies have the short stumps of the cord remaining. Because the umbilical cord stump is still connected to their blood and circulatory system, a catheter (small flexible tube) can be inserted into one of the two arteries or the vein of the umbilical cord. Medications, fluids, and blood can be given through this catheter. After placement of the umbilical catheter, x-rays are taken to check the location in the baby's body.
- Percutaneous line: A catheter is placed in a deep vein or artery in the baby's arm and is used for meeting a baby's longer-term needs than an IV in the hand or scalp.

A baby may need IV lines or catheters for just a short time or for many days. Once a baby is well enough to take milk feedings and is gaining weight, IV lines can often be removed. Sometimes, an IV may be needed for giving a baby antibiotics or other medication even when the baby can be fed normally.

INFECTION IN BABIES

Fighting infectious diseases today is much easier than in the past. Proper hygiene and proper precautions, along with numerous vaccines and rapidly advancing medical technology, help prevent many infections. However, a newborn baby has limited ability to prevent and fight infectious diseases. Special care may be needed for babies who develop an infection before, during, or after birth.

Prevention is the key to fighting many infectious diseases. At any time of life, but especially during pregnancy and after the birth of a baby, part of preventing the spread of an infectious disease includes the following:

- Receiving prenatal care from a qualified healthcare provider
- Proper hand washing techniques
- Taking certain precautions, depending on the disease
- Following the nationally recommended immunization schedule for children and adults
- Taking medication correctly

Even with proper prevention, sometimes a disease is unavoidable. Some reasons may be attributed to the following:

- Evolution of drug-resistant strains of a disease
- Changes in a person's environment
- Increased travel
- Inappropriate use of prescription drugs
- Lack of attention to proper personal hygiene

Infections in babies require clinical care by a physician or other healthcare professional. Listed below is some additional information regarding infections:

RESPIRATORY SYNCYTIAL VIRUS

RSV is the most common cause of bronchiolitis (inflammation of the lower airways) and pneumonia in babies. It is an illness that often occurs in yearly outbreaks in communities and in newborn intensive care units (NICUs). In the United States, RSV is more common in winter and spring months.

Causes

RSV is spread from respiratory secretions through close contact with infected persons or contact with contaminated surfaces or objects. Infection can occur when infectious material contacts mucous membranes of the eyes, mouth, or nose, and possibly through the inhalation of droplets generated by a sneeze or cough. The incubation period (time from exposure to symptoms) is about four days.

RSV does not usually occur until a baby is 4 to 6 weeks old. However, because premature babies are born before receiving all of the mother's immunities, they are more susceptible. Babies can also be reinfected with the virus. RSV is slightly more common in boys than girls. Babies with chronic lung disease (a condition that may develop following respiratory disease as premature infants) are also at increased risk of developing RSV.

Infection with the virus can lead to severe respiratory illness and pneumonia, and may become life threatening. RSV in infancy may be related to development of asthma later in childhood.

Symptoms

The following are the most common symptoms of RSV. However, each baby may experience symptoms differently. Symptoms may include:

- Runny nose
- Apnea
- Listlessness
- Fever
- Poor feeding
- Wheezing
- Retractions (pulling in) of the chest wall
- Rapid breathing
- Cough

Diagnosis

Diagnosis is sometimes difficult because the symptoms of RSV can resemble other infections. Illness in other family members, other babies in the hospital nursery, or the time of year may provide clues. In addition to a complete medical history and physical examination of child, a test of the baby's respiratory secretions may show the presence of a virus.

Treatment

Specific treatment for RSV will be determined by baby's physician based on:

- Baby's age, overall health, and medical history
- the extent of the condition
- Baby's tolerance for specific medications, procedures, or therapies
- expectations for the course of the condition
- Mother's opinion or preference

There are no medications used to treat the virus itself. Care of a baby with RSV involves treating the effects of the virus on the respiratory system. Because a virus causes the illness, antibiotics are not useful. Treatment may include:

- Supplemental oxygen
- Intravenous fluids (to prevent dehydration)
- Tube feedings (if the baby has difficulty sucking)
- Bronchodilator medications (to open the airways)
- Antiviral medications (for very sick or high-risk babies)

Prevention

Two medications are recommended for babies at high risk for RSV to protect them against the serious complications of the illness. One of the following medications is usually given monthly during the RSV "season" from late fall through spring:

- Respiratory syncytial virus immune globulin intravenous (RSV-IGIV)
- Palivizumab - an antibody against RSV.

These medications are not vaccines, and do not prevent the virus. But they do lessen the severity of the illness and may help shorten the hospital stay.

HUMAN IMMUNODEFICIENCY VIRUS

Human immunodeficiency virus (HIV) causes acquired immune deficiency syndrome (AIDS), which kills or impairs cells of the immune system and progressively destroys the body's ability to fight infections and certain cancers. The term AIDS applies to the most advanced stages of an HIV infection.

Causes

HIV is spread most commonly by sexual contact with an infected partner. HIV may also be spread through contact with infected blood, especially by sharing needles, syringes, or drug use equipment with someone who is infected with the virus. Most babies with HIV contract the infection from their HIV-infected mother during pregnancy. According to the National Institutes of Health (NIH), HIV transmission from mother to child during pregnancy, labour, and delivery, or by breastfeeding, has accounted for nearly all AIDS cases reported among US children.

Symptoms

The HIV virus may cause flu-like illness within a month or two after exposure, although there may not be any symptoms at all. Persistent or severe symptoms may surface within two years in babies born with an HIV infection.

The symptoms of HIV may resemble other conditions or medical problems. Always consult baby's physician for a diagnosis.

Health organizations recommend HIV testing of all pregnant women. Prenatal care that includes HIV counseling, testing, and treatment for infected mothers and their children saves lives and resources. Current recommendations are for HIV-positive women to take specific medications during pregnancy and during labour. Blood tests are also performed to check the amount of virus. Newborn babies of HIV-positive mothers may also receive medication. Studies have found this treatment can reduce the chance of a mother's transmission of HIV to her baby from 25 percent to less than 2 percent.

Cesarean delivery may be recommended for HIV-positive women. This also helps reduce the transmission of the virus to the baby, especially when the mother receives medications. HIV may also be transmitted through breast milk. A series of studies have determined that breastfeeding increases the risk of HIV transmission by about 14 percent. Currently, the Joint United Nations Programme on HIV/AIDS (UNAIDS) recommends that HIV-positive women be counseled so they can make an informed decision about how to best feed their children. Because breast milk contains the virus, HIV positive women should not breastfeed their babies.

CYTOMEGALOVIRUS

Cytomegalovirus (CMV) is a virus related to the herpes virus group of infections. Like herpes, it is inactive at times, but it is incurable and is a life-time infection. CMV may be passed from a mother to her baby during pregnancy and is the most common congenital viral infection. It is also called congenital cytomegalovirus or cytomegalovirus inclusion disease.

Causes

CMV without symptoms is common in babies and young children. It is found in saliva, urine, semen, and other body fluids. The virus is easily spread in households and in daycare centers. It can be transmitted to the foetus during pregnancy and to the baby during delivery or in breast milk.

Over half of women of childbearing age become infected with CMV at least six months before becoming pregnant. There appear to be few risks for complications of CMV for this group and only a few babies have the infection at birth. These babies appear to have no significant illness or abnormalities.

According to the Centers for Disease Control and Prevention (CDC), about 1 to 4 percent of women first become infected with CMV during pregnancy. With a first infection during pregnancy, there is a higher risk that after birth the baby may have CMV-related complications. About 5 to 10 percent of babies with congenital CMV will have signs of the infection at birth. Of these, over 90 percent will have serious complications including hearing loss, visual impairment, mental retardation, or epilepsy. Premature babies may be at increased risk for these problems.

Although CMV may be transmitted at delivery or through breast milk, these infections usually do not cause illness in the baby.

Symptoms

Most babies with congenital (present at birth) CMV do not have symptoms of the infection at birth However, each baby may experience symptoms differently. Symptoms may include:

- Premature birth
- Low birthweight
- Liver enlargement and jaundice
- Lung infection

- Anaemia
- Hearing loss

The symptoms of CMV may resemble other conditions or medical problems. Always consult baby's physician for a diagnosis.

Diagnosis

Most infections with CMV in the mother are not diagnosed because the virus produces few symptoms. A mother who has had CMV infection before may have antibodies present in her blood stream. The virus can also be cultured from the throat or urine of the mother or baby.

Treatment

Specific treatment for cytomegalovirus will be determined by baby's physician based on:

- Baby's gestational age, overall health, and medical history
- Extent of the disease
- Baby's tolerance for specific medications, procedures, or therapies
- Expectations for the course of the disease
- Opinion or preference

Research is underway to find antiviral drugs that might be effective against CMV. Other antiviral drugs and immunoglobulins may be of help in certain cases.

Prevention

Although an infected person may transmit the virus at any time, proper hand washing with soap and water is effective in removing the virus from the hands. Research is also underway to develop a vaccine to provide immunity to CMV.

GROUP B STREPTOCOCCUS

Group B streptococcus (GBS) is a bacterium that can be found in the digestive tract, urinary tract, and genital area of adults. Although GBS infection usually does not cause problems in healthy women before pregnancy, it can cause serious illness for the mother and baby during pregnancy and after delivery.

One out of every four or five pregnant women carries GBS in her rectum or vagina. In the pregnant mother, GBS infection may cause chorioamnionitis (a severe infection of the placental tissues) and postpartum (after birth) infection. Urinary tract infections caused by GBS can lead to preterm labour and birth.

Newborns can contract GBS during pregnancy, or from the mother's genital tract during labour and delivery. GBS is the most common cause of life-threatening infections in newborns, including pneumonia and meningitis. About one out of every 100 to 200 babies whose mothers carry GBS develop symptoms of GBS disease. Nearly 75 percent of the cases of GBS disease among newborns occur in the first week of life, called early-onset disease. Premature babies are more susceptible to GBS infection than full-term babies.

Although it is very rare, GBS infection may also develop in babies one week to several months after birth, called late-onset disease. Meningitis is more common with late-onset GBS disease. Only about half of late-onset GBS disease among newborns comes from a mother who is a GBS carrier. The source of infection for others with late-onset GBS disease is unknown.

Diagnosis

GBS can be cultured from the mother's vagina or rectum with a swab during a pelvic examination. GBS can also be cultured from a mother's urine. Cultures are usually done between 35 and 37 weeks of pregnancy and may take a few days to complete. Cultures collected earlier in pregnancy do not accurately predict whether a mother will have GBS at delivery.

In infants, GBS may be cultured from samples of sterile body fluids, such as blood or spinal fluid. Most newborns with GBS infection have symptoms in the first few hours after birth. Symptoms are related to the body systems that are affected by the infection and may include breathing problems, changes in blood pressure, or neurologic problems such as seizures.

Treatment

Treatment of GBS depends on when GBS infection is diagnosed - during pregnancy or after delivery. Specific treatment for GBS will be determined by physician based on:

- The pregnancy and birth history, overall health, and medical history
- Extent of the disease
- Baby's tolerance for specific medications, procedures, or therapies

- Expectations for the course of the disease
- Opinion or preference

If the mother has a positive GBS culture during pregnancy, the Centers for Disease Control and Prevention (CDC) and the American College of Obstetricians and Gynaecologists (ACOG) recommend treatment with intravenous (IV) antibiotics during labour to reduce the risk of transmission of the infection to the baby. Treatment may also be needed for women with certain risk factors, including the following:

- Fever during labour
- Rupture of membranes (bag of waters) for 18 hours or longer
- Labour or rupture of membranes before 37 weeks gestation
- History of GBS infection in a previous baby

Newborns who become ill with GBS infection may require care in the newborn intensive care unit (NICU). They are usually treated with intravenous (IV) antibiotics. Other treatments and specialized care may be needed depending on the severity of the infection and whether the infection causes serious problems such as meningitis or pneumonia.

Prevention

It is important to understand that, in spite of testing and treatment, some babies still develop GBS disease. Research is ongoing to develop vaccines to prevent GBS disease. In the future, women who are vaccinated against GBS may make antibodies that cross the placenta and protect the baby during birth and early infancy.

SEPSIS

Sepsis is a term for severe infection that is present in the blood and spreads throughout the body. In newborns, it is also called sepsis neonatorum or neonatal septicemia.

Causes

Sepsis can develop following infection by microorganisms including bacteria, viruses, fungi, and parasites. Infection in babies can be contracted during pregnancy, from the mother's genital tract during labour and delivery, or after birth from contact with others.

Sepsis in a newborn is more likely to develop when the mother has had pregnancy complications that increase the likelihood of infection. Such complications may include the following:

- Premature rupture of the membranes (amniotic sac), or membrane rupture for an extended length of time
- Bleeding problems
- A difficult delivery
- Infection in the uterus or placental tissues
- Fever in the mother

Babies can also develop sepsis by contracting infections after birth from infected persons or objects. Babies in the newborn intensive care unit (NICU) are at increased risk for acquiring nosocomial (hospital-acquired) infections. Many babies in the NICU are premature or have low birthweight which makes them more susceptible to infection and more likely to need invasive treatments and procedures. Microorganisms that normally live on the skin may cause infection if they enter the body through catheters and other tubes inserted into the baby's body.

Micro organisms causing infections and sepsis in babies

Prenatal	During Delivery	After Birth
rubella (German measles)	Group B streptococcus (GBS)	respiratory syncytial virus (RSV)
cytomegalovirus (CMV)	E. coli	Candida
varicella-zoster virus (chickenpox virus)	herpes simplex virus	Haemophilus influenzae type b (Hib)
Listeria monocytogenes	—	enterovirus

Sepsis can be life threatening for newborns, especially if the baby has a weakened immune system because of prematurity or another illness. When a baby's immature immune system cannot fight the microorganism, the infection can quickly spread and overtake the body, causing serious illnesses such as meningitis or pneumonia.

Symptoms

Sepsis in newborns is not always easy to identify since newborn babies often do not show symptoms of infections in the same way older babies and children may show symptoms. The following are some of the symptoms of infection in newborn babies. However, each baby may experience symptoms differently depending upon the type of organism causing the infection and the severity and location of the infection. Symptoms of infection may include the following:

- Apnea (stopping breathing) or difficulty breathing
- Bradycardia (decreased heart rate)
- Decreased temperature or temperature instability
- Weak suck
- Jaundice (yellow colouring of the skin and eyes)

Diagnosis

A sepsis workup may be needed to help identify the location of the infection and type of microorganism causing the infection. A sepsis workup may include the following procedures:

- Blood tests
- Lumbar puncture (Also called spinal tap.) - a special needle is placed into the lower back, into the spinal canal. This is the area around the spinal cord. The pressure in the spinal canal and brain can then be measured. A small amount of cerebral spinal fluid (CSF) can be removed and sent for testing to determine if there is an infection or other problems. CSF is the fluid that bathes child's brain and spinal cord.
- Blood cultures
- Urine culture (sometimes by suprapubic tap, insertion of a needle through the lower abdomen into the bladder)
- Culture of fluids from inside tubes and catheters that are inserted in the baby
- X-rays - a diagnostic test which uses invisible electromagnetic energy beams to produce images of internal tissues, bones, and organs onto film.

Procedures may also be performed to determine which antibiotics or medications are most effective for treating the specific microorganism.

Treatment

Specific treatment for sepsis will be determined by baby's physician based on:

- Baby's age, overall health, and medical history
- Extent of the disease
- Baby's tolerance for specific medications, procedures, or therapies

- Expectations for the course of the disease
- Opinion or preference

Early diagnosis and treatment of the infection are important in helping prevent sepsis from overwhelming a baby's body. However, cultures of blood and body fluids may take several days for the organism to grow and be identified. Because of this, babies who are at increased risk for sepsis, such as premature or low birthweight babies, may have preventive antibiotic treatment started as soon as cultures are taken. Most medications are given intravenously (IV).

Sepsis can be life threatening as the infection can affect several body systems at the same time. This can make providing treatment more difficult. Babies with sepsis will require care in the newborn intensive care unit (NICU), and may need antibiotics, other medications, and specialized treatment (such as a mechanical breathing machine). The healthcare team will be working to provide the best care to treat the infection and care for baby.

BLOOD DISORDERS

There are many blood disorders that place a newborn at higher risk and require clinical care by a physician or other healthcare professional. Listed below are the main one, for which we have provided a brief overview:

HAEMOLYTIC DISEASE OF THE NEWBORN

Hemolytic Disease of the Newborn is also called erythroblastosis foetalis. This condition occurs when there is an incompatibility between the blood types of the mother and baby.

- "Hemolytic" means breaking down of red blood cells
- "Erythroblastosis" refers to making of immature red blood cells
- "Foetalis" refers to foetus

Causes

HDN most frequently occurs when an Rh negative mother has a baby with an Rh positive father. When the baby's Rh factor is positive, like the father's, problems can develop if the baby's red blood cells cross to the Rh negative mother. This usually happens at delivery when the placenta detaches. However, it may also happen anytime blood cells of the two circulations mix, such as during a miscarriage or abortion, with a fall, or during an invasive prenatal testing procedure (i.e., an amniocentesis or chorionic villus sampling).

The mother's immune system sees the baby's Rh positive red blood cells as "foreign." Just as when bacteria invade the body, the immune system responds by developing antibodies to fight and destroy these foreign cells. The mother's immune system then keeps the antibodies in case the foreign cells appear again, even in a future pregnancy. The mother is now "Rh sensitized."

Although it is not as common, a similar problem of incompatibility may happen between the blood types (A, B, O, AB) of the mother and baby in the following situations:

Mother's Blood Type	O	A	B
Baby's Blood Type	A or B	B	A

In a first pregnancy, Rh sensitization is not likely. Usually it only becomes a problem in a future pregnancy with another Rh positive baby. During that pregnancy, the mother's antibodies cross the placenta to fight the Rh positive cells in the baby's body. As the antibodies destroy the red blood cells, the baby can become sick. This is called erythroblastosis foetalis during pregnancy. In the newborn, the condition is called hemolytic disease of the newborn.

Babies affected by HDN are usually in a mother's second or higher pregnancy, after she has become sensitized with a first baby. HDN due to Rh incompatibility is about three times more likely in Caucasian babies than African-American babies.

When the mother's antibodies attack the red blood cells, they are broken down and destroyed (hemolysis). This makes the baby anemic. Anaemia is dangerous because it limits the ability of the blood to carry oxygen to the baby's organs and tissues. As a result:

- The baby's body responds to the hemolysis by trying to make more red blood cells very quickly in the bone marrow and the liver and spleen. This causes these organs to get bigger. The new red blood cells, called erythroblasts, are often immature and are not able to do the work of mature red blood cells.
- As the red blood cells break down, a substance called bilirubin is formed. Babies are not easily able to get rid of the bilirubin and it can build up in the blood and other tissues and fluids of the baby's body. This is called hyperbilirubinemia. Because bilirubin has a pigment or colouring, it causes a yellowing of the baby's skin and tissues. This is called jaundice.

Complications of Hemolytic Disease

Complications of hemolytic disease of the newborn can range from mild to severe. The following are some of the problems that can result:

During Pregnancy

- Mild anaemia, hyperbilirubinemia, and jaundice: The placenta helps rid some of the bilirubin, but not all.
- Severe anaemia with enlargement of the liver and spleen: When these organs and the bone marrow cannot compensate for the fast destruction of red blood cells, severe anaemia results and other organs are affected.
- Hydrops foetalis: This occurs as the baby's organs are unable to handle the anaemia. The heart begins to fail and large amounts of fluid build up in the baby's tissues and organs. A foetus with hydrops is at great risk of being stillborn.

After Birth

- Severe hyperbilirubinemia and jaundice: The baby's liver is unable to handle the large amount of bilirubin that results from red blood cell breakdown. The baby's liver is enlarged and anaemia continues.
- Kernicterus: Kernicterus is the most severe form of hyperbilirubinemia and results from the buildup of bilirubin in the brain. This can cause seizures, brain damage, deafness, and death.

Symptoms

The following are the most common symptoms of hemolytic disease of the newborn. However, each baby may experience symptoms differently.

During Pregnancy

- With amniocentesis, the amniotic fluid may have a yellow colouring and contain bilirubin.
- Ultrasound of the foetus shows enlarged liver, spleen, or heart and fluid buildup in the foetus' abdomen.

After Birth

- A pale colouring may be evident, due to anaemia.
- Jaundice, or yellow colouring of amniotic fluid, umbilical cord, skin, and eyes may be present. The baby may not look yellow

immediately after birth, but jaundice can develop quickly, usually within 24 to 36 hours.

- The newborn may have an enlarged liver and spleen.
- Babies with hydrops foetalis have severe edema (swelling) of the entire body and are extremely pale. They often have difficulty breathing.

Diagnosis

Because anaemia, hyperbilirubinemia, and hydrops foetalis can occur with other diseases and conditions, the accurate diagnosis of HDN depends on determining if there is a blood group or blood type incompatibility. Sometimes, the diagnosis can be made during pregnancy based on information from the following tests:

- Testing the presence of Rh positive antibodies in the mother's blood
- Ultrasound - to detect organ enlargement or fluid buildup in the foetus. Ultrasound is a diagnostic imaging technique which uses high-frequency sound waves and a computer to create images of blood vessels, tissues, and organs. Ultrasound is used to view internal organs as they function, and to assess blood flow through various vessels.
- Amniocentesis - to measure the amount of bilirubin in the amniotic fluid. Amniocentesis is a test performed to determine chromosomal and genetic disorders and certain birth defects. The test involves inserting a needle through the abdominal and uterine wall into the amniotic sac to retrieve a sample of amniotic fluid.
- Sampling of some of the blood from the foetal umbilical cord during pregnancy to check for antibodies, bilirubin, and anaemia in the foetus.

Once a baby is born, diagnostic tests for HDN may include the following:

- Testing of the baby's umbilical cord blood for blood group, Rh factor, red blood cell count, and antibodies
- Testing of the baby's blood for bilirubin levels

Treatment

Once HDN is diagnosed, treatment may be needed. Specific treatment for hemolytic disease of the newborn will be determined by baby's physician based on:

- Baby's gestational age, overall health, and medical history
- Extent of the disease
- Baby's tolerance for specific medications, procedures, or therapies
- Expectations for the course of the disease
- Opinion or preference

During pregnancy, treatment for HDN may include:

- Intrauterine blood transfusion of red blood cells into the baby's circulation

This is done by placing a needle through the mother's uterus and into the abdominal cavity of the foetus or directly into the vein in the umbilical cord. It may be necessary to give a sedative medication to keep the baby from moving. Intrauterine transfusions may need to be repeated.

- Early delivery if the foetus develops complications

If the foetus has mature lungs, labour and delivery may be induced to prevent worsening of HDN.

After birth, treatment may include:

- Blood transfusions (for severe anaemia)
- Intravenous fluids (for low blood pressure)
- Help for respiratory distress using oxygen or a mechanical breathing machine
- Exchange transfusion to replace the baby's damaged blood with fresh blood

The exchange transfusion helps increase the red blood cell count and lower the levels of bilirubin. An exchange transfusion is done by alternating giving and withdrawing blood in small amounts through a vein or artery. Exchange transfusions may need to be repeated if the bilirubin levels remain high.

Prevention

Fortunately, HDN is a very preventable disease. Because of the advances in prenatal care, nearly all women with Rh negative blood are identified in early pregnancy by blood testing. If a mother is Rh negative and has not been sensitized, she is usually given a drug called Rh immunoglobulin (RhIg), also known as RhoGAM. This is a specially developed blood product that can prevent an Rh negative mother's antibodies from being able to react to Rh positive cells. Many women are given RhoGAM around the 28th week of pregnancy. After the baby is born, a woman should receive a second dose of the drug within 72 hours.

HEMORRHAGIC DISEASE OF THE NEWBORN

Hemorrhagic disease of the newborn is a bleeding problem that occurs in a newborn during the first few days of life.

Causes

Babies are normally born with low levels of vitamin K, an essential factor in blood clotting. A deficiency in vitamin K is the main cause of hemorrhagic disease of the newborn.

Vitamin K deficiency may result in bleeding in a very small percentage of babies. Babies at risk for developing hemorrhagic disease of the newborn include the following:

- Babies who do not receive preventative vitamin K in an injection at birth
- Exclusively breastfed babies (breast milk contains less vitamin K than cow's milk formula.)
- Babies whose mothers have seizure disorders and take anti-convulsant medications

Without the clotting factor, bleeding occurs, and severe bleeding or haemorrhage can result.

Symptoms

The following are the most common symptoms of hemorrhagic disease of the newborn. However, each baby may experience symptoms differently. Symptoms may include:

- Blood in the baby's bowel movements
- Blood in urine
- Oozing around the umbilical cord

The symptoms of hemorrhagic disease of the newborn may resemble other conditions or medical problems. Always consult baby's physician for a diagnosis.

Diagnosis

In addition to a complete medical history and physical examination, a diagnosis is based on the signs of bleeding and by laboratory tests for blood clotting times.

Treatment

Specific treatment for hemorrhagic disease of the newborn will be determined by baby's physician based on:

- Baby's gestational age, overall health, and medical history
- Extent of the disease
- Baby's tolerance for specific medications, procedures, or therapies
- Expectations for the course of the disease
- Opinion or preference

The Academy of Pediatrics recommends giving every newborn baby an injection of vitamin K after delivery to prevent this potentially life-threatening disease. If bleeding occurs, vitamin K is also given. Blood transfusions may also be needed if bleeding is severe.

HYPERBILIRUBINEMIA AND JAUNDICE

Hyperbilirubinemia is a condition in which there is too much bilirubin in the blood. When red blood cells break down, a substance called bilirubin is formed. Babies are not easily able to get rid of the bilirubin and it can build up in the blood and other tissues and fluids of the baby's body. This is called hyperbilirubinemia. Because bilirubin has a pigment or colouring, it causes a yellowing of the baby's skin and tissues. This is called jaundice. Depending on the cause of the hyperbilirubinemia, jaundice may appear at birth or at any time afterward.

Causes

During pregnancy, the placenta excretes bilirubin. When the baby is born, the baby's liver must take over this function. There are several causes of hyperbilirubinemia and jaundice, including the following:

- Physiologic jaundice: Physiologic jaundice occurs as a "normal" response to the baby's limited ability to excrete bilirubin in the first days of life.
- Breast milk jaundice: About 2 percent of breastfed babies develop jaundice after the first week. Some develop breast milk jaundice in the first week due to low calorie intake or dehydration.
- Jaundice from hemolysis: Jaundice may occur with the breakdown of red blood cells due to hemolytic disease of the newborn (Rh disease), having too many red blood cells, or bleeding.

- Jaundice related to inadequate liver function: Jaundice may be related to inadequate liver function due to infection or other factors.

About 60 percent of term newborns and 80 percent of premature babies develop jaundice. Infants of diabetic mothers and of mothers with Rh disease are more likely to develop hyperbilirubinemia and jaundice.

Although low levels of bilirubin are not usually a concern, large amounts can circulate to tissues in the brain and may cause seizures and brain damage. This is a condition called kernicterus.

Symptoms

The following are the most common symptoms of hyperbilirubinemia. However, each baby may experience symptoms differently. Symptoms may include:

- Yellow colouring of the baby's skin (usually beginning on the face and moving down the body)
- Poor feeding or lethargy: The symptoms of hyperbilirubinemia may resemble other conditions or medical problems. Always consult baby's physician for a diagnosis.

Diagnosis

The timing of the appearance of jaundice helps with the diagnosis. Jaundice appearing in the first 24 hours is quite serious and usually requires immediate treatment. When jaundice appears on the second or third day, it is usually "physiologic." However, it can be a more serious type of jaundice. When jaundice appears on the third day to the first week, it may be due to an infection. Later appearance of jaundice, in the second week, is often related to breast milk feedings, but may have other causes.

Diagnostic procedures for hyperbilirubinemia may include:

- Direct and indirect bilirubin levels: These reflect whether the bilirubin is bound with other substances by the liver so that it can be excreted (direct), or is circulating in the blood circulation (indirect).
- Red blood cell counts
- Blood type and testing for Rh incompatibility (Coomb's test)

Treatment for hyperbilirubinemia: Specific treatment for hyperbilirubinemia will be determined by baby's physician based on:

- Baby's gestational age, overall health, and medical history

- Extent of the disease
- Baby's tolerance for specific medications, procedures, or therapies
- Expectations for the course of the disease
- Opinion or preference

Treatment depends on many factors, including the cause of the hyperbilirubinemia and the level of bilirubin. The goal is to keep the level of bilirubin from increasing to dangerous levels. Treatment may include:

- Phototherapy: Since bilirubin absorbs light, jaundice and increased bilirubin levels usually decrease when the baby is exposed to special blue spectrum lights. Phototherapy may take several hours to begin working and it is used throughout the day and night. The baby's position is changed to allow all of the skin to be exposed to the light. The baby's eyes must be protected and the temperature monitored during phototherapy. Blood levels of bilirubin are checked to monitor if the phototherapy is working.
- Fiberoptic blanket: Another form of phototherapy is a fiberoptic blanket placed under the baby. This may be used alone or in combination with regular phototherapy.
- Exchange transfusion to replace the baby's damaged blood with fresh blood: Exchange transfusion helps increase the red blood cell count and lower the levels of bilirubin. An exchange transfusion is done by alternating giving and withdrawing blood in small amounts through a vein or artery. Exchange transfusions may need to be repeated if the bilirubin levels remain high.
- Ceasing breastfeeding for one or two days: Treatment of breast milk jaundice often requires stopping the breastfeeding for one to two days and giving the baby formula often helps lower the bilirubin levels. Breastfeeding can then be resumed.
- Treating any underlying cause of hyperbilirubinemia, such as infection

Prevention

While hyperbilirubinemia cannot be totally prevented, early recognition and treatment are important in preventing bilirubin levels from rising to dangerous levels.

HYPOGLYCEMIA

Hypoglycemia is a condition in which the amount of blood glucose (sugar) in the blood is lower than normal.

Causes

Hypoglycemia may be caused by conditions that:

- Lower the amount of glucose in the bloodstream
- Prevent or lessen storage of glucose
- Use up glycogen stores (sugar stored in the liver)
- Inhibit the use of glucose by the body

Many different conditions are associated with hypoglycemia, including the following:

- Inadequate maternal nutrition in pregnancy
- Excess insulin produced in a baby of a diabetic mother
- Severe hemolytic disease of the newborn (incompatibility of blood types of mother and baby)
- Birth defects and congenital metabolic diseases
- Birth asphyxia
- Cold stress (conditions that are too cold)
- Liver disease

Symptoms

Symptoms of hypoglycemia may not be obvious in newborn babies. The following are the most common symptoms of hypoglycemia. However, each baby may experience symptoms differently. Symptoms may include:

- Jitteriness
- Cyanosis (blue colouring)
- Apnea (stopping breathing)
- Hypothermia (low body temperature)
- Poor body tone
- Poor feeding
- Lethargy
- Seizures

The symptoms of hypoglycemia may resemble other conditions or medical problems. Always consult baby's physician for a diagnosis.

Diagnosis

A simple blood test for blood glucose levels can diagnose hypoglycemia. Blood may be drawn from a heel stick, with a needle from the baby's arm, or through an umbilical catheter (a tube placed in the baby's umbilical cord). Generally, a baby with low blood glucose levels will need treatment.

Treatment

Specific treatment for hypoglycemia will be determined by baby's physician based on:

- Baby's gestational age, overall health, and medical history
- Extent of the disease
- Baby's tolerance for specific medications, procedures, or therapies
- Expectations for the course of the disease
- Opinion or preference

Treatment includes giving the baby a rapid-acting source of glucose. This may be as simple as giving a glucose/water mixture or formula as an early feeding. Or, the baby may need glucose given intravenously. The baby's blood glucose levels are closely monitored after treatment to see if the hypoglycemia occurs again.

Prevention

There may not be any way to prevent hypoglycemia, only to watch carefully for the symptoms and treat as soon as possible. Mothers with diabetes with blood glucose levels in tight control can help minimize the amount of glucose that goes to the foetus.

HYPOCALCEMIA

Hypocalcemia is a condition in which there is too little calcium in the blood. A common form of hypocalcemia in babies is called neonatal hypocalcemia. This condition may occur at different times with different causes, including the following:

- Early hypocalcemia - occurs in the first three days of life.
- Late hypocalcemia - develops between the fifth to tenth days of life, usually after several days of formula feedings. Some

formulas have high levels of phosphate which can lower the blood calcium levels.

Causes

The causes of early hypocalcemia are unknown, while late hypocalcemia has a number of known causes, related primarily to calcium and phosphorus levels in the body as well as parathyroid hormone function.

Hypocalcemia is more common in premature and low birthweight babies, because their parathyroid glands are less mature. It can also occur in babies who have a difficult birth and in babies of diabetic mothers.

Symptoms

Symptoms of hypocalcemia may not be obvious in newborn babies. The following are the most common symptoms of hypocalcemia. However, each baby may experience symptoms differently. Symptoms may include:

- Irritability
- Muscle twitches
- jitterIness
- Tremors
- Poor feeding
- Lethargy
- Seizures

The symptoms of hypocalcemia may resemble other conditions or medical problems. Always consult baby's physician for a diagnosis.

Diagnosis

In addition to a complete medical history and physical examination, diagnosis of hypocalcemia is made by testing the blood for the amount of calcium.

Treatment

Hypocalcemia may get better without treatment in some cases, especially if there are no symptoms. However, specific treatment for hypocalcemia will be determined by baby's physician based on:

- Baby's gestational age, overall health, and medical history
- Extent of the disease
- Baby's tolerance for specific medications, procedures, or therapies

- Expectations for the course of the disease
- Opinion or preference

Treatment may include:

- Supplemental calcium gluconate (a form of calcium that is easily absorbed) given by mouth
- Intravenous (IV) calcium gluconate

POLYCYTHEMIA

Polycythemia is a condition in which there are too many red blood cells in the blood circulation. It is the opposite of anaemia, which results from too few red blood cells in the blood circulation. Polycythemia is also called plethora.

Causes

Polycythemia may be caused by the following:

- Increased red blood cell production:
  — A foetus with chronically lowered oxygen levels responds by producing extra red blood cells.
  — Some chromosomal abnormalities may cause increased red blood cell production.
- Extra blood cells enter the baby's circulation from another source:
  — A delay in clamping the umbilical cord after delivery results in blood from the placenta entering the baby's circulation.
  — Twin-to-twin transfusion, when the shared placenta of the two babies has a connecting circulation and blood flows from one baby to the other, may result in polycythemia.

Mild polycythemia may not cause problems. However, too many red blood cells can increase the blood volume or thicken the blood, making it harder to circulate through the blood system and to the organs. Babies can have difficulty breathing and their heart and blood vessels cannot compensate for the extra amount of blood. As the large numbers of cells begin to break down, a substance called bilirubin is produced. Increased bilirubin levels, called hyperbilirubinemia, can cause jaundice, a yellowing of the skin, eyes, and mucous membranes. Seizures can also occur with polycythemia.

Symptoms

Many babies with polycythemia have no visible symptoms of the condition. The following are the most common symptoms of polycythemia. However, each baby may experience symptoms differently. Symptoms may include:

- Deep reddish-purple colouring
- Poor feeding
- Lethargy
- Rapid breathing or respiratory distress
- Jaundice (yellowing of the skin, eyes, and mucous membranes)
- Low blood sugar

The symptoms of polycythemia may resemble other conditions or medical problems. Always consult baby's physician for a diagnosis.

Diagnosis

Laboratory tests show a high hematocrit (red blood cell count) when polycythemia is present. A high hemoglobin (protein in the blood that carries oxygen) level may also help diagnose polycythemia.

Treatment

Specific treatment for polycythemia will be determined by baby's physician based on:

- Baby's gestational age, overall health, and medical history
- Extent of the disease
- Baby's tolerance for specific medications, procedures, or therapies
- Expectations for the course of the disease
- Opinion or preference

Treatment may include:

- Removing some of the blood volume, thus, reducing the number of the red blood cells.
- Replacement of the withdrawn blood with fluids (to help dilute the red blood cell concentration).
- Partial exchange transfusion (slowly removing and replacing a large portion of the baby's blood volume).

These treatments are performed through a vein or artery, often the umbilical blood vessels.

THROMBOCYTOPENIA

Thrombocytopenia is a condition in which there are too few platelets - the cells produced in the bone marrow that are needed for clotting.

Causes

Thrombocytopenia may be caused by infections in the foetus or newborn such as rubella, syphilis, and bacterial or viral infections. It can also develop when a mother's immune system produces antibodies against the baby's platelets. Some medications taken by the mother or given to the baby can cause thrombocytopenia.

Symptoms

The following are the most common symptoms of thrombocytopenia. However, each baby may experience symptoms differently. Symptoms may include:

- Bruising or petechiae (small red spots on the skin)
- Signs of bleeding in other body systems
- Jaundice

The symptoms of thrombocytopenia may resemble other conditions or medical problems. Always consult baby's physician for a diagnosis.

Diagnosis

In addition to a complete medical history and physical examination, laboratory testing of the blood can show decreased platelet counts.

Treatment

Specific treatment for thrombocytopenia will be determined by baby's physician based on:

- Baby's gestational age, overall health, and medical history
- Extent of the disease
- Baby's tolerance for specific medications, procedures, or therapies
- Expectations for the course of the disease
- Opinion or preference

Treatment will often depend on the cause of the thrombocytopenia. Blood transfusion with platelets may be needed.

RESPIRATORY DISORDERS

There are many respiratory disorders that place a newborn at higher risk and require clinical care by a physician or other healthcare professional.

An important part of lung development in babies is the production of surfactant. This is a substance made by the cells in the small airways and consists of phospholipids and protein. It begins to be produced in the foetus at about 24 to 28 weeks of pregnancy. Surfactant is found in amniotic fluid between 28 and 32 weeks. By about 35 weeks gestation, most babies have developed adequate amounts of surfactant. Surfactant is normally released into the lung tissues where it helps lower surface tension in the airways. This helps keep the lung alveoli (air sacs) open. Premature babies may not have enough surfactant in their lungs and may have difficulty breathing.

Listed below are some, for which we have provided an overview:

RESPIRATORY DISTRESS SYNDROME

Hyaline membrane disease (HMD), also called respiratory distress syndrome (RDS), is one of the most common problems of premature babies. It can cause babies to need extra oxygen and help breathing. The course of illness with hyaline membrane disease depends on the size and gestational age of the baby, the severity of the disease, the presence of infection, whether or not a baby has a patent ductus arteriosus (a heart condition), and whether or not the baby needs mechanical help to breathe. HMD typically worsens over the first 48 to 72 hours, then improves with treatment.

Causes

HMD occurs when there is not enough of a substance in the lungs called surfactant. Surfactant is made by the cells in the airways and consists of phospholipids and protein. It begins to be produced in the foetus at about 24 to 28 weeks of pregnancy. Surfactant is found in amniotic fluid between 28 and 32 weeks. By about 35 weeks gestation, most babies have developed adequate amounts of surfactant.

Surfactant is normally released into the lung tissues where it helps lower surface tension in the airways. This helps keep the lung alveoli (air sacs) open. When there is not enough surfactant, the tiny alveoli collapse with each breath. As the alveoli collapse, damaged cells collect in the airways and further affect breathing ability. These cells are called hyaline membranes. The baby works harder and harder at breathing, trying to re-inflate the collapsed airways.

As the baby's lung function decreases, less oxygen is taken in and more carbon dioxide builds up in the blood. This can lead to increased acid in the blood called acidosis, a condition that can affect other body organs. Without treatment, the baby becomes exhausted trying to breathe and eventually gives up. A mechanical ventilator (breathing machine) must do the work of breathing instead.

- HMD occurs in over half of babies born before 28 weeks gestation, but only in less than one-third of those born between 32 and 36 weeks. Some premature babies develop HMD severe enough to need a mechanical ventilator (breathing machine). The more premature the baby, the higher the risk and the more severe the HMD.

Symptoms

The following are the most common symptoms of HMD. However, each baby may experience symptoms differently. Symptoms may include:

- Respiratory difficulty at birth that gets progressively worse
- Cyanosis (blue colouring)
- Flaring of the nostrils
- Tachypnea (rapid breathing)
- Grunting sounds with breathing
- Chest retractions (pulling in at the ribs and sternum during breathing)

The symptoms of HMD usually peak by the third day, and may resolve quickly when the baby begins to diurese (excrete excess water in urine) and begins to need less oxygen and mechanical help to breathe.

The symptoms of HMD may resemble other conditions or medical problems. Always consult baby's physician for a diagnosis.

Diagnosis

HMD is usually diagnosed by a combination of assessments, including the following:

- Appearance, colour, and breathing efforts (indicate a baby's need for oxygen).
- Chest x-rays of lungs - often show a unique "ground glass" appearance called a reticulogranular pattern. X-rays are electromagnetic energy used to produce images of bones and internal organs onto film.

- Blood gases (tests for oxygen, carbon dioxide and acid in arterial blood) - often show lowered amounts of oxygen and increased carbon dioxide.
- Echocardiography (EKG) - sometimes used to rule out heart problems that might cause symptoms similar to HMD. An electrocardiogram is a test that records the electrical activity of the heart, shows abnormal rhythms (arrhythmias or dysrhythmias), and detects heart muscle damage.

Treatment

Specific treatment for HMD will be determined by baby's physician based on:

- Baby's gestational age, overall health, and medical history
- Extent of the condition
- Baby's tolerance for specific medications, procedures, or therapies
- Expectations for the course of the condition
- Opinion or preference

Treatment for HMD may include:

- Placing an endotracheal (ET) tube into the baby's windpipe
- Mechanical breathing machine (to do the work of breathing for the baby)
- Supplemental oxygen (extra amounts of oxygen)
- Continuous positive airway pressure (CPAP) - a mechanical breathing machine that pushes a continuous flow of air or oxygen to the airways to help keep tiny air passages in the lungs open
- Surfactant replacement with artificial surfactant - most effective if started in the first six hours of birth. Surfactant replacement has been shown to reduce the severity of HMD. Surfactant is given as prophylactic (preventive) treatment for some babies at very high risk for HMD. For others it is used as a "rescue" method. The drug comes as a powder to be mixed with sterile water and then is given through the ET tube (breathing tube). Surfactant is usually given in several doses.
- Medications (to help sedate and ease pain in babies during treatment)

Prevention

Preventing a preterm birth is the primary means of preventing HMD. When a preterm birth cannot be prevented, giving the mother medications called corticosteroids before delivery has been shown to dramatically lower the risk and severity of HMD in the baby. These steroids are often given to women between 24 and 34 weeks gestation who are at risk of early delivery.

PNEUMOTHORAX

Pneumothorax is a lung disorder in which air in the lungs leaks out through holes in the lung tissue into the spaces outside the lung airways. Pneumothorax is one type of lung disorders called air leak syndrome. A baby can have more than one form of air leak. Types of air leaks include the following:

- Pneumothorax - air leaks into the space between the chest wall and the outer tissues of the lungs.
- Pneumomediastinum - air leaks into the mediastinum (the space in the thoracic cavity behind the sternum and between the two pleural sacs containing the lungs).
- Pneumopericardium - air leaks into the sac surrounding the heart.
- Pulmonary interstitial emphysema (PIE) - air leaks and becomes trapped between the alveoli, the tiny air sacs of the lungs.

Air leaks may occur suddenly or may develop gradually. The degree of illness depends on the location of the leak and the amount of air.

Causes

Air leaks occur when the alveoli (tiny air sacs) become overdistended and burst. Pressure of the air delivered by mechanical ventilators (breathing machines) is the most common cause. Meconium aspiration (inhalation of the first stools passed in utero) can also trap air and lead to overdistention (the lungs expand too much) and air leaks. Air leaks often occur in the first 24 to 36 hours when lung disease is at its peak. Some otherwise healthy babies can develop a "spontaneous" air leak that does not cause symptoms or distress.

Symptoms

The following are the most common symptoms of pneumothorax. However, each baby may experience symptoms differently. Symptoms may include:

- Increasing respiratory distress, including rapid breathing, grunting, nostril flaring, and chest wall retractions
- Difficulty hearing breath sounds when listening with a stethoscope
- Change in the location of heart or lung sounds when the organs are moved by the presence of air
- Changes in arterial blood gas levels

The symptoms of pneumothorax may resemble other conditions or medical problems. Always consult baby's physician for a diagnosis.

Diagnosis

In addition to a complete medical history and physical examination, diagnostic procedures for pneumothorax may include:

- Chest x-rays - a diagnostic test which uses invisible electromagnetic energy beams to produce images of internal tissues, bones, and organs onto film. X-rays may show the following:
  - — Air in places outside the normal lung airways
  - — Collapse of the lung
  - — Movement or shifting of other organs in the chest away from the air leak side
- Transillumination - a fiberoptic light probe placed on the baby's chest wall (the side of the chest with the air leak transmits brighter light). This procedure is often used in an emergency.

Treatment

Specific treatment for pneumothorax and air leak syndrome will be determined by baby's physician based on:

- Baby's gestational age, overall health, and medical history
- Extent of the condition
- Baby's tolerance for specific medications, procedures, or therapies
- Expectations for the course of the condition
- Opinion or preference

Treatment for pneumothorax may include:

- Supplemental oxygen

- Removal of the collected air by insertion of a chest tube (a needle or catheter placed through the chest wall into the air space). The air may be withdrawn with a syringe or the tube connected to a drainage system to help remove the air until the leak can seal.

Spontaneous air leaks that do not cause symptoms or distress may get better on their own without treatment. As the leak seals over, air is absorbed into the body.

There are no specific treatments for pneumomediastinum and pulmonary interstitial emphysema (PIE), as these air leaks are in spaces that cannot be treated with chest tubes. High frequency ventilation is sometimes used for babies with PIE.

Prevention

Despite careful regulation of the air pressure and the settings on mechanical ventilators, air leaks can still occur. Baby's physician and other healthcare providers in the newborn intensive care unit (NICU) will watch baby carefully for signs of air leak so that treatment can be started as quickly as possible.

BRONCHOPULMONARY DYSPLASIA

Chronic lung disease (CLD) is a general term for long-term respiratory problems in premature babies. It is also known as bronchopulmonary dysplasia (BPD).

Causes

CLD results from lung injury to newborns who must use a mechanical ventilator and extra oxygen for breathing. The lungs of premature babies are fragile and are easily damaged. With injury, the tissues inside the lungs become inflamed and can break down causing scarring. This scarring can result in difficulty breathing and increased oxygen needs. Some of the causes of lung injury include the following:

- Prematurity - the lungs, especially the air sacs, are not fully developed
- Low amounts of surfactant (a substance in the lungs that helps keep the tiny air sacs open)
- Oxygen use (high concentrations of oxygen can damage the cells of the lungs)
- Mechanical ventilation - the pressure of air from breathing machines, suctioning of the airways, use of an endotracheal

tube (ET tube - a tube placed in the trachea and connected to a breathing machine)

Symptoms

The following are the most common symptoms of CLD. However, each baby may experience different symptoms of the condition. Symptoms may include:

- Respiratory distress (rapid breathing, flaring of the nostrils, chest retractions)
- Continued need for mechanical ventilation or oxygen after a premature baby reaches 36 weeks gestation

The symptoms of CLD may resemble other conditions or medical problems. Always consult baby's physician for a diagnosis.

Diagnosis

Because CLD is a chronic disease and appears gradually, physicians must look at several factors. It is often diagnosed when a premature baby with respiratory problems continues to need additional oxygen after reaching 36 weeks gestational age. Chest x-rays compared with previous x-rays may show changes in the appearance of the lungs. The x-ray of lungs with CLD often have a bubbly, sponge-like appearance. X-rays are diagnostic tests which use invisible electromagnetic energy beams to produce images of internal tissues, bones, and organs onto film.

Treatment

Specific treatment for CLD will be determined by baby's physician based on:

- Baby's gestational age, overall health, and medical history
- Extent of the disease
- Baby's tolerance for specific medications, procedures, or therapies
- Expectations for the course of the disease
- Opinion or preference

Treatment of CLD may include:

- Extra oxygen (to make up for the decreased breathing ability of the damaged lungs)
- Mechanical ventilation with gradual weaning as the baby's lungs grow and can do more of the work of breathing

- Medications such as:
  - Bronchodilators (to help open the airways)
  - Steroids to help reduce inflammation)
- Limiting fluids and giving a medication (diuretic) to help reduce excess fluid which can worsen breathing ability
- Nutrition (to help the baby and the lungs grow)
- Immunization against lung infection by respiratory syncytial virus (RSV) and influenza

CLD can be a long-term condition. Some babies with CLD require mechanical ventilators for several months. Some babies will continue to require oxygen when they go home from the hospital, but most can be weaned from oxygen by the end of their first year. Babies with CLD may be at increased risk for respiratory infection and may have to be re-hospitalized.

REFERENCES

Carroll D, Tramer M, McQuay H, Nye B and Moore A (1997) Transcutaneous electrical nerve stimulation in labour pain: a systematic review British Journal of Obstetrics and Gynaecology 104 169-175

Walsh D (1999) Transcutaneous electrical nerve stimulation British Journal of Midwifery 7(7) 580

Johnson M I (1997) Transcutaneous electrical nerve stimulation in pain management British Journal of Midwifery 5(7) 400-405

Harrison R F, Woods T, Shore M, Mathews G and Unwin A (1986) Pain relief in labour using transcutaneous electrical nerve stimulation (TENS). A TENS/TENS placebo controlled study in two parity gourps British Journal of Obstetrics and Gynaecology 93 739-746

Garland D and Jones K (2000) Waterbirth: supporting practice with clinical audit MIDIRS Midwifery Digest 10(3) 333-336

Schorn M, McAllister J, Blanco J (1993) Water immersion and the effect on labour Journal of Nurse Midwifery 38(6) 336-342

Tawfik O, Badraoui M H H, El-Ridi F S (1982) The value of transcutaneous nerve stimulation (TNS) during labour in Egyptian mothers Scherz 2 98-195

Mander R (1997) Pethidine in childbirth MIDIRS Midwifery Digest 7(2) 202-203

11

Pharmaco-therapeutics

Drug use during pregnancy and lactation requires special consideration because both the mother and the foetus or nursing infant are affected. Few drugs are considered safe, and drug use is generally contraindicated. However, many pregnant or lactating women take drugs for various reasons, including acute disorders that may or may not be associated with pregnancy, chronic disorders that require continued treatment during pregnancy or lactation, and habitual use of nontherapeutic drugs (eg, alcohol, tobacco, others). The main purpose of this chapter is to describe potential drug effects on the foetus and maternal drug therapy to protect the foetus while providing therapeutic effects to the pregnant woman.

PREGNANCY AND LACTATION

Pregnancy is a dynamic state: Mother and foetus undergo physiologic changes that influence drug effects. In the pregnant woman, physiologic changes alter drug pharmacokinetics, and drug effects are less predictable than in the nonpregnant state. Most of the drugs in this chapter are described elsewhere; they are discussed here in relation to pregnancy and lactation. Other drugs are used mainly to influence some aspect of pregnancy. These drugs are discussed in greater detail and include those used to induce abortion (abortifacients), drugs used to stop preterm labour (tocolytics), and drugs used during labour and delivery.

MATERNAL-PLACENTAL- FOETAL CIRCULATION

Drugs ingested by the pregnant woman reach the foetus through the maternal-placental-foetal circulation, which is completed about the third week after conception. On the maternal side, arterial blood pressure carries blood and drugs to the placenta. In the placenta, maternal and foetal blood are separated by a few thin layers of tissue over a large surface area. Drugs readily cross the placenta, mainly by passive diffusion. Placental transfer begins approximately the fifth week after conception. When drugs are given on a regular schedule, serum levels reach equilibrium, with foetal blood usually containing 50% to 100% of the amount in maternal blood. After drugs enter the foetal circulation, relatively large amounts are pharmacologically active because the foetus has low levels of serum albumin and thus low levels of drug binding. Drug molecules are distributed in two ways. Most are transported to the liver, where they are metabolized. Metabolism occurs slowly because the foetal liver is immature in quantity and quality of drug-metabolizing enzymes.

Drugs metabolized by the foetal liver are excreted by foetal kidneys into amniotic fluid. Excretion also is slow and inefficient owing to immature development of foetal kidneys. In addition, the foetus swallows some amniotic fluid, and some drug molecules are recirculated. Other drug molecules are transported directly to the heart, which then distributes them to the brain and coronary arteries. Drugs enter the brain easily because the blood-brain barrier is poorly developed in the foetus. Approximately half of the drug-containing blood is then transported through the umbilical arteries to the placenta, where it reenters the maternal circulation. Thus, the mother can metabolize and excrete some drug molecules for the foetus.

DRUG EFFECTS ON THE FOETUS

The foetus, which is exposed to any drugs circulating in maternal blood, is very sensitive to drug effects because it is small, has few plasma proteins that can bind drug molecules, and has a weak capacity for metabolizing and excreting drugs. Once drug molecules reach the foetus, they may cause teratogenicity (anatomic malformations) or other adverse effects. The teratogenicity of many drugs is unknown. However, since 1984, Administration has required that new drugs be assigned a risk category. Drug teratogenicity is most likely to occur when drugs are taken during the first trimester of pregnancy, when foetal organs are formed. For drugs taken during the second and third trimesters, adverse effects are usually manifested in the neonate (birth to 1 month) or infant (1 month to 1 year) as growth retardation, respiratory problems, infection, or bleeding. Overall, effects are determined mainly by the type and amount of drugs, the duration of exposure, and the level of foetal growth and development when exposed to the drugs. Both therapeutic and nontherapeutic drugs may affect the foetus.

Alcohol is contraindicated during pregnancy; no amount is considered safe. Heavy intake may cause foetal alcohol syndrome, a condition characterized by multiple congenital defects and mental retardation.

Caffeine is the most commonly ingested nontherapeutic drug during pregnancy. It is present in coffee, tea, cola drinks, over-the-counter analgesics, antisleep preparations, and chocolate. Although ingestion of moderate amounts has not been associated with birth defects, spontaneous abortions, preterm births, and low birth weights have occurred. In addition, high doses may cause cardiac dysrhythmias in the foetus.

Cigarette smoking (nicotine and carbon monoxide ingestion) is one of the few preventable causes of perinatal morbidity and mortality and is contraindicated. Effects include increased foetal, neonatal, and infant mortality; decreased birth weight and length; shortened gestation; and increased complications of pregnancy (eg, placental abruption, spontaneous abortion; preterm delivery). These effects are attributed to decreased flow of blood and oxygen to the placenta and uterus. Nicotine causes vasoconstriction and decreases blood flow to the foetus; carbon monoxide decreases the oxygen available to the foetus. Chronic foetal hypoxia from heavy smoking has been associated with mental retardation and other long-term effects on physical and intellectual development. Overall, effects of smoking are dose related, with light smoking (<1 pack/day) estimated to increase foetal deaths by 20% and heavy smoking (1 or more packs/day) increasing deaths by 35%.

FOETAL THERAPEUTICS

Although the major concern about drugs ingested during pregnancy is adverse effects on the foetus, a few drugs are given to the mother for their therapeutic effects on the foetus. These include digoxin for foetal tachycardia or heart failure, levothyroxine for hypothyroidism, penicillin for exposure to maternal syphilis, and prenatal corticosteroids to promote surfactant production to improve lung function and decrease respiratory distress syndrome in preterm infants.

MATERNAL THERAPEUTICS

Thus far, the main emphasis on drug use during pregnancy has related to actual or potential adverse effects on the foetus. Despite the general principle that drug use should be avoided when possible, pregnant women may require drug therapy for various illnesses, increased nutritional needs, pregnancyassociated problems, chronic disease processes, treatment of preterm labour, induction of labour, and pain management during labour.

HERBAL AND DIETARY SUPPLEMENTS

Pregnancy increases nutritional needs and vitamin and mineral supplements are commonly used. Folic acid supplementation is especially important, to prevent neural tube birth defects (eg, spina bifida). Such defects occur early in pregnancy, often before the woman realizes she is pregnant. For this reason, it is recommended that all women of childbearing potential ingest at least 400 mcg daily from food and/ or a supplement. In addition, pregnancy increases folic acid requirements by 5- to 10-fold and deficiencies are common. A supplement is usually needed to supply adequate amounts. For deficiency states, 1 mg or more daily may be needed. Herbal supplements are not recommended during pregnancy. Ginger has been used to relieve nausea and vomiting during pregnancy, with a few studies supporting its use. Overall, it has not been proven effective, but is probably safe for use.

PREGNANCY-ASSOCIATED SYMPTOMS AND THEIR MANAGEMENT

Anaemias

Three types of anaemia are common during pregnancy. One is physiologic anaemia, which results from expanded blood volume. A second is iron-deficiency anaemia, which is often related to long-term nutritional deficiencies. Iron supplements are usually given for prophylaxis (eg, ferrous sulfate 300 mg or ferrous gluconate 600 mg three times daily). Iron preparations should be given with food to decrease gastric irritation. Citrus juices enhance absorption. A third type is megaloblastic anaemia, caused by folic acid deficiency. A folic acid supplement is often prescribed for prophylaxis.

Constipation

Constipation often occurs during pregnancy, probably from decreased peristalsis. Preferred treatment, if effective, is to increase exercise and intake of fluids and high-fibre foods. If a laxative is required, a bulk-producing agent (eg, Metamucil) is the most physiologic for the mother and safest for the foetus because it is not absorbed systemically. A stool softener (eg, docusate) or an occasional saline laxative (eg, milk of magnesia) may also be used. Mineral oil should be avoided because it interferes with absorption of fat-soluble vitamins. Reduced absorption of vitamin K can lead to bleeding in newborns. Castor oil should be avoided because it can cause uterine contractions. Strong laxatives or any laxative used in excess may initiate uterine contractions and labour.

Gastroesophageal Reflux Disease

Gastroesophageal reflux disease (GERD), of which heartburn (pyrosis) is the main symptom, often occurs in the later months of pregnancy. It develops when increased abdominal pressure and a relaxed esophageal sphincter allow gastric acid to splash into the esophagus and cause irritation, discomfort, and esophagitis. Nonpharmacologic interventions include eating small meals; not eating for 2 to 3 hours before bedtime; avoiding caffeine, gas-producing foods and constipation; and sitting in an upright position. For clients who do not obtain adequate relief with these measures, drug therapy may be needed. Antacids may be used if necessary. Because little systemic absorption occurs, the drugs are unlikely to harm the foetus if used in recommended doses. Cimetidine, ranitidine, or sucralfate may also be used.

Gestational Diabetes

Some women first show signs of diabetes during pregnancy.

This is called gestational diabetes. Women with risk factors (eg, obesity, family history of diabetes, being Hispanic, Native American, Asian, or African American) should be screened at the first prenatal visit. Most women without risk factors, or whose initial test was normal, should be tested between 24 and 28 weeks of gestation. For women with gestational diabetes, initial management includes nutrition and exercise interventions, calorie restriction for obese women, and daily self-monitoring of blood glucose levels. If these interventions are ineffective, recombinant human insulin is needed to keep blood sugar levels as nearly normal as possible. Oral antidiabetic drugs are generally contraindicated, although acarbose, metformin, and miglitol seem to cause minimal foetal risk. These women may revert to a nondiabetic state when pregnancy ends, but they are at increased risk for development of overt diabetes within 5 to 10 years. Gestational diabetes usually subsides within 6 weeks after delivery.

Nausea and Vomiting

Nausea and vomiting often occur, especially during early pregnancy. Dietary management (eg, eating a few crackers when awakening and waiting a few minutes before arising) and maintaining fluid and electrolyte balance are recommended. Antiemetic drugs should be given only if nausea and vomiting are severe enough to threaten the mother's nutritional or metabolic status. Meclizine, 25 to 50 mg daily, and dimenhydrinate, 50 mg every 3 to 4 hours, are thought to have low teratogenic risks. Pyridoxine (vitamin B6) also may be helpful. If used, recommended dosage is 10 to 25 mg daily.

Pregnancy-Induced Hypertension

Pregnancy-induced hypertension includes preeclampsia and eclampsia, conditions that endanger the lives of mother and foetus. Preeclampsia is most likely to occur during the last 10 weeks of pregnancy, during labour, or within the first 48 hours after delivery. It is manifested by edema, hypertension, and proteinuria. Drug therapy includes intravenous hydralazine or labetalol for blood pressure control and magnesium sulfate for prevention or treatment of seizures. Eclampsia, characterized by severe symptoms and convulsions, occurs if preeclampsia is not treated effectively. Delivery of the foetus is the only known cure for preeclampsia or eclampsia. For women at risk of developing preeclampsia, aspirin 60 mg daily, from 24 to 28 weeks of gestation until onset of labour, may be used for prophylaxis.

Selected Infections

Group B streptococcal Infections

Group B streptococcal infections may affect the pregnant woman and the neonate. During late pregnancy, urinary tract infections (UTIs) or amnionitis may occur. After cesarean delivery, endometritis, bacteremia, or wound infection may occur. In the infant, sepsis, meningitis, or pneumonia may occur. Because of the potentially serious consequences of infection with group B streptococci, pregnant women should have a vaginal culture at 35 to 37 weeks of gestation. A positive culture indicates infection that should be treated. However, antibiotics given at this time may not provide coverage during labour and delivery. Treatment should be initiated during labour, often with ampicillin 2 g intravenously (IV) as a loading dose, then 1 g IV every 4 hours until delivery.

HIV & AIDS

Human immunodeficiency virus (HIV) infection and acquired immunodeficiency syndrome (AIDS) can be transmitted to the foetus and neonate, and treatment is needed to reduce transmission. Oral zidovudine (AZT) monotherapy has been used for several years, after 14 weeks of gestation. During labour, IV AZT is given until delivery. After delivery, the infant should be given AZT for 6 weeks, with or without other anti-AIDS drugs. Increasingly, highly active antiretroviral therapy

(HAART) is being used for pregnant women. HAART is a combination of drugs that may include a nucleoside reverse transcriptase inhibitor (eg, zidovudine, lamivudine, or didansoine), a non-nucleoside reverse transcriptase inhibitor (eg, nevirapine) and a protease inhibitor (eg, ritonavir, saquinavir, nelfinavir). Women with HIV infection or AIDS should be encouraged to avoid pregnancy.

Urinary Tract Infections

Urinary tract infections commonly occur during pregnancy and may include asymptomatic bacteriuria, cystitis, and pyelonephritis. Although treatment of asymptomatic bacteriuria is controversial in some populations, the condition should be treated in pregnant women because of its association with cystitis and pyelonephritis. Asymptomatic bacteriuria and UTIs are also associated with increased preterm deliveries and low birth weights. Amoxicillin, cephalexin, and nitrofurantoin are commonly used drugs. Hospitalization and an IV cephalosporin may be needed for management of pyelonephritis.

MANAGEMENT OF CHRONIC DISEASES DURING PREGNANCY

Asthma

Asthma is associated with a variety of complications in pregnancy, including preeclampsia, perinatal death, low birth weights, and congenital malformations. Poor asthma control during pregnancy is considered more detrimental to a foetus than treatment with available drugs. Thus, good control is essential. Commonly used drugs include orally inhaled beta2 agonists (eg, albuterol or metaproterenol) and anti-inflammatory agents (eg, cromolyn or beclomethasone).

Diabetes Mellitus

Diabetes increases the risks of pregnancy for both mother and foetus, and the hormonal changes of pregnancy have diabetogenic effects that may cause or aggravate diabetes. Some women first show signs of diabetes during pregnancy (gestational diabetes). Others, who were previously able to control diabetes with diet alone, may become insulin dependent during pregnancy. Still others, already insulin dependent, are likely to need larger doses as pregnancy advances. Overall, pregnancy makes diabetes more difficult to control. In addition, insulin requirements fluctuate during pregnancy. For diabetic women who become pregnant, maintaining normal or near-normal blood sugar levels is required for successful outcomes because poor glycemic control increases the risks of birth defects. Recommendations for management include the following:

- If oral antidiabetic drugs are taken by a woman of childbearing potential, they should be discontinued before conception, if possible (eg, for a planned pregnancy attempt), or as soon as pregnancy is suspected. Oral antidiabetic drugs are contraindicated in pregnancy, mainly because of foetal hypoglycemia.

  This recommendation may change in the future, because acarbose, miglitol, and metformin are thought to have little risk for the foetus. Glyburide has been used in some women after 11 weeks of gestation. However, its use is not recommended during the last few weeks of pregnancy. Most oral agents have not been studied in pregnant women.

- Insulin is the antidiabetic drug of choice during pregnancy. Human insulin should be used because it is least likely to cause an allergic response. Because insulin requirements vary according to the stage of pregnancy, the diabetic client's blood glucose levels must be monitored closely and insulin therapy individualized. It is especially important that sufficient insulin is given to prevent maternal acidosis. Uncontrolled acidosis is likely to interfere with neurologic development of the foetus. At the same time, careful dietary control and other treatment measures are necessary.

- Insulin requirements usually decrease during the first trimester and increase during the second and third trimesters.

- During labour and delivery, short-acting insulin and frequent blood glucose tests are used to control diabetes, as during other acute situations.

- During the postpartum period, insulin requirements fluctuate because stress, trauma, infection, surgery, or other factors associated with delivery tend to increase blood glucose levels and insulin requirements. At the same time, termination of the pregnancy reverses the diabetogenic hormonal changes and decreases insulin requirements. Short-acting insulin is given, and dosage is based on frequent measurements of blood glucose. Once the insulin requirement is stabilized, the client may be able to return to the prepregnancy treatment program.

Hypertension

Chronic hypertension (hypertension beginning before conception or up to 20 weeks of pregnancy) is associated with increased maternal and foetal risks. Thus, appropriate management is mandatory. Nonpharmacologic interventions (e.g., avoiding excessive weight gain, sodium restriction, increased rest) should be emphasized. If drug therapy is required, methyldopa is the drug of first choice because it has not been associated with adverse effects on the foetus or neonate. Alternatives include labetalol and other beta blockers, clonidine, hydralazine, isradipine, nifedipine, and prazosin. With beta blockers, foetal and neonatal bradycardia, hypotension, hypoglycemia, and respiratory depression have been reported. As a result, some authorities recommend avoiding the drugs during the first trimester and stopping them 2 to 3 days before delivery. Opinions seem divided on the use of angiotensin-converting enzyme (ACE) inhibitors. Some sources say the drugs are contraindicated during pregnancy; others say they can be used during the first trimester but should then be discontinued because of potential renal damage in the foetus. The same effects would probably occur with angiotensin II receptor blockers (ARBs), because they also act on the renin-angiotensin system. Although diuretics are commonly used in the treatment of hypertension, they should not be given during pregnancy. They decrease blood volume, cardiac output, and blood pressure and may cause fluid and electrolyte imbalances, all of which may have adverse effects on the foetus.

Seizure Disorders

Although antiepileptic drugs (AEDs) are known teratogens, they must often be taken during pregnancy because seizures may also be harmful to mother and foetus. Fortunately, most pregnancies (90 to 95%) result in normal infants. Despite the usually good outcomes, the incidence of birth defects is 2 to 3 times higher in foetuses exposed to AEDs than in those not exposed. If an AED is required, monotherapy with the lowest dose that stops seizures should be used and plasma drug levels should be checked monthly. Women with epilepsy should take a folic acid supplement (at least 400 mcg daily) all the time and 800 mcg or more during pregnancy. Supplemental vitamin K is usually needed during the last month of pregnancy, to prevent bleeding in neonates. An injection of vitamin K is also given to the infant immediately after birth. There has been controversy as to whether teratogenic effects stemmed from epilepsy or AEDs. A newer study indicates that the drugs are responsible.

Moreover, the rate of birth defects in infants exposed to one AED was significantly higher than those not exposed (20.6% vs 8.5%) and 28% in infants exposed to two or more AEDs. Infants whose mothers took AEDs for bipolar disorder rather than epilepsy also had higher rates of birth defects.

ABORTIFACIENTS

Abortion is the termination of pregnancy before 20 weeks. It may occur spontaneously or be intentionally induced. Medical abortion may be induced by prostaglandins and an antiprogestin (Drugs at a Glance: Abortifacients, Prostaglandins, Tocolytics, and Oxytocics). Prostaglandins may be used to terminate pregnancy during the second trimester. In the female reproductive system, prostaglandins E and F are found in the ovaries, myometrium, and menstrual fluid. They stimulate uterine contraction and are probably important in initiating and maintaining the normal birth process. Drug preparations of prostaglandins are capable of inducing labour at any time during pregnancy. Misoprostol, a prostaglandin developed to prevent nonsteroidal anti-inflammatory drug-induced gastric ulcers, is being given orally or intravaginally for first or second trimester termination. It is not FDA approved for this use. Mifepristone is a progesterone antagonist used to terminate pregnancy during the first trimester. A prostaglandin is given approximately 48 hours after the mifepristone to augment uterine contractions and ensure expulsion of the conceptus.

TOCOLYTICS

Drugs given to inhibit labour and maintain the pregnancy are called tocolytics. Uterine contractions with cervical changes between 20 and 37 weeks of gestation are considered premature labour. Nonpharmacologic treatment includes bed rest, hydration, and sedation. Drug therapy is most effective when the cervix is dilated less than 4 cm and membranes are intact. Ritodrine, terbutaline, magnesium sulfate, and nifedipine are used as tocolytics. Ritodrine and terbutaline are beta-adrenergic agents that relax uterine smooth muscle and thereby slow or stop uterine contractions. Terbutaline is not FDA approved for use in premature labour, but is used widely for that purpose. Magnesium sulfate is most often used as an anticonvulsant in the treatment of preeclampsia, but it also inhibits preterm labour. Hypermagnesemia may occur because tocolytic serum levels (4 to 7 mEq/L) are higher than normal levels (1.5 to 2.5 mEq/L).

DRUGS USED DURING LABOUR AND DELIVERY AT TERM

At the end of gestation, labour usually begins spontaneously and proceeds through delivery of the neonate. In some instances, prostaglandin preparations (eg, Prepidil or Cervidil formulations of dinoprostone) are administered intravaginally to promote cervical ripening and induce labour. Drugs often used during labour, delivery, and the immediate postpartum period include oxytocics, analgesics, and anesthetics.

OXYTOCICS

Oxytocic drugs include oxytocin (Pitocin) and methylergonovine. Oxytocin is a hormone produced in the hypothalamus and released by the posterior pituitary gland. Oxytocin stimulates uterine contractions to initiate labour and promotes letdown of breast milk to the nipples in lactation. Pitocin is a synthetic form used to induce labour at or near full-term gestation and to augment labour when uterine contractions are weak and ineffective. It also can be used to prevent or control uterine bleeding after delivery or to complete an incomplete abortion. It is contraindicated for antepartum use in the presence of foetal distress, cephalopelvic disproportion, preterm labour, placenta previa, previous uterine surgery, and severe preeclampsia. Methergine is used for management of postpartum haemorrhage related to uterine atony.

ANALGESICS

Parenteral opioid analgesics are used to control discomfort and pain during labour and delivery. They may prolong labour and cause sedation and respiratory depression in the mother and neonate. Meperidine may cause less neonatal depression than other opioid analgesics. Butorphanol is widely used. If neonatal respiratory depression occurs, it can be reversed by naloxone (Narcan). Duramorph is a long-acting form of morphine that provides analgesia up to 24 hours after injection into the epidural catheter at the completion of a cesarean section. Regional analgesia is achieved by the epidural injection of opioids (eg, fentanyl) or preservative-free morphine. Possible side effects include maternal urinary retention, but no significant effects on the foetus.

ANAESTHETICS

Local anesthetics also are used to control discomfort and pain. They are injected by physicians for regional anaesthesia in the pelvic area. Epidural blocks involve injection into the epidural space of the spinal cord. Bupivacaine is commonly used. With regional anaesthesia, the mother is usually conscious and comfortable, and the neonate is rarely depressed. Fentanyl may be combined with a small amount of an anesthetic drug for both analgesia and anaesthesia. No significant effects on the foetus occurred in clinical studies.

NEONATAL THERAPEUTICS

In the neonate, any drug must be used cautiously. Drugs are usually given less often because they are metabolized and excreted slowly. Immature liver and kidney function prolongs drug action and increases risks of toxicity. Also, drug therapy should be initiated with low doses, especially with drugs that are highly bound to plasma proteins. Neonates have few binding proteins, which leads to increased amounts of free, active drug and increased risk of toxicity. When the health care provider is assessing the neonate, drugs received by the mother during pregnancy, labour and delivery, and lactation must be considered.

At birth, some drugs are routinely administered to prevent hemorrhagic disease of the newborn and ophthalmia neonatorum. Hemorrhagic disease of the newborn occurs because the intestinal tract lacks the bacteria that normally synthesize vitamin K. Vitamin K is required for liver production of several clotting factors, including prothrombin. Thus, the neonate is at increased risk of bleeding during the first week of life. One dose of phytonadione 0.5 to 1 mg is injected at delivery or on admission to the nursery.

Ophthalmia neonatorum is a form of bacterial conjunctivitis that may cause ulceration and blindness. It may be caused by several bacteria, most commonly Chlamydia trachomatis, a sexually transmitted organism. Erythromycin ointment 0.5% is applied to each eye at delivery. It is effective against both chlamydial and gonococcal infections.

PRINCIPLES OF THERAPY

PREGNANCY

Give medications only when clearly indicated, weighing anticipated benefits to the mother against the risk of harm to the foetus.

- When drug therapy is required, the choice of drug should be based on the stage of pregnancy and available drug information. During the first trimester, for example, an older drug that has not been associated with teratogenic effects is usually preferred over a newer drug of unknown teratogenicity.

- Any drugs used during pregnancy should be given in the lowest effective doses and for the shortest effective time.
- Counsel pregnant women about the use of immunizations during pregnancy. Live virus vaccines (eg, measles, mumps, polio, rubella, yellow fever) should be avoided because of possible harmful effects to the foetus. Inactive virus vaccines, such as influenza, rabies, and hepatitis B (if the mother is high risk and negative for hepatitis B antigen) and toxoids (eg, diphtheria, tetanus) are considered safe for use. In addition, hyperimmune globulins can be given to pregnant women who are exposed to hepatitis B, rabies, tetanus, or varicella.

LACTATION

Most systemic drugs taken by the mother reach the infant in breast milk. For some, the amount of drug is too small to cause significant effects; for others, effects on the nursing infant are unknown or potentially adverse.

Give medications only when clearly indicated, weighing potential benefit to the mother against possible harm to the nursing infant. For contraindicated drugs, it is usually recommended that the mother stop the drug or stop breast-feeding.

Any drugs used during lactation should be given in the lowest effective dose for the shortest effective time.

The American Academy of Pediatrics (AAP) supports breast-feeding as optimal nutrition for infants and does not recommend stopping during maternal drug therapy unless necessary. In some instances, mothers may pump and discard breast milk while receiving therapeutic drugs, to maintain lactation.

Women with human immunodeficiency virus (HIV) infection should not breast-feed. The virus can be transmitted to the nursing infant.

USE OF OXYTOCIN

Oxytocin is usually the drug of choice for induction or augmentation of labour because physiologic doses produce a rhythmic uterine contraction-relaxation pattern that approximates the normal labour process. It is also the drug of choice for prevention or control of postpartum uterine bleeding because it is less likely to cause hypertension than the ergot alkaloids.

HOME CARE

Many obstetric clients with conditions such as preterm labour, hyperemesis, and elevated blood pressure are now being managed in the home. The home care nurse who assists in managing these clients should be an obstetric specialist who is knowledgeable about normal pregnancy and potential complications. The nurse should be aware of the drugs being used to treat the complicated obstetric client as well as maternal use of any nonprescription and nontherapeutic drugs. A systematic assessment of maternal and foetal responses should be made on each visit. Home care visits also allow for assessment of compliance with the proposed management plan. Understanding of previous teaching should be evaluated on each visit. It is especially important for the client to know the danger signs and symptoms that may necessitate notifying a health care provider. The overall goal of home care is to maintain the pregnancy to the most advanced gestational age possible. Home care follow- up by a nurse has been demonstrated to positively affect the outcome of a high-risk pregnancy.

DRUG EFFECTS IN PREGNANCY

All drugs are relatively contraindicated and should be used only if necessary. For most drugs, adequate studies have not been done in pregnant women and effects on the foetus are unknown. They should be used only if potential benefit to the mother justifies potential harm to the foetus.

ADRENERGICS

Adrenergics are cardiac stimulants that increase rate and force of contractions and may increase blood pressure. Several were teratogenic and embryocidal in animal studies. These drugs are common ingredients in over-the-counter decongestants, cold remedies, and appetite suppressants. Oral and parenteral adrenergics may inhibit uterine contractions during labour; cause hypokalemia, hypoglycemia, and pulmonary oedema in the mother; and cause hypoglycemia in the neonate. These effects are unlikely with inhaled adrenergics (eg, albuterol). Oral albuterol and oral or intravenous terbutaline relax uterine muscles and inhibit preterm labour.

OPIOIDS

Opioids rapidly cross the placenta and reach the foetus. Maternal addiction and neonatal withdrawal symptoms result from regular use.

Use of codeine during the first trimester has been associated with congenital defects. When given to women in labour, opioids may decrease uterine contractility and slow progress toward delivery. They may also cause respiratory depression in the neonate.

Meperidine reportedly causes less neonatal respiratory depression than other opioids.

Butorphanol is also used. If respiratory depression occurs, it can be reversed by administration of naloxone, an opioid antagonist.

ANGIOTENSIN-CONVERTING ENZYME (ACE) INHIBITORS

These drugs can cause foetal and neonatal morbidity and death; several dozen cases have been reported worldwide. Adverse foetal effects apparently do not occur during first trimester exposure. With exposure during the second and third trimesters, however, effects may include foetal and neonatal injury such as hypotension, neonatal skull hypoplasia, anuria, renal failure, and death. As a result, the drugs should be discontinued as soon as pregnancy is detected. Infants exposed to the drugs in utero should be closely observed for hypotension, oliguria, and hyperkalemia.

ANGIOTENSIN II RECEPTOR BLOCKERS (ARBS)

These drugs should be discontinued when pregnancy is detected.

ANTIANGINAL AGENTS (NITRATES)

The drugs lower blood pressure and may decrease blood supply to the foetus. Thus, they should be used only if necessary.

ANTIANXIETY AND SEDATIVE-HYPNOTIC AGENTS (BENZODIAZEPINES)

These drugs should generally be avoided. They and their metabolites cross the placenta freely and accumulate in foetal blood. If taken during the first trimester, they may cause physical malformations. If taken during labour, they may cause sedation, respiratory depression, hypotonia, lethargy, tremors, irritability, and sucking difficulties in the neonate.

ANTIBACTERIALS

Penicillins cross the placenta but apparently produce no adverse effects on the foetus. They are considered safer than other antibiotics.

Cephalosporins cross the placenta and seem to be safe, although they have not been studied extensively in pregnancy. They have shorter half-lives, lower serum concentrations, and a faster rate of elimination in pregnancy.

Carbapenems and aztreonam have not been studied and foetal effects are unknown. Aminoglycosides cross the placenta and foetal serum levels may reach 15% to 50% of maternal levels. Ototoxicity may occur with gentamicin. Serious adverse effects on the foetus or neonate have not been reported with other aminoglycosides, but there is potential harm because the drugs are nephrotoxic and ototoxic.

Clindamycin (Cleocin) should be used only when infection with Bacteroides fragilis is suspected. Fluoroquinolones are contraindicated in pregnancy.

Erythromycin crosses the placenta to reach foetal serum levels up to 20% of maternal levels, but no foetal abnormalities have been reported. In animal studies, adverse foetal effects were reported with clarithromycin and dirithromycin but not with azithromycin.

Clarithromycin is contraindicated if a safer alternative is available.

Nitrofurantoin should not be used during late pregnancy because of possible hemolytic anaemia in the neonate.

Sulfonamides should not be used during the last trimester because they may cause kernicterus in the neonate.

Tetracyclines are contraindicated. They cross the placenta and interfere with development of teeth and bone in the foetus. Animal studies indicate embryotoxicity.

Trimethoprim, often given in combination with sulfamethoxazole (Bactrim), is contraindicated during the first trimester. It crosses the placenta to reach levels in foetal serum that are similar to those in maternal serum. It is a folate antagonist and may interfere with folic acid metabolism in the foetus. It was teratogenic in animals, but a few studies in pregnant women have not indicated teratogenic effects.

Vancomycin is not recommended because foetal effects are unknown.

ANTIFUNGALS

Systemic antifungals are generally contraindicated.

ANTICHOLINERGICS

Atropine crosses the placenta rapidly with IV injection; effects on the foetus depend on the maturity of its parasympathetic nervous system.

Scopolamine may cause respiratory depression in the neonate and may contribute to neonatal haemorrhage by reducing vitamin K-dependent clotting factors in the neonate.

ANTICOAGULANTS

Heparin does not cross the placenta and has not been associated with congenital defects. It is the anticoagulant of choice during pregnancy. However, its use has been associated with 13% to 22% unfavorable outcomes, including stillbirths and prematurity. Warfarin crosses the placenta and foetal haemorrhage, spontaneous abortion, prematurity, stillbirth, and congenital anomalies may occur. Approximately 31% of foetuses exposed to warfarin may experience a problem related to the anticoagulant. If a woman becomes pregnant during warfarin therapy, inform her of the potential risks to the foetus, and discuss the possibility of terminating the pregnancy.

ANTICONVULSANTS

Although more than 90% of women receiving antiseizure drugs deliver normal infants, the drugs (eg, carbamazepine, phenytoin, valproate) are known teratogens. After years of questioning whether teratogenesis resulted from epilepsy or antiepileptic drugs, a recent study confirms that anticonvulsant drug therapy in pregnant women causes physical abnormalities in their offspring. Moreover, infants exposed to one drug had a much higher rate of abnormalities than infants not exposed (20.6% vs. 8.5%) and infants exposed to two or more drugs had a still higher rate (28%). Infants whose nonepileptic mothers took the drugs for bipolar disorder also had higher rates of birth defects. In general, the foetal effects of newer drugs (eg, gabapentin, lamotrigine, oxcarbazepine, tiagabine, and topiramate) (Topamax) are unknown.

ANTIDEPRESSANTS

Tricyclic antidepressants (eg, amitriptyline) have been associated with teratogenicity and embryotoxicity when given in large doses, and there have been reports of congenital malformations and neonatal withdrawal syndrome. Monoamine oxidase inhibitors (eg, phenelzine), were associated with fewer viable offspring and growth retardation in animal studies with large doses. The selective serotonin reuptake inhibitors were teratogenic in animals and, in one study of 228 women who took fluoxetine during the first trimester, 5.5% of the infants had major birth defects. In addition, late exposure to fluoxetine resulted in more preterm births than early exposure (14.3% vs. 4.1%).

ANTIDIABETIC DRUGS

Insulin is the only antidiabetic drug recommended for use during pregnancy. Sulfonylureas except glyburide are teratogenic in animals; foetal effects of other oral agents are largely unknown.

ANTIEMETICS

None of the available antiemetic drugs has been proven safe for use and nondrug measures are preferred for controlling nausea and vomiting when possible. If drug therapy is necessary, some antihistamines (eg, cyclizine, dimenhydrinate) are considered safer for the foetus than other drugs.

ANTIHISTAMINES

Histamine-1 receptor blocking agents (eg, diphenhydramine), have been associated with teratogenic effects, but the extent is unknown. The drugs should generally not be used during the third trimester because of possible adverse effects in the neonate. With histamine-2 receptor blocking agents, cimetidine and ranitidine are considered acceptable for treatment of gastroesophageal reflux disease that does not respond to dietary and other lifestyle changes.

ANTIHYPERTENSIVES

Methyldopa crosses the placenta and reaches foetal concentrations similar to those of maternal serum. However, no teratogenic effects have been reported despite widespread use during pregnancy. Neonates of mothers receiving methyldopa may have decreased blood pressure for about 48 h. Hydralazine is considered safe. Clonidine, guanabenz, and guanfacine are not recommended because effects in pregnant women are unknown.

ANTIMANIC AGENT

Lithium crosses the placenta and foetal concentrations are similar to those of the mother. Cardiac and other birth defects may occur. In the neonate, lithium is eliminated slowly and may cause bradycardia, cyanosis, diabetes insipidus, hypotonia, hypothyroidism, and electrocardiogram (ECG) abnormalities. Most of these effects resolve within 1 to 2 wk.

ANTIPSYCHOTICS

Phenothiazines (eg, chlorpromazine) readily cross the placenta. Studies indicate that the drugs are not teratogenic, but animal studies indicate potential embryotoxicity, increased neonatal mortality, and decreased performance. The possibility of permanent neurologic damage cannot be excluded. Use near term may cause abnormal movements, abnormal reflexes, and jaundice in the neonate and hypotension in the mother. Foetal effects of newer drugs are unknown.

ANTITUBERCULAR DRUGS

These drugs are recommended for treatment of active tuberculosis; use for prophylaxis can usually be delayed until after delivery. Isoniazid, ethambutol, and rifampin were embryocidal or teratogenic in animal studies. The effects of drug combinations on the foetus are unknown.

ANTIVIRALS

Most systemic antivirals were teratogenic in animal studies. No well-controlled studies support their use in pregnancy, except for zidovudine and other anti-human immunodeficiency virus (HIV) drugs to prevent transmission of HIV infection to the foetus.

ASPIRIN

Aspirin is contraindicated because of potential adverse effects on the mother and foetus. Maternal effects include prolonged gestation, prolonged labour, and antepartum and postpartum haemorrhage. Foetal effects include constriction of the ductus arteriosus, low birth weight, and increased incidence of stillbirth and neonatal death.

BETA-ADRENERGIC BLOCKING AGENTS

Safety for use of these drugs (eg, propranolol) has not been established. Teratogenicity has not been reported in humans, but problems may occur during delivery. These include maternal bradycardia and neonatal bradycardia, hypoglycemia, apnea, low Apgar scores, and low birth weight. Neonatal effects may last up to 72 h.

CALCIUM CHANNEL BLOCKING AGENTS

Teratogenic and embryotoxic effects occurred in small animals given large doses. Diltiazem caused foetal death, skeletal abnormalities, and increased incidence of stillbirths. Nifedipine caused developmental toxicity in animals. Foetal effects of most of the drugs are unknown. Because the drugs decrease maternal blood pressure, there is a potential risk of inadequate blood flow to the placenta and the foetus.

CORTICOSTEROIDS

Systemic corticosteroids cross the placenta. Animal studies indicate that large doses of cortisol early in pregnancy may produce cleft palate, stillbirths, and decreased foetal size. Chronic maternal ingestion during the first trimester has shown a 1% incidence of cleft palate in humans. Infants of mothers who received substantial amounts of corticosteroids during pregnancy should be closely observed for signs of adrenal insufficiency.

Betamethasone is used to promote foetal production of surfactant to increase lung maturity in the preterm infant. Inhaled corticosteroids (eg, those used to treat allergic rhinitis or asthma) are less likely to cause adverse effects in the foetus because of less systemic absorption.

DIGOXIN

Digoxin is apparently safe for use during pregnancy. It crosses the placenta to reach foetal serum levels that are 50% to 80% those of maternal serum. Foetal toxicity and neonatal death have occurred with maternal overdose. Dosage requirements may be less predictable during pregnancy, and serum drug levels and other assessment parametres must be closely monitored. Digoxin also has been administered to the mother for treatment of foetal tachycardia and heart failure.

DIURETICS

Thiazides (eg, hydrochlorothiazide) cross the placenta. They are not associated with teratogenesis, but they may cause other adverse effects. Because the drugs decrease plasma volume, decreased blood flow to the uterus and placenta may occur with resultant impairment of foetal nutrition and growth.

Other adverse effects may include foetal or neonatal jaundice, thrombocytopenia, hyperbilirubinemia, hemolytic jaundice, fluid and electrolyte imbalances, and impaired carbohydrate metabolism. These drugs are not indicated for treatment of dependent oedema caused by uterine enlargement and restriction of venous blood flow. They also are not effective in prevention or treatment of pregnancy-induced hypertension (preeclampsia).

They may be used for treatment of pathologic oedema. Loop diuretics (eg, furosemide) are not considered teratogenic, but animal studies indicated foetal toxicity and death. Like the thiazides, loop diuretics may decrease plasma volume and blood flow to the placenta and foetus. Potassium-conserving diuretics (eg, triamterene, an ingredient in Dyazide and Maxide) cross the placenta in animal studies, but effects on the human foetus are unknown.

DYSLIPIDEMICS

Cholestyramine and colestipol are considered safe because they are not absorbed systemically. HMG-CoA reductase inhibitors or "statins" are contraindicated during pregnancy. They should be given to women of childbearing age only if they are highly unlikely to become pregnant and are informed of potential hazards. If a woman becomes pregnant while taking one of these drugs, the drug should be stopped and the patient informed of possible adverse drug effects on the foetus.

NONSTEROIDAL ANTI-INFLAMMATORY DRUGS

Use of NSAIDs (eg, ibuprofen) should generally be avoided, especially during the third trimester. If these drugs are taken in the third trimester, effects on human foetuses include constriction of the ductus arteriosis prenatally, nonclosure of the ductus arteriosius postnatally, impaired function of the tricuspid valve in the heart, pulmonary hypertension, degenerative changes in the myocardium, impaired platelet function with resultant bleeding, intracranial bleeding, renal impairment or failure, oligohydramnios, gastrointestinal (GI) bleeding or perforation, and increased risk of necrotizing enterocolitis, a life-threatening disorder. If taken near delivery, maternal effects include delayed onset of labour and delivery and increased risk of excessive bleeding. The newer COX-2 inhibitors (eg, celecoxib) have not been studied in pregnant women; diclofenac is contraindicated in pregnant women.

THYROID HORMONE

Levothyroxine does not readily cross the placenta and it seems safe in appropriate dosages. However, it may cause tachycardia in the foetus. When given as replacement therapy in hypothyroid women, the drug should be continued through pregnancy.

REFERENCES

Posner, Judith. It's all in your head: feminist and medical models of menopause (strange bedfellows). Sex Roles. 5:170- 190.

Rothman, Barbara Katz. In Labor: Women and Power in the Birthplace 1991.

Smith-Rosenberg, Carroll. The Hysterical Women: Sex Roles in Nineteenth Century America. Social Research. 39. Winter 1972: 652-78.

Steiger, Carolyn. Becoming a Midwife Hoogan House Publishing, 1987.

Ulrich, Laurel Thatcher. A Midwife's Tale . Vintage Books, New York, 1990.

Varney, Helen. Nurse Midwifery . 2nd Edition. Blackwell Scientific Publications. 1987.

Buchan, William., Advice to Mothers. Philadelphia: 1804.

Culpeper, Nicholas., Directory for Midwives., London: 1651-1777.

Blunt, John., Man-Midwifery Dissected., London: 1763.

Hunter, William., The Anatomy of the Human Gravid Uterus., Birmingham: 1774.

Raynalde, Thomas., The Byrth of Mankynd., London: 1545.

Sharp, Jane., The Midwives Book, Or the Whole Art of Midwifery Discovered., London: 1671.

Smellie, William., An Abridgement of the Practice of Midwifery: and a Set of Anatomical Tables with Explanations., Worcester: 1786.

12

Abortion

An abortion is the termination of a pregnancy by the removal or expulsion of an embryo or foetus from the uterus, resulting in or caused by its death. An abortion can occur spontaneously due to complications during pregnancy or can be induced. Abortion as a term most commonly refers to the induced abortion of a human pregnancy, while spontaneous abortions are usually termed miscarriages.

Abortion has a long history and has been induced by various methods including herbal abortifacients, the use of sharpened tools, physical trauma and other traditional methods. Modern medicine utilizes medications and surgical procedures to induce abortion. The legality, prevalence, and cultural views on abortion vary substantially around the world. In many parts of the world there is a divisive public debate over the ethical and legal aspects of abortion between the pro-life and pro-choice movements. The approximate number of induced abortions performed worldwide in 2003 was 42 million, which declined from nearly 46 million in 1995.

TYPES OF ABORTION

SPONTANEOUS ABORTION

Spontaneous abortion (also known as miscarriage) is the expulsion of an embryo or foetus due to accidental trauma or natural causes before the 20th week of gestation. Most miscarriages are due to incorrect replication of chromosomes; they can also be caused by environmental factors. A pregnancy that ends between 20 and 37 weeks of gestation, if it results in a live-born infant, is known as a "premature birth". When a foetus dies in utero after about 20 weeks, or during delivery, it is usually termed "stillborn". Premature births and stillbirths are generally not considered to be miscarriages although usage of these terms can sometimes overlap.

Most miscarriages occur very early in pregnancy. Between 10% and 50% of pregnancies end in clinically apparent miscarriage, depending upon the age and health of the pregnant woman. In most cases, they occur so early in the pregnancy that the woman is not even aware that she was pregnant. One study testing hormones for ovulation and pregnancy found that 61.9% of conceptuses were lost prior to 12 weeks, and 91.7% of these losses occurred subclinically, without the knowledge of the woman.

The risk of spontaneous abortion decreases sharply after the 10th week from the last menstrual period (LMP), with a loss rate between 8.5 weeks LMP and birth of about two percent; pregnancy loss is "virtually complete by the end of the embryonic period."

This risk of spontaneous abortion is greater in those with a known history of several spontaneous abortions or an induced abortion, those with systemic diseases, and those over the age 35. Other causes can be infection (of either the woman or foetus), immune response, or serious systemic disease. A spontaneous abortion can also be caused by accidental trauma; intentional trauma or stress to cause miscarriage is considered induced abortion or feticide.

INDUCED ABORTION

A pregnancy can be intentionally aborted in many ways. The manner selected depends chiefly upon the gestational age of the embryo or foetus, in addition to the legality, regional availability, and doctor-patient preference for specific procedures. Reasons for procuring induced abortions are typically characterized as either therapeutic or elective. An abortion is medically referred to as therapeutic when it is performed to:

- Save the life of the pregnant woman;
- Preserve the woman's physical or mental health;
- Terminate pregnancy that would result in a child born with a congenital disorder that would be fatal or associated with significant morbidity; or
- Selectively reduce the number of fetuses to lessen health risks associated with multiple pregnancy.

ABORTION METHODS

SURGICAL

In the first 12 weeks, suction-aspiration or vacuum abortion is the most common method. Manual Vacuum aspiration (MVA) abortion consists of removing the foetus or embryo by suction using a manual syringe, while electric vacuum aspiration (EVA) abortion uses an electric pump. These techniques are comparable, and differ in the mechanism used to apply suction, how early in pregnancy they can be used, and whether cervical dilation is necessary. MVA, also known as "mini-suction" and "menstrual extraction", can be used in very early pregnancy, and does not require cervical dilation. Surgical techniques are sometimes referred to as 'Suction (or surgical) Termination of Pregnancy' (STOP). From the 15th week until approximately the 26th, dilation and evacuation (D&E) is used. D&E consists of opening the cervix of the uterus and emptying it using surgical instruments and suction.

Dilation and curettage (D&C), the second most common method of abortion, is a standard gynecological procedure performed for a variety of reasons, including examination of the uterine lining for possible malignancy, investigation of abnormal bleeding, and abortion. Curettage refers to cleaning the walls of the uterus with a curette. The World Health Organization recommends this procedure, also called sharp curettage, only when MVA is unavailable. The term D and C, or sometimes suction curette, is used as a euphemism for the first trimester abortion procedure, whichever the method used.

Other techniques must be used to induce abortion in the second trimester. Premature delivery can be induced with prostaglandin; this can be coupled with injecting the amniotic fluid with caustic solutions containing saline or urea. After the 16th week of gestation, abortions can be induced by intact dilation and extraction (IDX) (also called intrauterine cranial decompression), which requires surgical decompression of the foetus' head before evacuation. A hysterotomy abortion is a procedure similar to a caesarean section, and is performed under general anesthesia because it is considered major abdominal surgery. It requires a smaller incision than a caesarean section and is used during later stages of pregnancy.

From the 20th to 23rd week of gestation, an injection to stop the foetal heart can be used as the first phase of the surgical abortion procedure to ensure that the foetus is not born alive.

MEDICAL

Effective in the first trimester of pregnancy, non-surgical abortions (referred to as 'medical abortions') comprise 10% of all abortions. Combined regimens include methotrexate or mifepristone, followed by a prostaglandin. When used within 49 days gestation, approximately 92%

of women undergoing medical abortion with a combined regimen completed it without surgical intervention. Misoprostol can be used alone, but has a lower efficacy rate than combined regimens. In cases of failure of medical abortion, vacuum or manual aspiration is used to complete the abortion surgically.

OTHER METHODS

Historically, a number of herbs reputed to possess abortifacient properties have been used in folk medicine: tansy, pennyroyal, black cohosh, and the now-extinct silphium. The use of herbs in such a manner can cause serious - even lethal - side effects, such as multiple organ failure, and is not recommended by physicians.

Abortion is sometimes attempted by causing trauma to the abdomen. The degree of force, if severe, can cause serious internal injuries without necessarily succeeding in inducing miscarriage. Both accidental and deliberate abortions of this kind can be subject to criminal liability in many countries. In Burma, Indonesia, Malaysia, the Philippines, and Thailand, there is an ancient tradition of attempting abortion through forceful abdominal massage.

Reported methods of unsafe, self-induced abortion include misuse of misoprostol, and insertion of non-surgical implements such as knitting needles and clothes hangers into the uterus. These methods are rarely seen in developed countries where surgical abortion is legal and available.

LEGISLATIONS

Abortion in India has been legal since 1971 and there are about 11 million abortions performed per year. Legalizing abortion has not ensured its accessibility to the poor nor been an effective method for curtailing population growth. Legal abortion was introduced in 1971, when concern about burgeoning population growth became an issue for India. Although abortion is legal, it is estimated that four million Indian women a year still resort to illegal abortions because of social taboos, misconceptions about the law, and the lack of skilled practitioners and medical facilities.

Giving or taking prenatal tests solely to determine the sex of the foetus is being criminalized by the Indian parliament. Female children are still widely considered to be a social and financial liability in a country where the dowry system is still a part of marriage. The prenatal tests have been used to detect female fetuses, which are then aborted. Under Indian law, ending a pregnancy only because a foetus is female has already been outlawed, although the practice is common. Poor women who cannot afford the cost of either prenatal testing or abortion often resort to female infanticide.

Abortion became legal in India in 1971 in order to prevent overpopulation. However, this appears to have been unsuccessful as India now has 1.1 billion people and is the second most populous country in the world, after China. In 1994, under pressure from a coalition of activists, the Indian government changed course, outlawing the use of ultrasound machines to reveal foetus gender. In 2002, the penalties were stiffened: up to three years in jail and a $230 fine for the first offence and five years imprisonment and $1, 160 for the second.

STATISTICS

Abortions are a major cause of maternal morbidity and mortality in India. Because most of the abortions are not reported and the sex selective abortions are carried out secretly the statistics of abortions in India is of varying reliability. The available statistic is grossly in adequate as the hospitals keep records of only legal and reported abortions.

Number of Abortions in India

According to the Consortium on National Consensus for Medical Abortion in India, every year an average of about 11 million abortions take place annually and around 20, 000 women die every year due to abortion related complications. Most abortion-related maternal deaths are attributable to illegal abortions. In the following table Number of abortions reported includes legal reported induced abortions.

Year	1972	1975	1980	1985	1990	1995	2000
Number of abortions reported	24300	214197	388405	583704	581215	570914	723142

Abortion by Selection of Gender

The Lancet study seemed to confirm that laws were not deterring families from sex selection. By analyzing national birth records and fertility histories from a 1998 Indian government survey of 1 million households, the study estimated that at least 500, 000 female fetuses in 1997 were aborted. Based on that one year, they came to the 10 million figure. The study also found that families whose first child was a girl were 30 percent less likely overall to produce another girl. And if the mothers had at least a 10th-grade education, the gap was twice as large as that for illiterate mothers. having gender-based abortions have been illegal since 1994.

FEMALE ABORTION

A lot of people in India are turning more towards abortion for girls because In India, there are less than 93 women for every 100 men in the population. The accepted reason for such a disparity is the practice of female infanticide in India, prompted by the existence of a dowry system which requires the family to pay out a great deal of money when a female child is married. For a poor family, the birth of a girl child can signal the beginning of financial ruin and extreme hardship. Which then they choose to have an ultrasound so they can make sure if they are having a male or female. The implication is that by avoiding a girl, a family will avoid paying a large dowry on the marriage of her daughter. According to UNICEF, the problem is getting worse as scientific methods of detecting the sex of a baby and of performing abortions are improving. Experts say that sex-selective abortions in India reduced the number of girls per 1, 000 boys from 945 in 1991 to 927 in 2001.

MEDICAL ABORTION AND THE LAW

In order to prevent the misuse of induced abortions, most countries in the world have created strict abortion laws and so has India. As per India's abortion laws only qualified doctors, under stipulated conditions, can perform abortion on a woman in a clinic or a hospital that has been approved of doing so. The Indian abortion laws fall under the Medical Termination of Pregnancy (MTP) Act, which was enacted by the Indian Parliament in the year 1971. The MTP Act came into effect from April 1st, 1972 and was once amended in 1975. The Medical Termination of Pregnancy (MTP) Act of India clearly states the conditions under which a pregnancy can be ended or aborted, the persons who are qualified to conduct the abortion and the place of implementation.

INDICATIONS FOR EARLY MEDICAL ABORTION

All women coming to a health facility seeking termination of pregnancy up to 7 weeks period of gestation (49 days from the first day of the last menstrual period in women with regular cycle of 28 days) provided the following aspects have been assessed and found appropriate:

- Frame of the mind of patient and her acceptability of minimum three follow-up visits
- Ready for surgical procedure if failure or excessive bleeding occurs
- Family support

- Permission of guardian in case of minor as per MTP Act 1971 easy access to appropriate health care facility

Only registered medical practitioners as prescribed by the MTP Act are authorized to prescribe mifepristone with misoprostol for medical abortion (Definition 2(d) of section 2 and MTP rule 3). Mifepristone with misoprostol for termination of early pregnancy not exceeding seven weeks, may be prescribed by a registered medical practitioner as prescribed under section 2 (d) and rule 3, having access to a place approved by the Government under section 4 (b) and rule (1), for surgical and emergency back-up when such a back-up is indicated. This may include primary health care-clinic or hospital-based set-up. Initial workup, counseling, prescription and administration could be in a clinic or in the consulting room. Home administration of misoprostol may be advised at discretion in certain cases with an access to 24-hours emergency services.

Choice between Medical and Surgical Abortion

- Vacuum Aspiration (Suction evacuation) is the most commonly-used method for termination of early pregnancies. However, being a surgical technique, it is associated with risks of infection, perforation of uterus, incomplete abortion and post-procedure uterine synechiae formation (Asherman's Syndrome).
- The success of abortion with drugs depends on multiple factors including the regimen used, dosage schedule, route of administration and gestational age. However, after counseling, the woman should be allowed to make an informed decision.
- Mifepristone with misoprostol is favourable if pregnancy is = 7 weeks.
- Surgical abortion is preferred if patient desires concurrent tubal ligation.
- If a woman fulfills the criteria for selecting either method, final choice to be given to the woman.

CONTRAINDICATIONS FOR MEDICAL ABORTION

Where a pregnant woman has a serious medical disease and continuation of pregnancy could endanger her life. Indian MTP act lay a clear guideline under which medical abortion is contra indicated

Contraindications Due to Medical Reasons

- Smoking > 35 years
- Anaemia - hemoglobin < 8 gm %

- Suspected /confirmed ectopic pregnancy/undiagnosed adnexal mass
- Coagulopathy or women on anticoagulant therapy
- Chronic adrenal failure or current use of systemic corticosteroids
- Uncontrolled hypertension with BP >160/100mmHg
- Cardio-vascular diseases such as angina, valvular disease, arrhythmia
- Severe renal, liver or respiratory diseases
- Glaucoma
- Uncontrolled seizure disorder
- Allergy or intolerance to mifepristone/misoprostol or other prostaglandins
- Lack of access to 24-hours emergency services.

Psycho-social Situations

This includes the cases when:

- Women unable to take responsibility
- Anxious women wanting quick abortion
- Language or comprehension barrier
- Not willing for surgical abortion in case of failure

COMPLICATIONS

IMMEDIATE COMPLICATIONS

Approximately 10% of women undergoing elective abortion will suffer immediate complications, of which approximately one-fifth (2%) are considered life threatening. The nine most common major complications which can occur at the time of an abortion are: infection, excessive bleeding, embolism, ripping or perforation of the uterus, anesthesia complications, convulsions, haemorrhage, cervical injury, and endotoxic shock. The most common "minor" complications include: infection, bleeding, fever, second degree burns, chronic abdominal pain, vomiting, gastro-intestinal disturbances, and Rh sensitization.

DEATH

According to the best record based study of deaths following pregnancy and abortion, a 1997 government funded study, women who abort are approximately four times more likely to die in the following year than women who carry their pregnancies to term. In addition, women who carry to term are only half as likely to die as women who were not pregnant.

The Finland researchers found that compared to women who carried to term, women who aborted in the year prior to their deaths were 60 percent more likely to die of natural causes, seven times more likely to die of suicide, four times more likely to die of injuries related to accidents, and 14 times more likely to die from homicide. Researchers believe the higher rate of deaths related to accidents and homicide may be linked to higher rates of suicidal or risk-taking behaviour.

The leading causes of abortion related maternal deaths within a week of the surgery are haemorrhage, infection, embolism, anesthesia, and undiagnosed ectopic pregnancies. Legal abortion is reported as the fifth leading cause of maternal death in the United States, though in fact it is recognized that most abortion related deaths are not officially reported as such.

BREAST CANCER

The risk of breast cancer almost doubles after one abortion, and rises even further with two or more abortions.(3)

CERVICAL, OVARIAN, AND LIVER CANCER

Women with one abortion face a 2.3 relative risk of cervical cancer, compared to non-aborted women, and women with two or more abortions face a 4.92 relative risk. Similar elevated risks of ovarian and liver cancer have also been linked to single and multiple abortions. These increased cancer rates for post-aborted women are apparently linked to the unnatural disruption of the hormonal changes which accompany pregnancy and untreated cervical damage.

UTERINE PERFORATION

Between 2 and 3% of all abortion patients may suffer perforation of heir uterus, yet most of these injuries will remain undiagnosed and untreated unless laparoscopic visualization is performed. Such an examination may be useful when beginning an abortion malpractice suit. The risk of uterine perforation is increased for women who have previously given birth and for those who receive general anesthesia at the time of the bortion. Uterine damage may result in complications in later pregnancies and may eventually evolve into problems which require a hysterectomy, which itself may result in a number of additional complications and injuries including osteoporosis.

CERVICAL LACERATIONS

Significant cervical lacerations requiring sutures occur in at least one percent of first trimester abortions. Lesser lacerations, or micro fractures, which would normally not be treated may also result in long term reproductive damage.

Latent post-abortion cervical damage may result in subsequent cervical incompetence, premature delivery, and complications of labour. The risk of cervical damage is greater for teenagers, for second trimester abortions, and when practitioners fail to use laminaria for dilation of the cervix.

PLACENTA PREVIA

Abortion increases the risk of placenta previa in later pregnancies (a life threatening condition for both the mother and her wanted pregnancy) by seven to fifteen fold. Abnormal development of the placenta due to uterine damage increases the risk of foetal malformation, perinatal death, and excessive bleeding during labour.

COMPLICATIONS OF LABOUR

Women who had one, two, or more previous induced abortions are, respectively, 1.89, 2.66, or 2.03 times more likely to have a subsequent pre-term delivery, compared to women who carry to term. Prior induced abortion not only increased the risk of premature delivery, it also increased the risk of delayed delivery.

Women who had one, two, or more induced abortions are, respectively, 1.89, 2.61, and 2.23 times more likely to have a post-term delivery (over 42 weeks). Pre-term delivery increases the risk of neo-natal death and handicaps.

HANDICAPPED NEWBORNS IN LATER PREGNANCIES

Abortion is associated with cervical and uterine damage which may increase the risk of premature delivery, complications of labour and abnormal development of the placenta in later pregnancies. These reproductive complications are the leading causes of handicaps among newborns.

ECTOPIC PREGNANCY

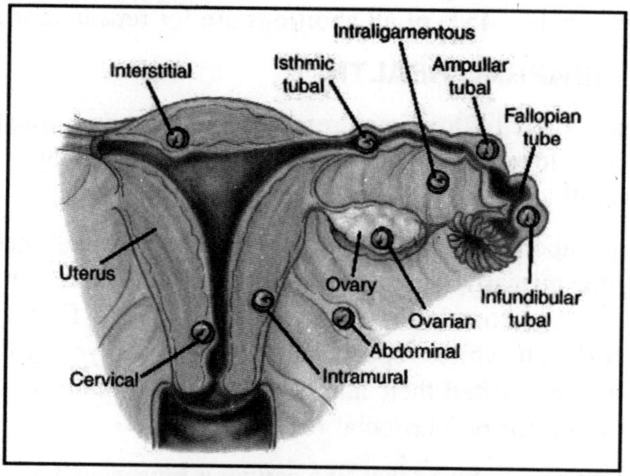

Fig. Ectopic Pregnancy

Abortion is significantly related to an increased risk of subsequent ectopic pregnancies. Ectopic pregnancies, in turn, are life threatening and may result in reduced fertility.

PELVIC INFLAMMATORY DISEASE (PID)

PID is a potentially life threatening disease which can lead to an increased risk of ectopic pregnancy and reduced fertility. Of patients who have a chlamydia infection at the time of the abortion, 23% will develop PID within 4 weeks. Studies have found that 20 to 27% of patients seeking abortion have a chlamydia infection. Approximately 5% of patients who are not infected by chlamydia develop PID within 4 weeks after a first trimester abortion. It is therefore reasonable to expect that abortion providers should screen for and treat such infections prior to an abortion.

ENDOMETRITIS

Endometritis is a post-abortion risk for all women, but especially for teenagers, who are 2.5 times more likely than women 20-29 to acquire endometritis following abortion.

INCREASED RISKS FOR WOMEN SEEKING MULTIPLE ABORTIONS

In general, most of the studies cited above reflect risk factors for women who undergo a single abortion. These same studies show that women who have multiple abortions face a much greater risk of experiencing these complications. This point is especially noteworthy since approximately 45% of all abortions are for repeat aborters.

LOWER GENERAL HEALTH

In a survey of 1428 women researchers found that pregnancy loss, and particularly losses due to induced abortion, was significantly associated with an overall lower health.

Multiple abortions correlated to an even lower evaluation of "present health." While miscarriage was detrimental to health, abortion was found to have a greater correlation to poor health. These findings support previous research which reported that during the year following an abortion, women visited their family doctors 80% more for all reasons and 180% more for psychosocial reasons.

The authors also found that "if a partner is present and not supportive, the miscarriage rate is more than double and the abortion rate is four times greater than if he is present and supportive. If the partner is absent the abortion rate is six times greater."

This finding is supported by a 1984 study that examined the amount of health care sought by women during a year before and a year after their induced abortions. The researchers found that on average, there was an 80 percent increase in the number of doctor visits and a 180 percent increase in doctor visits for psychosocial reasons after abortion.

INCREASED RISK FOR CONTRIBUTING HEALTH RISK FACTORS

Abortion is significantly linked to behavioral changes such as promiscuity, smoking, drug abuse, and eating disorders which all contribute to increased risks of health problems. For example, promiscuity and abortion are each linked to increased rates of PID and ectopic pregnancies.

Which contributes most is unclear, but apportionment may be irrelevant if the promiscuity is itself a reaction to post- abortion trauma or loss of self esteem.

INCREASED RISKS FOR TEENAGERS

Teenagers, who account for about 30 percent of all abortions, are also at much high risk of suffering many abortion related complications. This is true of both immediate complications, and of long-term reproductive damage.

NURSING MANAGEMENT

There are many professional components required in enabling nurses to plan, deliver, develop and evaluate abortion services within their scope of practice, and within the limits of the MTP Act. Nursing needs to be dynamic and respond to the changing needs of our country. Nurses have developed new roles, are working across traditional boundaries, and have been instrumental in setting up new services to meet health needs in a variety of health settings.

Recent and anticipated future developments in abortion services will continue to provide both challenges and opportunities for nurses practising at every level. The need for organizational support and robust clinical governance mechanisms is fundamental to assist nurses who are individually accountable for their professional practice and to ensure their legal duty of care to patients and clients is fulfilled. The current climate of change in health care provides an ideal opportunity for clinical leaders to shape the way abortion services are provided in the future. The development of a designated resource to achieve this (for example, consultant nurse, clinical nurse specialist and nurse practitioner roles) has been successful in shaping local, regional and national nursing practice in caring for women undergoing abortion. All nurses have an opportunity to lead from a clinical perspective and can be empowered to influence change in service provision and practice development, ensuring improved services for women undergoing abortion within the legal framework

NURSING ROLES

Since 1972, the authorisation and provision of abortion has been the legal responsibility of a registered medical practitioner, and the strict requirements are set out in the MTP Act 1971. The role of the nurse was historically to provide general nursing care. However, recent advances in abortion methods, particularly medical abortion (abortion stimulated by drugs rather than surgical removal), have led to the development of innovative nursing roles and a more holistic provision of nursing care. Nurses are now planning, leading, and managing a significant proportion of care for women undergoing medical abortion, under the guidance of a registered medical practitioner.

The requirements of the MTP Act 1971 mean that in this guidance, the phrase 'Nurse led' means that nurses are taking delegated responsibility from a registered medical practitioner. The role of nurses in abortion services has developed in response to a number of internal and external drivers. The legal requirements of Act do not allow nurses to authorise an abortion and the need for a doctor's involvement will limit the extent of nursing activity in abortion services. The inquiry was completely focused on scientific developments and did not look at ethical or moral arguments. The nursing profession endeavours to develop more responsive, patient-centred services.

In addition, the increasing number of doctors 'opting out' of providing abortion services has resulted in gaps in service provision, which has led to further opportunities for enhanced development nursing roles in providing medical termination of pregnancy. The principles of role development should be focused upon clinical need. They should empower nurses to develop their knowledge and skills for the benefit of patient care, rather than involve the ad hoc acquisition of technical skills or the inappropriate delegation of unpleasant or unwanted tasks by other professional groups. Role development should occur after a health care provider has identified the need for, and potential benefits from, development, and should be given organizational support and built into planning for sustainability.

Providers should work in partnership with commissioners and institutes of higher education to enable robust service and practice development. Employers must ensure that role, purpose and responsibilities are clearly specified. Individuals should ensure that they identify the professional competencies, additional knowledge and skills they will need, and that they have access to appropriate education, training, competency assessment and continuing support/supervision. Once they have achieved competency, nurses should be able to practise within agreed protocols and under the guidance of a registered medical practitioner. Examples of role development to date may include:

- Performing a pregnancy test and communicating the results to the woman.
- Pre-admission assessment.
- Pre- and post-abortion counselling.
- Participation in the process of obtaining consent for abortion procedures.
- Administration of abortificient drugs.
- Vaginal and speculum examination.
- Screening or testing for sexually transmitted Infections.
- Ultrasound assessment of gestational age, implantation site and viability.

- Insertion of osmotic cervical dilators.
- Assessment and provision of contraception via nurse independent prescribing or patient group directions.
- Discharge following medical and surgical procedures.
- Ability to make an assessment and take appropriate action based upon the assessment framework for children in need and use of domestic abuse pathways.
- Provision of care for the mature minor/vulnerable woman.
- Leading on service and practice development.
- Developing political awareness, advocacy and influencing skills.

To develop such roles, nurses need:

- To be accountable for their own practice
- To identify a medical champion who shares the "vision" and supervises and supports the nursing team
- A sound knowledge base and be appropriately educated and trained. (This may include undertaking an accredited training course e.g. sonography, counselling, Practice of Family
- Planning and Sexual Health course, Faculty of Sexual and Reproductive Health (FSRH) abortion modules)
- Up-to-date knowledge of evidence based practice
- Robust competency assessment ensuring confidence in performing practical skills (e.g. pelvic examination)
- Understanding and implementation of the principles of risk management
- Opportunities to develop and practice leadership, mentoring and supervisory skills
- Thorough working knowledge of the law on abortion.

REFERENCES

Gould D (2000) Normal Labour: a concept analysis Journal of Advanced Nursing 31(2) 418-427

Harris T (2001) Changing the focus for the third stage of labour British Journal of Midwifery 9(1) 7-11

Jamie E Bolane How will I know if I'm in labour? Childbirth Graphics

Klein M, Lloyd I, Redman C, Bull M and Turnball A C (1983)

Bibliography

Albers L L (1999) The duration of labor in healthy women Journal of Perinatology 19(2) 114-119

Albers L L, Schiff M and Gorwoda J G (1996) The length of active labor in normal pregnancies Obstetrics and Gynaecology 87(3) 355-359

Ament LA and Hanson L. A Model for the Future: Certified nurse-midwives replace residents and house staff in hospitals. Nursing and Health Care Prospectives 1998;19:1 26-33.

Brown SA and Grimes DE. A meta-analysis of nurse practitioners and nurse-midwives in primary care. Nursing Research 1995;44:332-39.

Buchan, William., Advice to Mothers. Philadelphia: 1804.

Capan P, et al. Nurse-managed clinics provide access and improved health care. Nurse practitioner 1993; 18:50-5.

Carroll D, Tramer M, McQuay H, Nye B and Moore A (1997) Transcutaneous electrical nerve stimulation in labour pain: a systematic review British Journal of Obstetrics and Gynaecology 104 169-175

Cherry J, Foster J. Comparison of hospital charges generated by certified nurse-midwives' and physicians' clients. Journal Nurse-Midifery 1982; 27:7-11.

Courter, Gay. The Midwife's Advice. Penguin. 1992. Paperback 1994.

Davis, Elizabeth. Heart and Hands. 2nd. Edition. Celestial Arts, 1992. A Midwife's guide to pregnancy, childbirth and the art and science of midwifery.

Davis-Floyd, Robbie. Birth as an American Rite of Passage. 1992.

Donnison, Jean. Midwives and Medical Men: A History of Inter-Professional Rivalries and Women's Rights. Schocken books, 1977.

Edwards, Margot and Waldorf, Mary. Reclaiming Birth: History and Heroines of American Childbirth Reform. The Crossing Press, 1984

Ehrenreich, Barbara and English, Derdre. Witches, Midwives and Nurses: A History of Women Healers. The Feminist Press, 1973.

Enkin, Murray, Keirse, Marc J.N.C., Renfrew, Mary and Neilson, James. 2nd Edition. A Guide to Effective Care in Pregnancy and Childbirth. Oxford University Press, 1995.

Featherstone I E (1999) Physiological third stage of labour British Journal of Midwifery 7(4) 216-221

Fleming V and Hagen S (1998) To suture or not to suture British Journal of Midwifery Letters 6(11) 737

Gabay M and Wolfe SM. Nurse-Midwifery, the Beneficial Alternative. Public Health Reports 1997; 112(5): 386-395.

Garland D and Jones K (2000) Waterbirth: supporting practice with clinical audit MIDIRS Midwifery Digest 10(3) 333-336

Goer, Henci. Obstetric Myths Versus Research Realities Bergin & Garvey, 1995.

Gordon, Linda. Woman's Body, Woman's Right: A Social History of Birth Control in America. New York: Grossman, 1977.

Haire D and Elsberry C. Maternity care and outcomes in a high-risk service: the North Central Bronx Hospital experience. Birth 1991; 18:33-7.

Harris T (2001) Changing the focus for the third stage of labour British Journal of Midwifery 9(1) 7-11

Hartley, Carla. Helping Hands: The Apprentice Workbook.

Harvey S, et al. A randomized controlled trial of nurse-midwifery care. Birth 1996; 23:128-35

Hellman L and O'Brien F. Nurse-midwifery-an experiment in maternity care. Obstetrics and Gynecology 1964; 24:343-49.

Jamie E Bolane How will I know if I'm in labour? Childbirth Graphics

Kilpatrick S J and Laros R K (1989) Characteristics of normal labor Obstetrics and Gynaecology 74(1) 85-87

Kitzinger, Sheila. Homebirth. 1991. A commonsense guide to the alternatives to giving birth in the hospital.

Kitzinger, Sheila. The Midwife Challenge. Pandora, 1991.

Klein M, Lloyd I, Redman C, Bull M and Turnball A C (1983)

Lee B (1999) Royal Society of Medicine forum: what is normal birth? RCM Midwives Journal 2(2) 386-387

Leep, Nicky, and Hunter, Billie. The Midwife's Tale. The untold story of birth in the 1920's , 1930's and 1940's in Britain.

Mander R (1997) Pethidine in childbirth MIDIRS Midwifery Digest 7(2) 202-203

Mann RJ, San Francisco General Hospital nurse-midwifery practice: the first thousand births. American Journal of Obstetrics and Gynecology 1981;140:676-82.

Midwifery Perspectives Vienna Midwifery Seminar College of Midwifery Southern Health Board June 2002

Midwifery Today. Getting an Education: Paths to Becoming a Midwife 1995 (Midwifery Today, PO Box 2672-350, Eugene, OR, 97402. USA.

Mitford, Jessica. The American Way of Birth The Penguin Group, 1993.

Nielsen I. A midwife-physician team in private practice. American Journal of Nursing 1975; 75:1693-95.

Nihell, Elizabeth., A Treatise on the Art of Midwifery: Setting Forth Various Abuses Therein, Especially as to the Practice with Instruments., London: 1760.

Oakley D, et. al. Processes of care: comparisons of certified nurse-midwives and obstetricians. Journal of Nurse-Midwifery 1995; 40:399-409.

Oakley D, et. al. Processes of care: comparisons of certified nurse-midwives and obstetricians. Journal of Nurse-Midwifery 1995; 40:399-409.

O'Connell, R (2002) Midwives and Maternity Care in Ireland Opportunities to move ahead? Midwifery Matters 92: 9-10

Odent, Michel. Birth Reborn . Pantheon Books. New York, 1984 and 1990.

Odibo L (1997) Suturing of perineal trauma: how well are we doing - an audit British Journal of Midwifery 5(11) 690-692

O'Donnell, C., O'Connell, R., (2007) Natural Benefits: Making Breastfeeding Easier World of Irish Nursing 15 (7) 18-19

O'Driscoll K, Meagher D with Boylan P (1993) Active Management of Labor 3rd ed Mosby:London

Olofsson C, Ekblom A, Ekman-Ordeberg G, Hjelm A and Irestedt L (1996)

Posner, Judith. It's all in your head: feminist and medical models of menopause (strange bedfellows). Sex Roles. 5:170- 190.

Raynalde, Thomas., The Byrth of Mankynd., London: 1545.

Robinson J (1996) What is normal labour? MIDIRS Midwifery Digest 6:1 56-58

Safriet BJ. Health care dollars and regulatory sense: the role of advanced practice nursing. Yale Journal of Regulation Summer 1992; 9:149-220.

Schorn M, McAllister J, Blanco J (1993) Water immersion and the effect on labour Journal of Nurse Midwifery 38(6) 336-342

Steiger, Carolyn. Becoming a Midwife Hoogan House Publishing, 1987.

Stone, Sarah., A Complete Practice of Midwifery., London: 1737.

Tawfik O, Badraoui M H H, El-Ridi F S (1982) The value of transcutaneous nerve stimulation (TNS) during labour in Egyptian mothers Scherz 2 98-195

Turnbull D, et. al. Randomized, controlled trial of efficacy of midwife-managed care. Lancet 1996; 348:213-18.

Ulrich, Laurel Thatcher. A Midwife's Tale . Vintage Books, New York, 1990.

Varney, Helen. Nurse Midwifery . 2nd Edition. Blackwell Scientific Publications. 1987.

Walsh D (1999) Transcutaneous electrical nerve stimulation British Journal of Midwifery 7(7) 580

Weaver, Pam and Evans, Sharon K. Practical Skills Guide. Morningstar Publications. 1994.

O'Driscoll K, Meagher D with Boylan P (1993) Active Management of Labor 3rd ed Mosby:London

Robinson J (1996) What is normal labour? MIDIRS Midwifery Digest 6:1 56-58

Lee B (1999) Royal Society of Medicine forum: what is normal birth? RCM Midwives Journal 2(2) 386-387

Kilpatrick S J and Laros R K (1989) Characteristics of normal labor Obstetrics and Gynaecology 74(1) 85-87

Index

G

H

I

J

L

M

N

O

P

Q

R

S

T

U